Clinical Surgical Skills Made Easy

Ahmed Farag • Ehab A. Mansour
Desmond C. Winter
Editors

Clinical Surgical Skills Made Easy

Springer

Editors
Ahmed Farag
Kasr Al Ainy-Faculty of Medicine
Cairo University hospitals
Cairo, Egypt

Ehab A. Mansour
General and Colorectal Surgery
St. Vincent's University Hospital
Dublin, Ireland

Desmond C. Winter
St Vincent's University Hospital
Dublin, Ireland

ISBN 978-3-031-69157-7 ISBN 978-3-031-69158-4 (eBook)
https://doi.org/10.1007/978-3-031-69158-4

This Springer imprint is published by the registered company Springer Nature Switzerland AG
The registered company address is: Gewerbestrasse 11, 6330 Cham, Switzerland

Preface

A lot of the excellent books in clinical surgery have been written all over the world, but to the best of my knowledge none of them have helped the student or even the practicing physician to understand the philosophy of why they are taking a patient's history or performing the clinical examination in an orthodox way, and why we examine them and even may fail them in the exam if they ignore basic steps? Why despite being swellings, we have a separate sheet for thyroid and hernia and don't include them in the general sheet for swellings? Is there a different way for clinical examination than what we have to do in our practice later on? Is there a common goal for clinical examination, labs, and X-rays? Why do we have a separate sheet for neck swellings, chest, and abdomen but we don't have a comprehensive sheet to examine a limb? This book includes a sheet for the examination of a limb in order to avoid the common mistakes during examination of a limb swelling or ulcer, both by students and by young practicing clinicians.

From my experience, the answer is simple, and it is that every single step in history taking and clinical, laboratory, radiologic, instrumental (e.g., endoscopic and others), and pathologic examination has to reach a clinical diagnosis that rests on two pillars:

1. Anatomical diagnosis
2. Pathologic diagnosis

in the milieu of the general condition of the patient, which may affect the decision-making or help in tailoring the treatment according to their general condition.

We are treating the patient in general not only the disease.

Cairo, Egypt — Ahmed Farag
Dublin, Ireland — Ehab A. Mansour
Dublin, Ireland — Desmond C. Winter

Contents

1 **Introduction** 1
Ahmed Farag, Ehab A. Mansour, and Desmond C. Winter

2 **A Qualifying Statement** 3
Ahmed Farag, Ehab A. Mansour, and Desmond C. Winter

3 **General Examination Sheet** 7
Ahmed Farag and Ehab A. Mansour

4 **Examination of Swellings** 23
Mohamed Yehia Elbarmelgi and Mahmoud Mostafa

5 **DD. of Swelling in the Femoral Triangle** 31
Ahmed Farag

6 **Swelling in the Popliteal Fossa** 41
Ahmed Farag

7 **Examination of an Ulcer** 49
Mohamed Yehia Elbarmelgi and Mahmoud Mostafa

8 **Lymphadenopathy Sheet and D.D. of Multiple Swellings** 55
Ahmed Farag

9 **General Limb Sheet** 63
Ahmed Farag

10 **DD. of Limb Edema** 67
Ahmed Farag

11 **Limb Pain Sheet** 71
Ahmed Farag

12 **Examination of the Thyroid** 79
Alexandra M. Zaborowski and Ruth S. Prichard

13 **Abdominal Examination Sheet** ... 87
Ahmed Farag and Reem Awad Alharbi

14 **Digital Rectal Examination "DRE"** ... 123
Shimaa Alkhaldi

15 **Pelvic and Rectal Clinical Examination** ... 127
Ilario Froehner Junior and Peter Petros

16 **Acute Abdomen** ... 137
Kimberley Logbochi Olivia Mvetimbo Tamb and Audrius Dulskas

17 **Urology Sheet** ... 149
Steven Anderson, Elsayed M. Salih, and Mohammed Aboelmaged

18 **Hernia Sheet** ... 169
Ahmed Farag, Asif Mehraj, and Patrick Jordan

19 **D.D. of Inguinoscrotal Swelling** ... 179
Ahmed Farag, Asif Mehraj, and Patrick Jordan

20 **Vascular Examination Sheet** ... 185
Mohammed Elkassaby

21 **Breast Examination Sheet** ... 203
Tim Harding

22 **Examination of the Axilla** ... 215
Alexandra M. Zaborowski and Arnold D. K. Hill

23 **Examination of the Head and Neck** ... 219
Husam Hosny and Ahmed Farag

24 **Examination of a Mass in the Head and Face** ... 235
Ahmed Farag, Amr Kamel Elfeky, and Nicholas Johnson

25 **Clinical Examination of Thoracic Surgery** ... 259
Sandhya Chalasani

26 **Peripheral Nerve and Hand Examination** ... 271
Husam Hosny

27 **Neurological Examination** ... 281
Ahmed Adel Mohamed Ezzat and Hazem Abdel Badie Ahmed Gouda

28 **Examination of the Spine** ... 289
Khaled Saoud

29 Orthopedic Examination 299
Mahmoud Massoud and Ashraf Mohey

30 Sheet for of a Swelling from the Bone 321
Ashraf Mohey and Ahmed Hassan Amin

31 Peri-Operative Care 329
Lauren O'Connell

32 Management of the Patient in the Post-Operative Setting 337
Lauren O'Connell

33 Stoma Examination 349
Enda Hannan, Nicholas Johnson, Tim Harding,
and Ehab A. Mansour

34 Conclusion 361
Ahmed Farag

Chapter 1
Introduction

Ahmed Farag, Ehab A. Mansour, and Desmond C. Winter

Abstract Clinical diagnosis, as well as, interpretation of X-Rays and Surgical Jars represent the final common pathway of medical education. Clinical diagnosis is a part of applied Medical Science which is based on the basic sciences namely Anatomy, Histology, physiology, Biochemistry, pathology, Parasitology and Bacteriology…. etc. In fact diagnosis is based on two Pillars namely: Anatomical Diagnosis and Pathologic diagnosis. Clinical examination is never complete without thorough though swift General examination.

Keywords Diagnosis · Clinical · Anatomical · Pathologic · General · Examination · Pillars · Thorough

Clinical diagnosis, as well as, interpretation of X-Rays and Surgical Jars represent the final common pathway of medical education. Clinical diagnosis is a part of applied Medical Science which is based on the basic sciences namely Anatomy, Histology, physiology, Biochemistry, pathology, Parasitology and Bacteriology…. etc.

In fact diagnosis is based on two Pillars namely: **Anatomical Diagnosis and Pathologic diagnosis.** Clinical examination is never complete without **through though swift General examination.**

Diagnoses such as liver Cirrhosis, Cancer stomach or Ulcerative Colitis includes the name of the organ affected and the Pathology responsible for the Patients' Symptoms.

In Fact from my more than 40 years of Clinical Practice and 35 years of teaching Clinical skills to Medical students. I can claim that the knowledge of the anatomic

A. Farag (✉)
Kasr Alainy Hospital, Cairo University, Cairo, Egypt

E. A. Mansour
General and Colorectal Surgery, St. Vincent's University Hospital, Dublin, Ireland

D. C. Winter
St Vincent's University Hospital, Dublin, Ireland

A. Farag et al. (eds.), *Clinical Surgical Skills Made Easy*,
https://doi.org/10.1007/978-3-031-69158-4_1

diagnosis (the organ affected) represents a more difficult question than the diagnosis of the pathology in that organ.

This explains why the Medical student is subconsciously happy if he knows that he will take the sheet of Thyroid or the sheet of a hernia because he had one of the questions already answered namely the anatomic diagnosis. Similarly if he knows that the case is Hepato-splenomegaly or Varicose Veins. Accordingly the most difficult sheet to take is the case of Abdominal examination where a lot of organs are closely packed in this single space which makes the anatomic diagnosis and accordingly the final diagnosis, the most difficult to achieve which make this examination from my point of view "The Mark of A Good Clinician".

This book which I had decided to write in order to serve both functions of passing the clinical examination and optimizing our diagnostic skills. In fact both tasks are intimately related as we will see through the rest of the book. *Authors*

"Clinical skills save Lives. Clinical skills save resources" Authors.

"**The Key for correct treatment is correct diagnosis**". I keep telling my patients that "Even the medical student knows the treatment of any disease when he is asked about it in the examination. Diagnosis may be the major challenge to reach the diagnosis even for the most Challenging task even for the most talented doctor". "Authors".

"**A good Clinician who detects more (Symptoms)** and signs
Than others do". **Norman Browse** modified by authors.

"**Eyes Don't See what Mind doesn't Know** (only gifted people Do)" **Unknown wise man** modified by Authors.

"**Clinical Diagnosis is like the detective work in CSI"**. A good Clinician can reach the diagnosis because he asked a question or found a clue that others failed to do" Authors.

"**Clinical Diagnosis is like us walk on two limbs** or rests on Two Pillars namely **Anatomical and Pathologic Diagnosis** in a milieu of associated disease and **General Condition** of the patient". "Authors."

"The Brain of the Clinician is like a CPU of a computer which literally allocates all the data taken in the Clinical Sheet in one of 3 Categories namely anatomical diagnosis, Pathologic diagnosis and/or the General Condition of the patient". Failing to do such allocation with each single item can risk losing the diagnosis or doing a medical Error. "Authors."

"**Clinical signs should be done exactly in the same way it had been described otherwise we can miss the diagnosis**" Authors.

"**The Key for proper treatment is proper Clinical diagnosis which has to guide our Further Investigations**". "Authors".

Complete and swift Clinical Examination not only saves Health care resources by avoiding unnecessary Investigations or interventions but also it can save lives and decreases the Preventable health care Errors "i.e. Morbidity and Mortality". "Authors".

Chapter 2
A Qualifying Statement

Ahmed Farag, Ehab A. Mansour, and Desmond C. Winter

Abstract Human learning is mainly categorized into:

1. Skill Based Learning: which will be a life–long Memory which will be performed even subconsciously. Like Driving and Many of the Clinical examination Skills.
2. Rule Based Learning: Which is a Life-long Memory which will be practice Consciously Like—Swelling in the Lower part of the front of the Neck is Thyroid Swelling till Prove Otherwise|| or—A Swelling in the Parotid area is a Parotid swelling till Prove Otherwise|| and—A Cystic Swelling along the course of an Artery which look like an abscess should be aspirated first before Surgical drainage||.
3. Knowledge based Learning: Is a Short term memory which is done consciously and —frequently forgotten||.

Keywords Learning · Skill · Rule · Knowledge · Memory · Swelling · Clinical · Examination

Human Learning is Mainly Categorized into

1. **Skill Based Learning:** which will be a life–long Memory which will be performed even subconsciously. Like Driving and Many of the Clinical examination Skills.

A. Farag (✉)
Kasr Alainy Hospital, Cairo University, Cairo, Egypt

E. A. Mansour
General and Colorectal Surgery, St. Vincent's University Hospital, Dublin, Ireland

D. C. Winter
St Vincent's University Hospital, Dublin, Ireland

A. Farag et al. (eds.), *Clinical Surgical Skills Made Easy*,
https://doi.org/10.1007/978-3-031-69158-4_2

2. **Rule Based Learning:** Which is a Life-long Memory which will be practice Consciously Like "Swelling in the Lower part of the front of the Neck is Thyroid Swelling till Prove Otherwise" or "A Swelling in the Parotid area is a Parotid swelling till Prove Otherwise" and "A Cystic Swelling along the course of an Artery which look like an abscess should be aspirated first before Surgical drainage".
3. **Knowledge based Learning**: Is a Short term memory which is done consciously and "frequently forgotten".

The Aim of this book is to Develop **reflexes** in Clinical examination through conversion most of the Knowledge based learning in the traditional Clinical teaching into a **Rule-Based Learning which will be hard to Forget.**

RCSI General Rules in the Clinics and During Clinical Examination

WIPE Mnemonic for Beginning a Clinical Exam OSCE

Wash your hands (and consider need for transmission based precautions*).

Introduce yourself and Identify the patient Permission (explain what you are going to do and gain consent), **P**ain (ask if any) and **P**osition the patient.

Expose patient appropriately (& consider if chaperone required) & relevant Equipment.

Equipment Required for Clinical Exam

- White coat.
- Appropriately dressed.
- Bare below the elbow (sleeves rolled up, no wrist watches, Rings, etc.).
- Stethoscope.
- Reflex hammer.
- Tuning forks (128 Hz & 256 Hz).
- Pen torch.
- Neurotip/monofilament.
- Cotton wool bud.
- Measuring tape.
- Stopwatch.
- Snellen chart.
- Pen & paper.

Upon Completion of OSCE Station/Long Case Clinical Exam

- Thank the patient.
- Inform them that they can redress, or cover them with a blanket if appropriate.
- Check end of bed notes.
- Wash your hands.
- Offer to present your findings.
- Consider your differentials.

Chapter 3
General Examination Sheet

Ahmed Farag, and Ehab A. Mansour

Abstract One of the causes of difficulties for students to understand, remember and perform proper clinical diagnosis is the lack of an answer to his question—why we take the sheet in a certain pattern and why we are punished by losing marks if we ignore or forget certain parts of the history taking and Clinical examination.

As explained in the Introduction Clinical Examination rests on two Pillars namely.

Keywords Students · Proper · Clinical · Examination · Sheet · Examination · History · Anatomy · Pathology

General Plan (Fig. 3.1)

Box 3.1 Anatomical Diagnosis Means an Area or Organ

- Areas such as the Axilla Cubital Fossa, Femoral triangle or popliteal fossa.
- And by Organs we mean every single organ, Cavity "like peritoneal cavity" or Skin, Subcutaneous, Deep fascia, Muscle, Bone, Artery, Vein, Nerve or Lymphatic vessel.

A. Farag (✉)
Kasr Alainy Hospital, Cairo University, Cairo, Egypt

E. A. Mansour
General and Colorectal Surgery, St. Vincent's University Hospital, Dublin, Ireland

A. Farag et al. (eds.), *Clinical Surgical Skills Made Easy*,
https://doi.org/10.1007/978-3-031-69158-4_3

Box 3.2 Pathologic Diagnosis Which Includes

- **Congenital:**
- **Traumatic:** Direct e.g. Sharp "Penetrating or None penetrating a Cavity" or Blunt, indirect such as a Twist or Psychic trauma in autoimmune disease.
- **Inflammatory:** Acute or chronic each can be Specific or non-specific.
- **Neoplastic:** Benign, Locally malignant or Malignant "Primary or Secondary".
- **Auto-Immune:**
- **Degenerative:** e.g. Osteo-arthritis.
- **Others: e.g.** Allergic, metabolic Drug induced ...etc.

Box 3.3 Rule Based Learning in Clinical Examination

- Always remember in Local examination the Head, Neck and Mouth rather than the traditional Head and Neck.
- Also remember the Examination of the Chest is "Chest Front, Back and Breast in males and females" rather that chest and breast separately.
- Remember Examination of the Abdomen is Examination of the Abdomen Front and Back, Perineum, Gluteal region and Upper thighs.
- In Limb examination don't forget Examination of Limb distal for compression effect on the Arteries, Veins, nerves, or Primary focus "e.g. Inflammation or Malignancy" and the Limb proximally for L.Ns or Masses.

One of the causes of difficulties for students to understand, remember and perform proper clinical diagnosis is the lack of an answer to his question "why we take the sheet in a certain pattern and why we are punished by losing marks if we ignore or forget certain parts of the history taking and Clinical examination".

As explained in the Introduction Clinical Examination rests on two Pillars namely

1. **Anatomical Diagnosis** "The organ which harbors the disease".
2. **Pathologic Diagnosis** "classified as Congenital, Traumatic, Inflammatory, neoplastic, Autoimmune, degenerative ....etc."
3. In a milieu of **general** fitness of the patient and associated disease.

   It has to be born in mind that **every Item** in the sheet adds to the **anatomical** or **pathologic** diagnosis as will be explained as follows:

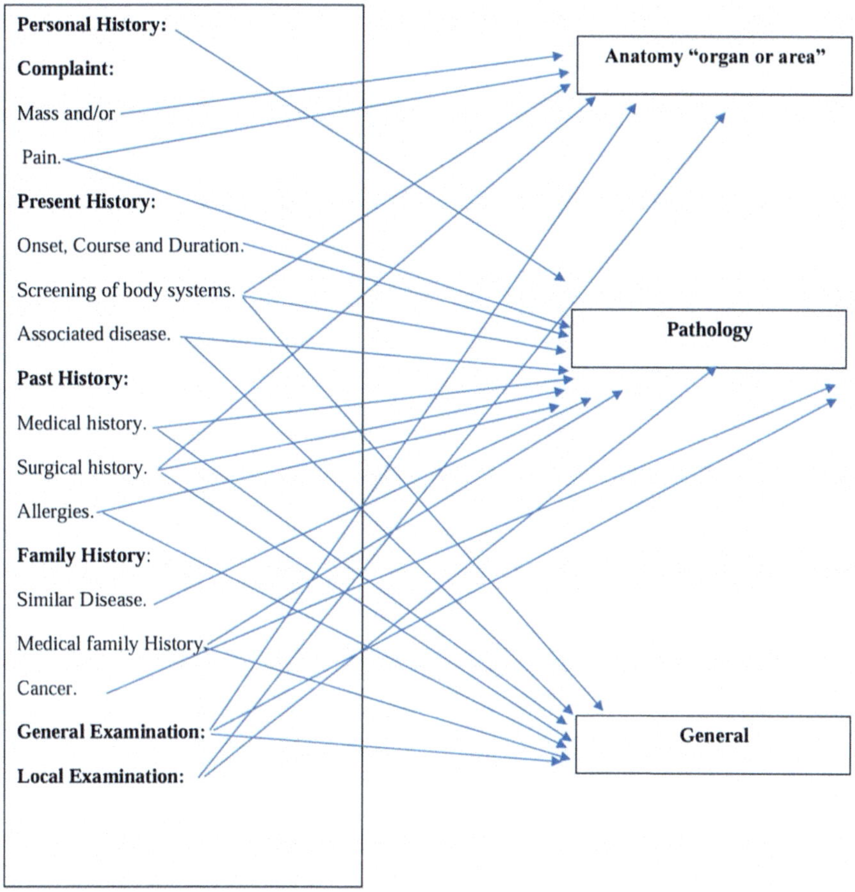

Fig. 3.1 General plan of clinical surgical examination

Personal History (Fig. 3.2)

This includes: Name, Sex, Age, religion, Race, Occupation, Residency, marital status, Number of Children and their age and Sex, Menstrual History in Females and History of intake of contraceptive Pills, Special habits of Medical importance and right or left handedness.

The personal history is important for filling the records and starting the patient doctor relationship yet the Personal history is of paramount importance for **the pathologic** diagnosis because it is related to the **Epidemiology of the disease**.

Age: congenital diseases present mainly in the infancy or childhood but some of them present later such as congenital hernia.

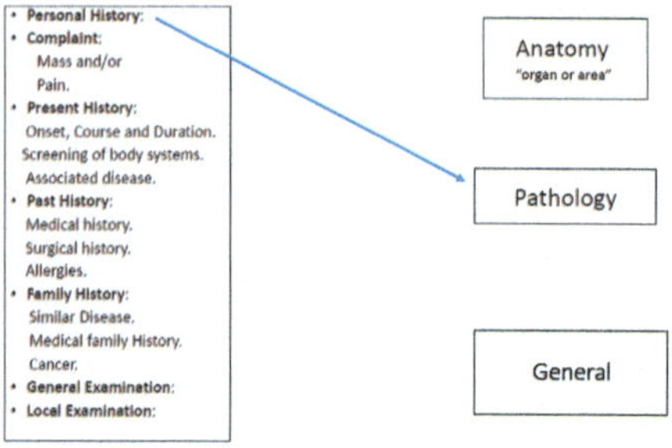

Fig. 3.2 Relation between personal history and pathology

Sex: Sex related disorders are clear example but the prevalence of certain diseases in certain sex may have the probability in certain pathologic diagnosis e.g. A benign looking parotid swelling in females most probably a mixed parotid tumor "which is more common in females", but in males the most probable is warthin tumor "being more common in males than females".

Religion: Gaucher disease "A lipid storage disease leading to massive splenomegaly" is more common in Jews and cancer Penis and cervix are more common in uncircumcised males and their wives respectively.

Race: Sickle disease is more common in black "African" race and Cooley's anemia is more common in Mediterranean race.

Occupation:

- Some diseases are more common in certain occupations such as Bilharziasis and Anklystoma in Peasants in Egypt due to their contact with water channels. Cancer bladder is more common in patients working in aniline dye. Cancer of the skin of the scrotum in chimney sweepers and Mule spinners in the past.
- On the other hands a second opinion is needed before thyroid surgery for benign disease in teachers, Lawyers and singers with the risk of losing the high pitched voice.
- Surgery for moderately severe lower limb ischemia may be indicated in a peddler who needs to walk for long distances to earn living but not in a General Director.

Residency: limb swelling in patients living at Fayoum in Egypt raises the possibility of Filariasis and Neck swelling in patients living at Oasis raises the possibility of Endemic Goiter.

Special habits of Medical importance:

- Liver Cirrhosis and Chronic Pancreatitis are more common in Alcoholics
- Chronic Obstructive Airway disease (COPD) and Bronchogenic carcinoma are causally related to Cigarette smoking which is also approved adverse risk factor after treatment in vascular disease and in reconstructive Surgery such as skin and other types of flaps.

Marital status and number and age of children: in sex transmitted diseases.

Menstrual History and history of intake of Contraceptive Pills:

- Cancer breast is more common in Early Monarchy and Late Menopause and in Nulliparous females or those who didn't' breast feed their children.
- Benign breast disease and Deep Vein Thrombosis (DVT) is more common in those receiving contraceptive pills and is a contraindication to injection sclerotherapy in the treatment of varicose veins for fear of inducing DVT.

Handedness: A nerve injury in the left hand of a right handed worker is less serious than a nerve injury in his dominant hand while both hands are of equal importance in a pianist.

Complaint (Fig. 3.3)

In the patients' own words Such as pain in the right side of the abdomen or by Quadrants, "rather than pain in the right iliac fossa"

- The Site of the complaint suggests the **Anatomical Diagnosis** e.g. *swelling* in the lower part of the front of the neck is thyroid till prove otherwise and a swelling in the palm of the hand cannot be a lymph node because it is not the anatomical site of such structure (Fig. 3.3).
- The Situation is little bit different if the complaint is *pain* because it may be a referred pain from another site e.g. upper abdominal pain may be referred from the chest "Always remember that inferior myocardial infarction presents as upper abdominal pain" (Fig. 3.4).
- Also remember in the case of swelling to ask if *the swelling is Painful or Painless*? Is important from the **pathologic** point of view Painful swellings are most probably benign but some malignant tumors cause pain such as oral cancer, those causing bowel obstruction, Ulcerating lesions and those infiltrating nerves such as advanced pancreatic cancers and pelvic Malignancies while painless rapidly growing lesions carries the possibilities of being malignant.
- ***TIME OUT:*** at this point start to think of the most probable diagnosis or Diagnoses based on which organ is affected "the Anatomical Diagnosis" and

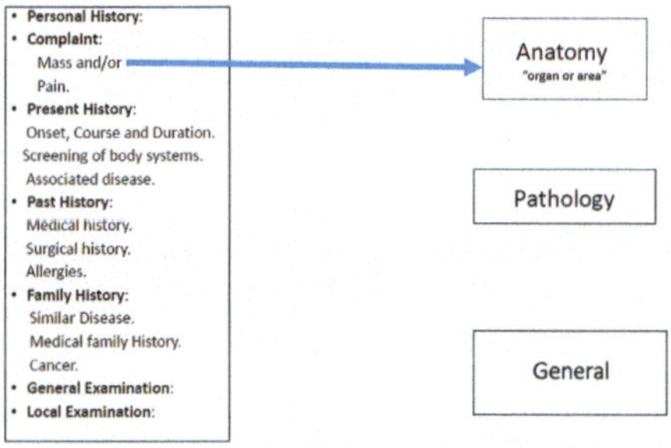

Fig. 3.3 Relation between complaint (mass) and anatomy

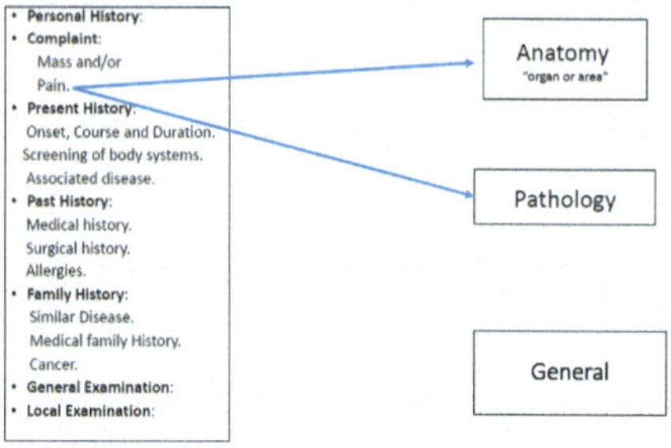

Fig. 3.4 Relation between complaint (pain) and both anatomy and pathology

what is the possible disease affecting that organ based on the type of the patient as was taken in the personal history "The Pathologic Diagnosis".

"I.e. The Type of the patient helps to suggest the list of possibilities concerning the ***pathology*** *according to the patient's complaint".*

Present History (Fig. 3.5)

Onset, Course and Duration

All the three items refer to **the pathology** putting in mind being categorized into congenital, traumatic, inflammatory, neoplastic, autoimmune… etc. as follows:

Onset: (Mode of onset + was it associated with trauma or inflammation?)

Mode of onset:

- Instantaneous or sudden i.e. within seconds or minutes refers to trauma (e.g. hematoma or fracture).
- Acute i.e. within hours or days refer to acute inflammations such as cellulitis, Abscesses or other acute inflammations either specific such as mumps or non-specific inflammation.
- Gradual Onset i.e. within weeks or months, which suggests sub-acute or chronic inflammations (Mostly painful or tender) or raises the possibility of neoplastic (usually but not always painless).
- Accidental Discovery.

Was the associated with trauma or inflammation?

This question is of paramount importance to exclude two of the main pathologies seen in surgical practice and failure to ask such question will lead to missing the diagnosis.

Example: A 50 years old lady presenting with a hard mass in the breast with dimpling of the skin and nipple retraction will be considered as being malignant by most clinicians but a good clinician will ask about the history of trauma (direct

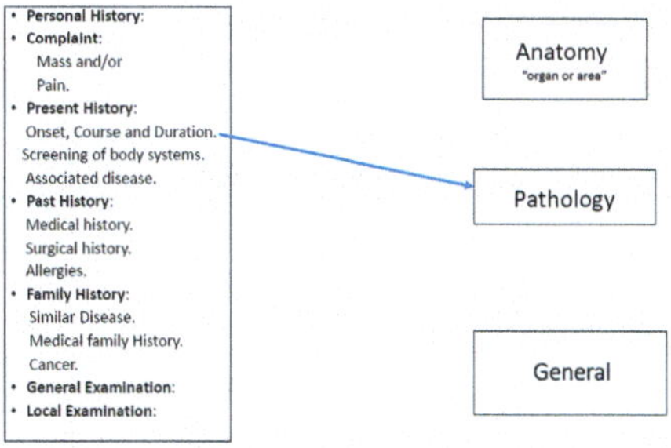

Fig. 3.5 Correlation between onset, course and duration and pathology

violent trauma or repeated minor traumata with an ill-fitting bra) or symptoms suggestive of inflammation (pain, redness, hotness, swelling, fever and rigors) at the onset. Direct violent trauma can lead to hematoma which can become organized and even calcified mimicking cancer breast, similarly minor repeated traumata can lead to fat necrosis and untreated or inadequately treated breast abscess associated with the onset can become calcified over months and years presenting like a breast cancer and the patient has to be asked directly about them.

Trauma of surgical importance is either direct (Penetrating or non-penetrating) or indirect like twisting movements leading to fracture or rupture of a muscle or a tendon and Psychic trauma precipitating autoimmune disease (e.g. immediately preceding the onset of primary thyrotoxicosis "Grave's disease").

Course:

Types:

- Rapidly Progressive (minutes, hours, weeks or months).
- Slowly Progressive (over years).
- Stationary.
- Regressive.
- Intermittent (returning to the base line i.e. normal, between attacks). E.g. autoimmune disorders and repeated cellulitis in a normal limb)
- Remittent (leaves the organ or the patient in a worse situation after each attack. E.g. attacks of cellulitis on top of Lymphedema where the limb is in a worse situation after each attack.

An intelligent clinicians make use of this item in the pathologic diagnosis especially in excluding certain pathologies and proving others.

E.g. regressive, stationary, slowly progressive, intermittent and remittent course can exclude malignancy except in the case of Jaundice due to peri-ampullary carcinoma which can have a single remission followed by progressive course. Also some malignant tumors like some cases of breast cancer are slowly progressive.

Duration:

A long duration over years usually exclude malignancy.

Analysis of the Complaint

Common complaints should be analyzed systemically as will be presented in each sheet. **Analysis of the complaint is useful in either anatomical diagnosis or pathologic diagnosis** e.g.

Pain: Type, site, referral, what brings, what relieves and associated symptom. Examples:

Type of pain helps in anatomical diagnosis (Colicky pain occurs in hollow organs such as GI, biliary or urinary systems and non-colicky pain is in solid organs).

Site of pain helps in anatomical diagnosis putting in mind that it may be related to an organ at the site of pain or referred from another site e.g. Epigastric pain may originate from Anterior abdominal wall, stomach, Transverse colon, Pancreas, Aorta or posterior abdominal wall mainly vertebrae or may be referred from inferior infarction or Myocardial ischemia.

Referral of pain: helps in anatomical diagnosis but may be helpful in pathologic diagnosis. E.g. A pain in the epigastrium which refers to the back suggests the pancreas or aorta as a source of pain. In cases diagnosed as gastric pain or known gastric ulcer, pain referred to back suggests a posterior penetration of the ulcer or gastric cancer invading the pancreas.

What brings pain: helps in anatomical diagnosis e.g. fatty dyspepsia suggests a biliary pathology, while acid dyspepsia suggests a gastric pathology?

What relieves pain: suggests anatomical diagnosis. E.g. pain which is relieved by vomiting and alkalis suggests stomach as a source of pain and pain which is relieved by defecation of passage of gas suggest the colon as an anatomical diagnosis.

Associated symptoms: Suggests Anatomical diagnosis where nausea and vomiting suggest Stomach and small bowel. Bloating refers to the colon and jaundice suggests Hepato-bilio-pancreatic system or blood "in hemolytic crises as a source of pain, while simple regurgitation of undigested food suggests esophagus as an anatomic diagnosis….etc.

Similarly analysis of complaints like **vomiting** may suggest pathologic diagnosis. E.g. forceful vomiting suggests mechanical obstruction while regurgitated vomiting suggests adynamic obstruction.

Screening Questions for the Body Systems (Fig. 3.6)

This helps in assessment of:

1. The general condition of the patient which is important to tailor treatment for each patient **"we are treating the patient not the disease".** E.g. the decision to treat a hernia in a normal patient is different from the decision to treat hernia in a child grade C liver failure or will have an impact on choosing the type of Anesthesia if surgery is a must.

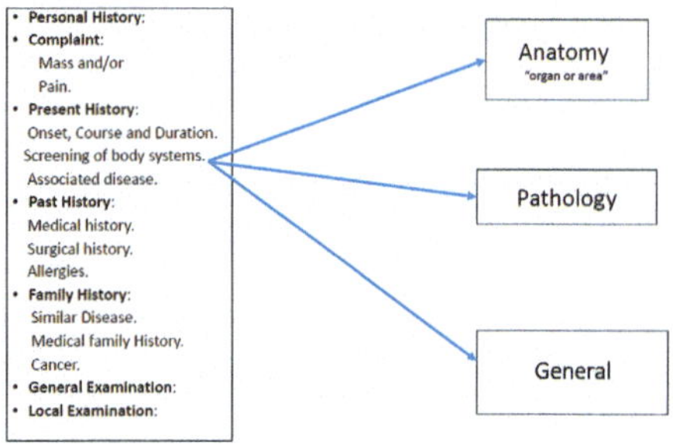

Fig. 3.6 Correlation between screening of the body systems and the categories of anatomy, pathology and general condition

2. The clue for the diagnosis may be only uncovered by systematic General examination
   - Can help in the anatomical diagnosis of the disease such as in metastases of unknown Primary and in Fever of unknown Origin.
   - Can Help in diagnosis the pathologic diagnosis, (e.g. xanthomas and xanthelasmas refers to atherosclerosis as a cause of arterial obstruction or aneurysms, while rheumatoid arthritis may refer to the cause of splenomegaly ….etc.). In addition presence of generalized lymphadenopathy may refer to the cause of abdominal complaints such as abdominal masses or Jaundice e.g. Lymphoma).
3. Helps to stage the disease such as in cancer or in Organ failure (pathologic diagnosis). The clue for the diagnosis may be only uncovered by systematic General examination

Screening Questions of the body Systems:

- **GIT:**
- **General** such as appetite and recent change in body weight.
- **Upper GI Symptoms**: Dysphagia, regurgitation, Heart-burn, hyperacidity, Dyspepsia, nausea, Vomiting, satiety, Colics, Hematemesis and or Melena.
- **Lower GI:** Colonic distension, Colonic pain, Diarrhea, Constipation, Bleeding or Mucous per rectum.
- **Anal and rectum:** Tenismus, bleeding, mucous or discharge per anus, swelling, prolapse or pain and its relation to defecation.
- **Hepato-Biliary**: Pain and/or swelling in the upper right quadrant of the abdomen. Jaundice.
- **Spleen:** Pain and/or swelling in the Left upper quadrant of the abdomen. +/− Manifestations of hypersplenism.
- **Urinary Symptoms:**
- **Upper Urinary**: Loin pain, Renal Colics, Mass or Symptoms suggestive of Uremia.

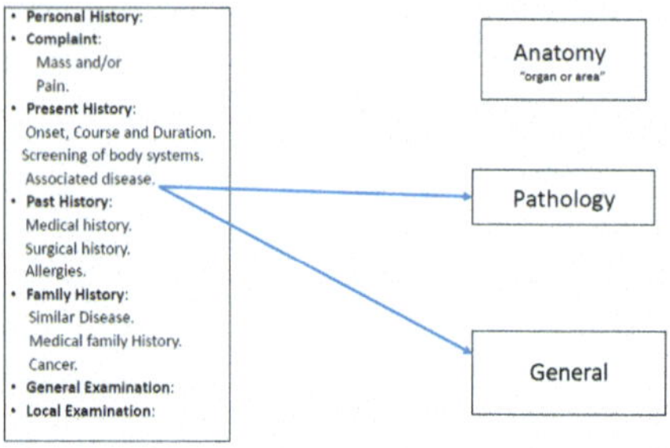

Fig. 3.7 Correlation between associated disease/s and both pathology and general condition

- **Lower Urinary which includes:**
- **Urine Color: Amber or normal, red due to blood jaundice or dye, white due to** phosphaturia or Chyluria or Prune Colored due to vitamin A or B12", **abnormal contents** "Air or Pneumaturia, crystals or Crystaluria, Stones or Necrotic tissue or Necroturia" **and act of micturition:** Frequency, urgency, precipitancy, urge incontinence, Start of the act, stream of urine, Termination of the act, post-operative dripping, and double micturition.
- **Chest symptoms**: Cough, wheezes, Expectoration and hemoptysis.
- **Cardiac Symptoms**: Palpitation, chest pain during exercise or during rest may present as pain in the upper abdomen, Left shoulder, inside the left arm or left sided neck or signs of heart failure such as Dyspnea, orthopnea or Paroxysmal nocturnal Dyspnea.
- **Neurologic Symptoms:**
- **Central:** Such as Insomnia, change in mood, change in behavior. **Or peripheral:** Such as Tremors, Anesthesia, and Paresthesia.
- **Musculoskeletal:** Such as Weakness, Spasm, abnormal movement.

History of associated Diseases (Fig. 3.7): e.g. Diabetes Mellitus, Hypertension, Tuberculosis …etc. They help in the pathology of the current disease and in General condition of the patient which may affect the decision for the management of the patient including investigations and treatment.

Past Medical History (Fig. 3.8)

Like T.B, Cancer, Infectious mononucleosis etc. They can help in the current pathologic diagnosis or in the General condition of the patient. An abdominal pain and or masses in the abdomen in a patient with past history of proved TB is tuberculous peritonitis till prove otherwise.

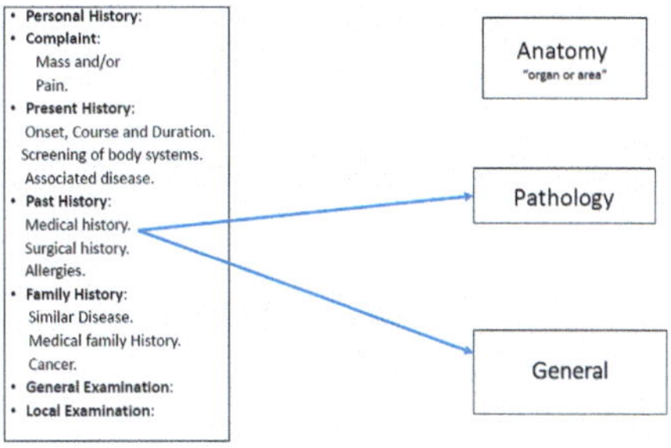

Fig. 3.8 Correlation between medical history and both pathology and general condition

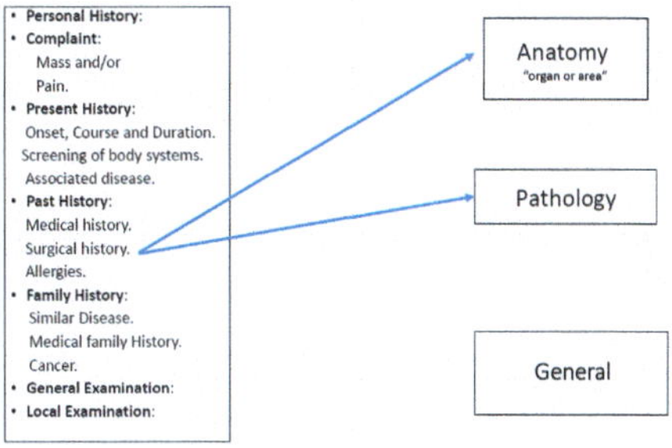

Fig. 3.9 Correlation between surgical history and both anatomy and pathology

Past History of Surgeries (Fig. 3.9)

It can help in Anatomical diagnosis e.g. to exclude appendicitis in Acute abdomen or to suggest ectopic pregnancy in a female in the childbearing period who had an operation for an ectopic pregnancy on one side before.

It can help in pathologic diagnosis in a patient with pain and swelling in the right hypochondrium who had a surgery for G.IL cancer before, "? Metastases" or adhesive etiology of Intestinal obstruction or vague abdominal pain after abdominal exploration.

History of Allergies to Medications or General Allergies (Fig. 3.10)

This is a vital part of any sheet in the General condition of the patients and failure to record this in the patient sheet may lead to Medico-legal issues to the doctor if this patient is given the medication he is allergic to it. It is also important to suggest the pathology of some complaints like joint pains in a patient known to be allergic in General to food or pollutants,

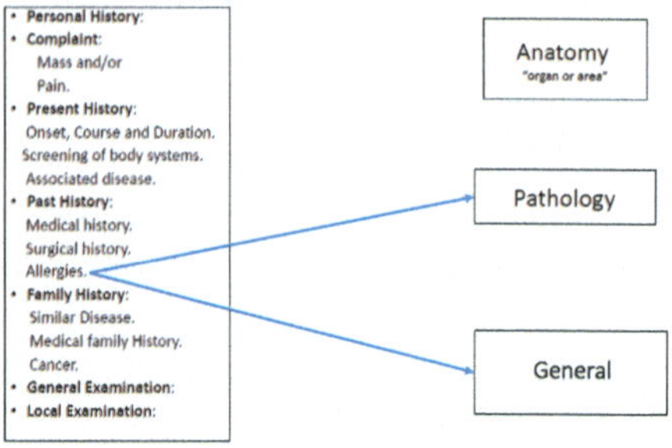

Fig. 3.10 Correlation between history of allergies and both pathology and general condition

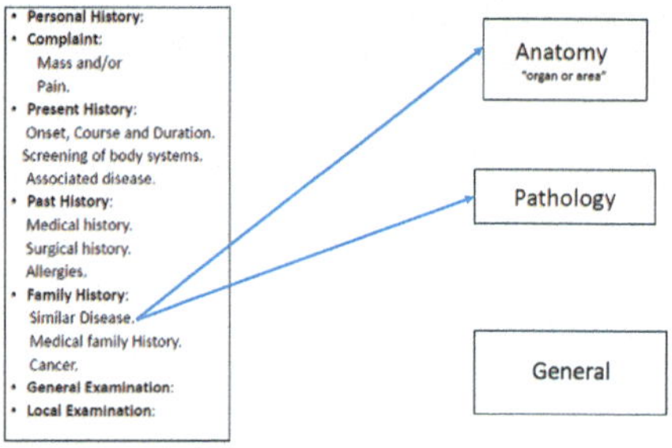

Fig. 3.11 Correlation between family history and both anatomy and pathology

Family History

Family History of Similar Disease (Fig. 3.11)

It helps in the Pathologic diagnosis. Family history of Colorectal Cancer or breast Cancer are Common example.

Family History of Medical Diseases (Fig. 3.12)

It helps in Anatomical diagnosis such as Thyroid disease "Goiter" which will be verified by examination and may suggest the pathology of the current disease with familial predilection such as cancer, DM and/or Hyperlipidemia. The last two may accelerate the incidence of vascular disease at a younger age such as Ischemia or aneurysm.

Family History of Cancer (Fig. 3.13)

Mentioned separately due to its importance not only for specific organ cancers but for the familial types of cancers such as HNPCC or "Hereditary Non-Polyposis Colorectal cancers".

Second Time-Out: Provisional diagnosis at the end of History taking.

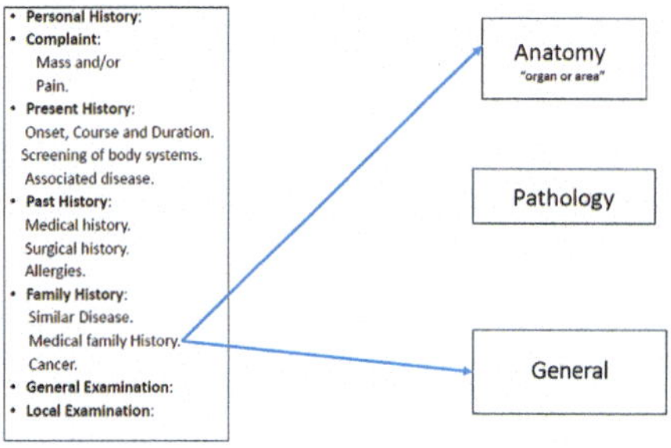

Fig. 3.12 Correlation between family history of medical disease and both anatomy and general condition +/− pathology

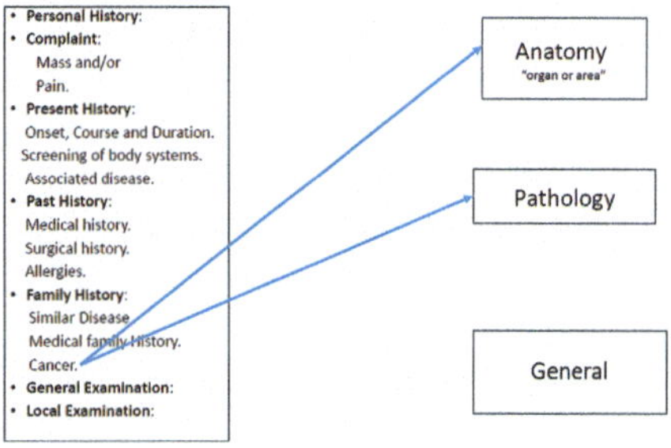

Fig. 3.13 Correlation between family history of cancer and both anatomy and pathology

General Examination (Fig. 3.14)

General Principles in General Examination:

1. Areas to be examined:
   - The body areas can be divided as areas above the diaphragm and areas below the diaphragm.
   - Areas above the diaphragm include General Look, head and Neck, both upper limbs, Chest front and back (Heart, Lungs and <u>both breasts</u> in males and females).
   - Areas Below the diaphragm include both lower limbs, abdomen front and back including buttocks and the Perineum.
   - In short case with a complaint in any area above the diaphragm all the areas above the diaphragm should be examined + a minimum of one area below the diaphragm namely the liver. (e.g. in thyroid swelling the local examination is the head and neck together with general look, both upper limbs, chest specially both breasts and the liver reserving the local examination (H & N) to the end. While in short cases with unilateral edema, both lower limbs should be examined together with the Abdomen front and back, the perineum and at least the Virchow and the left supraclavicular lymph nodes. The cause of the unilateral edema may be due to compression of the ipsilateral iliac vein by a metastatic lymph nodes from a squamous cell carcinoma in the buttocks or carcinoma of the anal Canal for example.

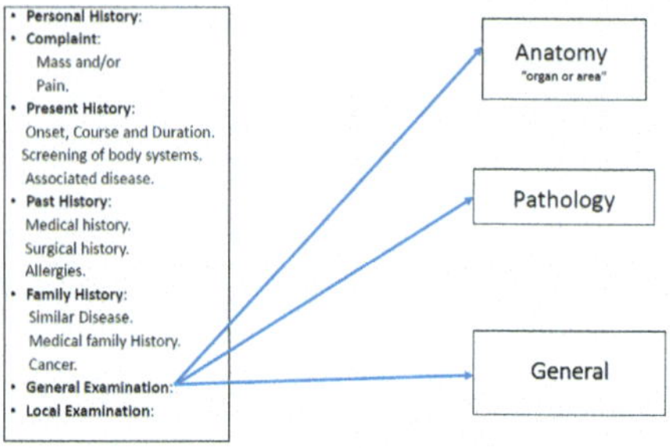

Fig. 3.14 Correlation between general examination and all categories "Anatomy, Pathology and General condition"

2. In Long Cases a recommended sequence of examination <u>**(March of Examination)**</u> is recommended to achieve the 3 goals of General examination:

   N.B. <u>The items mentioned in general examination are for screening of the patient in general examination but never enough for local examination</u>.

   - **General look**: Normal or Abnormal "e.g. Toxic, earthy, anxious, Apathetic look …etc."
   - **Decubitus in Bed**: Elevated leg in DVT, hanging limb beside the bed near a fan in critical ischemia, folded on himself in pancreatic pains and aortic aneurysm.
   - **Upper Limb** in the following sequence: Fine <u>tremors</u>, Flapping tremors, <u>Nails</u> (Clubbing, vertical ridging, spooning …etc.), <u>Palm of the hand</u> (warmth, color, sweating), <u>Pulse</u> on both sides for equality in volume and arrival) delayed pulse in one side compared to the other is pathognomonic of a proximal aneurysm. Then sampling of pulse on one of them for rate and rhythm if they are equal on both sides. <u>Water Hummer</u> Pulse and <u>Blood pressure</u>.
   - Then we complete the **Vital Signs** namely <u>Temperature</u> and <u>Respiratory rate</u>.
   - **Head and Neck:** Jaundice, Pallor, Central cyanosis, Supraclavicular and Virchow Lymph node +/− thyroid gland and the main group of the deep cervical lymph nodes deep to the sternomastoid on both sides.
   - **Chest:** front and back including the heart and lungs and both breasts in males and females.
   - **Both Lower Limbs:** for pedal pulse, edema "Unilateral or bilateral, Pitting or Non-pitting" and tender calf muscles.
   - **Abdominal examination:**

   - Examination includes examination of the Liver and spleen in lesions in the upper half of the body and full abdominal examination specially both inguinal and iliac lymph nodes in lesions of the lower limbs and perineum.

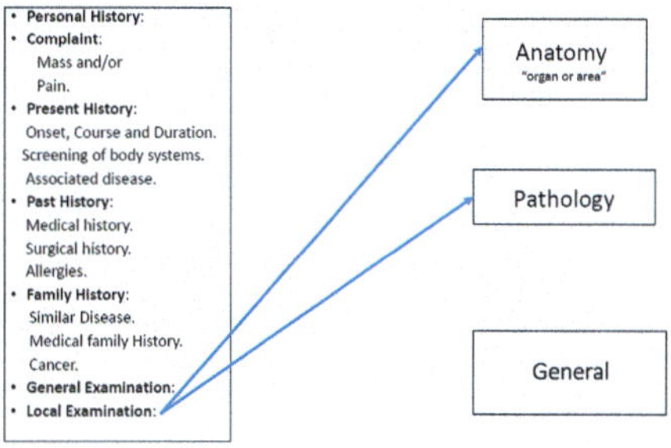

Fig. 3.15 Correlation between local examination and both anatomy and pathology

Local Examination (Box 3.4 and Fig. 3.15)

Will be addressed in the relevant section it includes

Box 3.4 Important Points to Remember

- Always remember in Local examination the Head, Neck and Mouth rather than the traditional Head and Neck.
- Also remember the Examination of the Chest is "Chest Front, Back and Breast" rather that chest and breast separately.
- Remember Examination of the Abdomen is Examination of the Abdomen Front and Back, Perineum, Gluteal region and Upper thighs.

- **Inspection:** "No touch to the patient with few exceptions"
- **Palpation:** e.g. "Superficial and deep" in the abdomen or by tips of the fingers and Flat of the hand in the breast.
- **Percussion:** For resonance or dullness.
- **Auscultation:** for sounds using the stethoscope.

It helps in Anatomical and pathologic diagnosis.

Investigations

Should be guides by the sound Clinical history taking and Clinical examination "both General and Local" they are directed to achieve:

1. Confirmation of the diagnosis If not already confirmed by Clinical sheet "i.e. No investigation is needed for a confirmed Lipoma, Haemangioma or Ingrowing toe nail.
2. To determine the disease not only in cancer but also for suspected organ dysfunction "Liver, Kidney, lung, heart or Brain dysfunctions' as a part of complete

assessment of the patient condition and tailoring the treatment for each individual patient.
3. To discover a suspected more serious disease discovered by the complete though swift general examination such as hidden thyrotoxicosis or arrhythmias in a cardiac patient presenting with a simple hernia or other common surgical complaints.
4. As a routine preoperative Investigations as suggested by the hospital or national Guidelines.

Investigations can be categorized into 4 main categories for the purpose of memorization for the undergraduate and postgraduate students during examination in that order of invasiveness.

1. Lab tests:
2. Radiology:
3. Instrumental: like endoscopy "+/− biopsies" or manometry.
4. Pathologic diagnosis: which may be

   - Needle biopsies:

     - Fine needle for cytology "or aspiration of fluids for cytology, to study the characters of the cells including the mitotic figures and the nuclear-cytoplasmic ratio suggestive of malignancy.
     - Tru-Cut needle biopsy for Histopathology
     - Endoscopic biopsies.

   - Surgical Biopsies:

     - Incisional: a Small wedge of the lesion.
     - Excisional: the lesion is removed totally and sent for pathology.

The Histopathology can be examined as:

- Frozen section "Immediate"
- Paraffin blocks.

Sections from Paraffin blocks are examined with Haematoxyline and Eosin or specific stains.

Chapter 4
Examination of Swellings

Mohamed Yehia Elbarmelgi and Mahmoud Mostafa

Abstract Examination of a swelling related to an organ such as Thyroid or parotid swelling and not related to an anatomical area such as Groin, Popliteal fossa, femoral triangle, axilla for example is discussed in their relevant chapters in this book. By Examination of a swelling in this Chapter we mean a swelling in the Skin, Subcutaneous tissue related to deep Fascia, Muscle or bone. Over a cavity or in a limb. By a Cavity we mean, the Cranium, spinal Cord.

Keywords Swelling · Examination · Organ · Skin · Subcutaneous · Fascia · Muscle · Cavity

Examination of a swelling related to an organ such as Thyroid or parotid swelling and not related to an anatomical area such as Groin, Popliteal fossa, femoral triangle, axilla for example is discussed in their relevant chapters in this book. By Examination of a swelling in this Chapter we mean a swelling in the Skin, Subcutaneous tissue related to deep Fascia, Muscle or bone. Over a cavity or in a limb. By a Cavity we mean, the Cranium, spinal Cord "e.g. Meningocele and its variant", Chest Cavity which extends into the Lowe Neck "e.g. Empyema necessitans (EN) and Pneumatocele in the Posterior triangle of the Neck", Abdominal Cavity which extends to the front, back, Perineum and femoral triangle "e.g. Hernia".

The same principles apply to the swellings in other sheets except the Abdominal Cavity, Thyroid and Lymph nodes and in the Anatomical areas of surgical importance mentioned above.

Components of the sheet includes (Tables 4.1 and 4.2):

M. Y. Elbarmelgi (✉)
Cairo University, Cairo, Egypt

M. Mostafa
Arab Contractors Medical Centre ACMC, Cairo, Egypt

A. Farag et al. (eds.), *Clinical Surgical Skills Made Easy*,
https://doi.org/10.1007/978-3-031-69158-4_4

Table 4.1 Understanding history taking of a mass

Item of the history taking	Anatomy	Pathology	General
Personal history		+	+
Complaint			
Mass	+		
Pain	+	+	
Onset		+	
Course		+	
Duration		+	
Screening of body systems	+	+	+
Past history of medical importance		+	
Family history		+	+

Table 4.2 Understanding examination of a mass

	Anatomy	Pathology	General
General		+	+
Site	+		
Size			
Shape	+	+	
Surface		+	
Surrounding structures	+	+	
Special signs		+++	
Other swellings	+	++	
Temperature		+	
Tenderness		+	
Edge	+	+	
Consistency		++	
Mobility	+	+	
Percussion		+	
Auscultation		+	
Limb distal, limb proximal, catchment area	+	+	

History Taking

Personal History: As Mentioned Before in the General Sheet is important in the epidemiology "pathology".

Complaint: It is important in the anatomical diagnosis but we have to ask at this point 2 main questions both are important for pathologic diagnosis namely: Painful or painless and single or Multiple. Both are important in the pathology.

From the pathologic point of view painful is mostly but not always benign swelling while painless is not pathognomonic "or diagnostic" of Malignant swelling.

Multiple swellings includes a narrow differential diagnosis namely: Multiple lipomatosis, multiple neurofibromatosis, Pyaemic abscesses, Hiradenitis suppurativa, Multiple Fistulae "T.B or Crohn's disease" Multiple Lymphadenopathy, Multiple warts or papillomas, Multiple exostosis and Multiple metastases.

Present History: Which is important in the pathology

- Onset:

  1. Mode of onset:

     Catastrophic onset which is immediate within seconds or minutes due to trauma or acute bleeding in a cyst.
     Acute: over hours "acute inflammation".
     Recent: over Weeks or Months such as tumors or chronic inflammations.
     Insidious: over years: Mostly benign.

  2. Was it associated with trauma or inflammation? Failure to ask this question may lead to loss of diagnosis.

- Course:

  Progressive: Increases in severity or size.
  Regressive: Decreases in severity or size.
  Stationary: Stable.
  Intermittent: May increase in severity or size but return to baseline.
  Remittent: May increase or decrease in size but do not return to baseline.

- Duration:

  Short: hours, days, weeks, months.
  Long: years.

In Short case Examination we go directly to examination after this brief history or take this history during examination of the swelling due to short time allocated for each case but in Long case examination and in our clinics specially in the first visit we have to ask the screening questions for each system in the body.

Similarly we have to remember the areas to be examined mentioned in the General sheet but in Long case and in our Clinics we have to apply the Marsh of General examination mentioned in the General sheet "2 min of Swift but structured G. Examination.

Local examination of a Swelling includes Inspection, Palpation, Percussion, and Auscultation if it apply. Some swellings will not be needed be examined by percussion and/or auscultations as will be seen in details later-on.

1. **<u>Inspection</u>:** for **7 S**:

   - **Site:** Describe the anatomical site (e.g., Swelling in the left arm).
   - **Size:** width x length x height cm in dimensions.
   - **Shape:** Rounded "equal in all directions", oblong One direction is more than the other 2 dimensions" Irregular or otherwise.
   - **Surface:** Regular (smooth) or showing irregularity (e.g., nodular or lobulated).

- **Surrounding structures "Skin, Muscle Fascia, Vessels and organs":** By inspection we examine the overlying skin for ulcers, dilated veins, or scars (We describe the healing of that scar either healed by primary or secondary intention), any tethering or dimpling which indicates attachment to skin. Deep or superficial to the nearby muscle or fascia, and nearby structures such as a vessel or an organ like trachea "Displacement from the normal position".
- **Special Signs:**

  Pulsating: The Mass should be inspected tangentially "Transmitted pulsations from a nearby artery such as Carotid Body tumor or expansile pulsations like an Aneurysm or A-V fistula where the latter is associated with dilated pulsating Veins, or a highly vascular solid tumors. It can be a pulsating artery "Visible on the surface of a non-pulsating tumor".
  Impulse on Cough "e.g. Hernia, Empyema Necessitates or Meningocele".

- **Other Swellings:** This is a very important item. Searching for other similar swelling should be done especially in bilateral conditions (e.g., bilateral inguinal hernia). Also, it is very important to look for the draining lymph nodes site (e.g., axilla in breast swelling).

2. **Palpation:** for **7 S T,T E,C and M**:
   N.B Palpation is by the palmer aspect of the examining hand and fingers not the tip of fingers.

- **Temperature:** By the dorsum of the fingers, you should start with the normal side comparing it to the affected side and report if the surface of the swelling is warmer than the normal side.
- **Tenderness:** By the palmer aspect of the examining hand or fingers, you should palpate the swelling gently asking the patient if it is tender, you should also look at the facies of the patient while palpating to elicit tenderness over the swelling.
- **Site:** We describe the anatomical site (e.g., Swelling in the left arm) and which part of the arm Upper, mid or Lower and which aspect Medial, Lateral, Volar "Anterior" or dorsal aspect of the arm
- **Size:** width x length x height cm in dimensions by a ruler or your fingers.
- **Shape:**
- **Surface:**
- **Edge:** By the side of the examining fingers from the normal area moving towards the mass from all directions, palpating the edge of the swelling, the edge may be:

(a) Well defined edge "I can sharply demarcate where the pathology starts" in which the examining fingers can elicit a true edge. They are usually benign except in the Breast where cancer breast have a well-defined edge though may be irregular but may be smooth like medullaruy carcinoma of the breast.
(b) Ill-defined edge in which the fingers cannot detect a true edge. Usually with cancer and Inflammations, where an intermediate zone is infiltrated with

malignant or inflammatory cells. N.B. It is not pathognomonic "Diagnostic" of cancer.

(c) Slippery edge where the edge can be pushed away (this is pathognomonic for lipomas due to very soft consistency and melting of fat that may occur)

- **Consistency: "Consistency = Fluctuation test"**
- Except the thyroid swellings who are not amenable to Fluctuation test.
- **Fluctuation** can be tested by placing the index and middle finger of the one hand (somewhat apart) on the swelling downwards pressure over the lesion with these fingers. Fluctuation occurs when the finger of the one hand is forced upwards when pushing downwards with the fingers of the other hand. Use a balloon partially filled up with water to practice this technique "Should be done in a Cross direction".
- Alternate in small swelling (<2 cm), apply pressure by index finger of the other hand placed in between these two fingers (**Paget's test**).
- **Bipolar Fluctuation test**: in Vaginal hydrocele or its variants where 2 fingers are located at the anterior and posterior surface of the upper pole of the swelling as receiving fingers and the other hand index and thumb pressing and releasing the fluid at the lower pole of the swelling.
- **Cross Fluctuation test** where two cystic swellings are close to each other and separated by a band e.g. an Ileo-psoas abscess which is under the sheath of the muscle and crossing under the inguinal Ligament. The left hand compresses and empties one swelling e.g. above the inguinal ligament, whilst the right hand straddles the front of the others welling i.e. below the inguinal ligament. Each hand is squeezed alternately, while the other hand receives the pulse. "Though called Cross Fluctuation test it is done in one direction".
- **For Solid lesions "Non Fluctuant"** It may be:
- Hard: like bone "Malignant, Boney swelling or Calcification".
- Firm: Like the tip of the nose.
- Soft: Like the lobule of the ear.
- **Important pitfalls**:

1. Muscles such as the thigh muscle may feel fluctuant in the transverse direction but it is fluctuant in the vertical direction which shows the importance of doing the fluctuation test in both directions.
2. Tense cystic lesions look hard on palpation and soft cystic lesions look like soft solid lesions that's why we prefer to start with the fluctuation test.
3. Lipomas may give a positive fluctuation test since the fat is semifluid in the body temperature but it has a slippery edge and fine tethering to the skin on movement of the lesion under the overlying skin.

- **Mobility:**

1. Examining the swelling mobility over the underlying muscle is by moving the swelling in 2 perpendicular directions while the muscle is resting and contracting if you can move it in both directions, so the swelling is mobile "A skin or a subcutaneous swelling".

2. If the swelling is attached to the fascia over the muscle: The swelling may be freely mobile before contraction of the muscle and on the contraction of the muscle it has a limited mobility in all directions.
3. A swelling which arises from the muscle: If the swelling is mobile in one direction and has a limited mobility in the vertical direction before contraction of the muscle and becomes fixed in All directions after the contraction of the muscle.
4. A swelling which is arises from or attached to a vertical structure "e.g. Vessel, Nerve or an organ such as trachea: the swelling is mobile in one direction and has a limited mobility in the vertical direction.
5. A swelling which is attached to the periosteal or bone or arises from them: Its **base** is fixed in all directions "D.D. is rocking where the tip of such lesion may show some degree of mobility in all or some directions while the base is fixed".

- **Surrounding structures:**
- The surrounding structures of each swelling depend on its anatomical site (hence the importance of anatomy for surgical practice). However, in all swelling you should examine the:

(a) The overlying skin to detect if the swelling is attached to the skin or not, pinching test is a preferable test for this. It is performed by pinching the skin over swelling in different sites if you can hold a fold of skin over the swelling, so it is not attached to the swelling and vice versa.

Gliding test: which is the ability of the skin to glide freely on the surface of the swelling.

Moving the swelling under the skin: which is moving the swelling and noticing the skin for dimpling "which indicates attachment to the skin" or fine multiple dimples in case of lipomas being attached to the skin by normal strands.

Elevation of the hand: is a special type of examining the attachment of the breast mass to the skin which will be mentioned in the Chapter on breast examination.

(b) Underlying Fascia, muscle or bone: Vide supra in the mobility section.

A special form of that examination is in the breast masses which is the dependency test mentioned in the Chapter on breast examination.

- **Special Signs:**

1. Pulsations: Using the Two fingers at s opposite ends of the mass to differentiate Expansile "increased distance between the examining fingers during each pulsation" or transmitted "A constant distance between the examining fingers during pulsations:
2. Impulse on Cough: and direction of descend in cases of inguinal hernia "DD direct in direct hernia or downwards, Forwards and medially in cases of indirect hernia"

3. Compressibility and refill in 2 or 3 pulsations: Pathognomonic of Haemangioma.
4. Partial compressibility: Lymphangioma "Such as Cystic Hygroma" or Haemangio-Lipoma.
5. Indentibilty: The swelling retains the site of the pressing finger after removing the examining hand, where the content is dough like such as a fecal mass in the colon or Sebum in a large sebaceous cyst.
6. Reducibility: Uncomplicated hernia with a notice on direction of reduction in inguinal hernia examination "Direct posterior in direct hernia and backwards, upwards and laterally in indirect inguinal hernia".
7. Slippery Edge: Lipoma.
8. Trans-illumination test: in vaginal hydrocele, Spermatocele, Meningocele and Cystic Hygroma for example.

- **Other Swellings:** Similar swellings "D.D. of Multiple swellings" or draining Lymph nodes.

3. **Percussion:** Percussion over the swelling is usually not helpful, however percussion should be done over the cavity of the swelling as in chest and abdominal swelling which will be discussed in detail in relevant chapters.
4. **Auscultation:** Auscultation over the swelling may detect thrill or venous hum if it is a vascular swelling. (e.g., aneurysm).

Limb Distal and Limb Proximal for Limb swellings:
Distal Limb examination: for pulsation, sensations, passive, active movements, color changes, Edema, Varicose veins.
Proximal limb examination: for Lymph nodes, Masses in the Femoral triangle or abdomen.
Full Abdominal examination if it Lies on the.
Abdominal Cavity: such as hernias, Masses, abscesses. They shouldn't be considered as a primary pathology except after excluding being an extension of intra-abdominal pathology or caused by intra-abdominal pathology.
Catchment area If in the Neck or the swelling is a Lymph nodes swelling:
Full examination of the head including the mouth in Neck swellings or examination of the Limbs, Chest and abdomen including front and back, breast, Perineum, P.R. and P.V. according to the group of the LN enlarged in axillary or inguinal Lymph nodes.

Chapter 5
DD. of Swelling in the Femoral Triangle

Ahmed Farag

Abstract Together with DD. Of a mass in the right iliac fossa, it is also one of the differential diagnosis of a mass in the Groin. Like the general approach in Clinical diagnosis DD. Of a mass in the Femoral triangle includes Anatomy and Pathology and General examination.

Keywords Differential · Diagnosis · Femoral · Triangle · Mass · Anatomy · Pathology · General examination

Together with DD. Of a mass in the right iliac fossa, it is also one of the differential diagnosis of a mass in the Groin.

Like the general approach in Clinical diagnosis DD. of a mass in the femoral triangle includes anatomy and pathology and general examination:

Anatomy (Table 5.1)

1. Skin: Sebaceous cysts, inflammations, papillomas or Carcinoma.
2. Subcutaneous Tissue: Haemangioma, Lymphangioma or Lipomas.
3. Lymph Nodes: “contrary to the neck the superficial inguinal LNs are more Important.”
4. Varicose Veins “Saphena Varix”.
5. Femoral Hernia.
6. Thrombosis of the femoral vein.
7. Aneurysm of the Femoral artery.
8. Traumatic A-V fistula “Bucher’s thigh.”
9. Neurofibroma of the femoral nerve.
10. Psoas bursa and Ileo-Psoas Abscess.
11. Ectopic testis “rare”.
12. Bone tumor from the upper end of the femur.

A. Farag (✉)
Kasr Alainy Hospital, Cairo University, Cairo, Egypt

A. Farag et al. (eds.), *Clinical Surgical Skills Made Easy*,
https://doi.org/10.1007/978-3-031-69158-4_5

Table 5.1 DD. of a mass in the femoral triangle

Organ affected	Lesion	General examination	Local examination
1. Skin	Sebaceous cysts:	Similar Lesions, Dandruff	Cyst with a black punctum which moves with the skin
	Inflammations:	Fever, rigors and malaise	Warm, red hot and tender
	Papillomas:	Similar lesions	Soft skin appendage
	Carcinoma:	Mets to LNs	Usually an Ulcer with raised everted edge and necrotic floor
2. Sub-cutaneous tissue	Haemangioma:	Similar Lesions	Bluish red or blue which is soft and compressible and refills in 1–2 s
	Lymphangioma:	Similar lesions	Partially compressible
	Lipomas	Similar lesions "if painful i.e. multiple painful lipomatosis "Dercum's disease"	Subcutaneous, may be attached to the skin with fine strands, soft Pseudo-cystic "Fat is fluid in the body temperature", with slippery edge. Some Lipomas have ill-defined edges
3. Lymph Nodes.	Inflammatory:	Signs of Acute inflammation, other LNs, Hepato-splenomegaly "HSM"	Local signs of inflammation
	Secondary malignant	Primary in the Perineum, Anal Canal, Vagina, Prostate and LLs "e.g. melanoma of the big toe"	Hard irregular or rounded with or without pressure symptoms causing edema of the LLs or secondary Varicose Veins
	Lymphoma and Leukemia:	Other Lymph node groups with or without HSM	Discrete, rounded, large, Rubbery in Hodgkin's L. but irregular and amalgamated in Non HL
4. Saphena Varix	Primary V.Vs:	Congenitally weak mesenchyme: such as Varicocele, piles, hernias and Flat foot	VVs affection of the Short, long, or both venous System. Minimal or no edema, pigmentation, cyanosis or ulcerations
	Secondary VV:	Right lower quadrant Abdominal mass with pressure on the iliac veins	Veins crossing the Groin and lower abdomen with direction of flow away from the Sapheno-femoral junction. Edema, pigmentation, cyanosis or ulcerations are common "Post- postphlebitic Limb"

(continued)

Table 5.1 (continued)

Organ affected	Lesion	General examination	Local examination
5. Femoral Hernia	Primary or secondary to increase intra-abdominal pressure	Other hernias, COPD, Intra-abdominal mass or ascites	Swelling with shows an impulse on cough and usually partially reducible during Lying down "unless complicated" with its neck below and lateral to the Pubic tubercle[a]
6. Femoral vein thrombosis	Usually post-delivery or post-operative rarely spontaneous	Signs suggestive of Pulmonary embolism or abdominal mass causing compression	A Cord like structure with tenderness in the course of the femoral and or iliac veins. Edema or cyanosis of the ipsilateral LL with or without signs of impending venous gangrene "An emergency Limb threatening situation"
7. Aneurysm of the femoral artery	Atherosclerosis:	Other Aneurysms and other ischemias in old patients. "Cardiac Cerebral, renal or Abdominal anginas	Swelling in the course of the artery which gives Expansile pulsations pressure on the artery proximally the swelling decrease in size distal edema may develop due to pressure on the vein. Signs of distal embolization "Blue toe syndrome
	Accelerated Atherosclerosis:	As above but in the 50's of age with history of DM and heavy smoking	As above
	Arteritis:	In the 40 years of age and Smoking	As Above
8. Traumatic A-V fistula	History of a penetrating trauma to the femoral triangle	Usually a butcher trying to debone a piece of meat resting on his thigh using a sharp knife	The same as aneurysm but there is an associated pulsating Varicose veins with tachycardia due to increased venous return through the fistula with positive Branham's sign[b]
9. Neurofibroma of the femoral nerve		An Isolated swelling or associated with multiple neurofibromatosis with Café au-lait patches over the trunk	Oval swelling, firm in consistency which moves from side-to side but not longitudinally Warning signs of tenderness, sensory or motor changes in the distribution of the femoral nerve raises the possibility of malignant transformation

(continued)

Table 5.1 (continued)

Organ affected	Lesion	General examination	Local examination
10. Ileo-Psoas Abscess	T.B. or Complicated Ileo-caecal Crohn's	Signs and Symptoms of T.B. and Signs of T.B. of the spine. Or signs and Symptoms of CD recurrent diarrhea, operations and loss of weight	Cystic mass partly above and partly below the inguinal ligament with Cross Fluctuation between the 2 swellings. "See examination of a Mass"
11. Ectopic testis (Rare)	Congenital	May be Bilateral	An empty ipsilateral scrotum May be associated with inguinal hernia
12. Bone tumor from the upper end of the femur	Benign or Malignant	Other swellings or metastases from a malignant tumor	The Swelling characteristically does not move in relation to bone[c]

[a]If you doubt from the first sight during inspection if it is femoral or inguinal hernia you have to suspect a femoral hernia. If you move your finger over the inguinal ligament between the Pubic tubercle and the ASIS the femoral hernia will be always or mostly below the inguinal ligament. In strangulated femoral hernia an external ring test will detect an empty inguinal canal

[b] Branham's Sign is when the artery proximal to it was compressed. In modern medicine, the sign is elicited when pressure is applied to an artery proximal to an arteriovenous fistula and said to be positive if the following occurs:

- Swelling reduces in size
- Bruit and thrill disappears
- Blood pressure rises
- Pulse rate and heart rate return to normal

[c]The mobility should be tested at the base of the swelling Sine the upper part of the swelling will show some rocking movement if there is a degeneration in the tumor

Personal History

- Age: Metastatic LNs from pelvic or Lower Limb Malignancies are more common in old age, while Lymphomas are more common in younger age group. The cause of Arterial aneurysm is suggested by age "Atherosclerosis in older age groups i.e. >60 years, while arteritis is suggested in young age groups i.e. 40's or less, while accelerated atherosclerosis due to DM are in the 50's".
- Sex: Cancer Prostate as a cause of enlarged inguinal LNs in males. Femoral hernia is more common in Females.
- Occupation: Butchers in traumatic A-V fistula and Prolonged standing "Teachers and Surgeons" for Varicose Veins.
- Smoking: for worsened arterial disease.

Complaint: Mass "Painful or Painless"

Present History

- Onset: catastrophic onset "in traumatic femoral aneurysm or A.V fistula called Bucher's thigh", Acute such as acute Lymphadenopathy, Subacute such as chronic lymphadenopathy or insidious or accidentally discovered "such as Saphena Varix and neuromas"
- Course: Rapidly progressive such as acute inflammatory LNs, rapidly progressive "Such as metastatic Lymph nodes from carcinoma of the Anal canal or Vulva or Lymphoma" very slowly progressive or stationary "such as Lipoma"
- Duration: long duration usually indicates benign lesions.
- Limb distal: For pulses, Veins, Lymphatic edema, sensation and motor power "Active and passive".
- Perineum: For primary tumor or inflammation.
- Abdominal and Pelvic Symptoms: For other hernias in case of hernias, other arterial diseases or aneurysms, other lymph node enlargements and/or hepatosplenomegaly.
- Other swellings in the body: for other aneurysms or associated ischemias in the other parts of the body in cases of femoral aneurysm or for Generalized lymphadenopathy in cases of Inguino-iliac lymphadenopathy or for COPD as a cause of increased intra-abdominal pressure as a cause for an inguinal or femoral hernia.

Personal History

- Age is important to differentiate between the etiologies of P.A. aneurysm due to arteritis and atherosclerosis "Old age". Ectopic testis usually in infancy, Childhood or in young males. Inguinal Lymphadenopathy due to malignant lesions is most probably is due to Lymphoma in young age or due to Secondaries from a Lower Limb Melanoma or SCC or from Pelvic malignancy in older age group.
- Sex: Femoral Hernia is more common in females but it can occur in males.
- Occupation: Saphena Varix due to Varicose veins are more common among teachers, Surgeons and Sellers.
- Habits of Medical importance: Such as smoking in aneurysms.
- Contraceptive pills: Are contraindication to use injection sclerotherapy to treat Varicose veins for dear of spreading thrombosis into the deep system of veins.

- **Complaint:**

- Swelling in the Femoral triangle "Upper part of the front of the thigh" which may be:

  - Painless.
  - Painful:

1. In acute or associated with pain such Acute Lymphadenitis, complicated Femoral Hernia,
2. Pain not related to the swelling may be:
   - Due to Varicose Veins in cases of affected long saphenous System.
   - Acute Ilio-Femoral Thrombosis.
   - Due to distal ischemia associated with Femoral artery aneurysm.
   - Due to Nerve pain in cases of Neurofibrosarcoma of the Femoral nerve affecting mainly the front of the thigh "Distribution of the femoral nerve".
   - Due to a primary inflammatory or painful malignant lesion in the limb distally metastasizing into the Vertical group of the superficial inguinal LNs.
   - Bone pain from Primary or secondary bone tumor with or without pathologic fracture.
   - Acute inflammation in the skin or subcutaneous tissue.

Present History

- Onset:
  1. Trauma?
  2. Inflammation?
  3. Mode of Onset?
     - Immediate in Bucher's thigh, Strangulated Hernia or pathologic fracture of the upper end of the femur.
     - Acute "Hours" in Acute abscess, Cellulitis or Acute Lymphadenitis.
     - Gradual or accidentally identified in the rest of swellings.
- Course:
  - Progressive "Rapid or Slow progression". Rapidly progressive like expanding hematoma after traumatic femoral artery Aneurysm. Or Slowly progressive "over Hours or days" like acute inflammatory lesions.
  - Regressive "spontaneous or on treatment such as in cases of inflammation".
- Duration: Very short "Rupture aneurysm or traumatic A-V fistula or Femoral hernia complicated by obstruction or strangulation", short "Inflammation" Weeks, months or years in the rest of pathologies"
- Associated Symptoms:
  - Of a primary focus "Neoplastic or inflammatory in the ipsilateral LL or in the Pelvis or perineum.
  - Acute Limitation of the movement of the hip joint "with flexion" due to an Ileopsoas abscess or in acute appendicitis with retrocaecal Position.

- Distal LL edema in cases of Varicose veins with skin pigmentation and ulcerations in secondary varicose veins.
- Claudication pains or rest pain if PA aneurysm is associated with distal arterial disease or Blue toe Syndrome from repeated distal embolization in cases of mural thrombosis in PA aneurysm.
- Acute distal critical ischemia "Pain, Pallor, pulseless distal limb with acute loss of function which may show later mottling, Cyanosis and acute gangrene from acute thrombosis of a Femoral artery aneurysm" with edema in cases of acute rupture of PAA.
- Multiple similar Swellings in the same limb "Popliteal LN" in cases of inflammatory or neoplastic "Secondaries from squamous cell carcinoma or Melanoma "Black colored LNs with or without in-transit black metastases at the medial aspect of the thigh Lymphatics" or primary neoplastic cause such as Lymphoma or Leukemia"
- Multiple lipomas.
- Boney swellings like exostosis or metastases.
- Systemic manifestations of inflammations, other Lymph node affection, Hepatosplenomegaly in cases of Lymphoma/Leukemia, Systemic allergies autoimmune diseases, Neurofibromatosis with Café-au-Lait patches, Allergies including Urticaria, scratch marks, serum Sickness or metastases to the Lung, Liver, brain or bones or the source of metastases in the upper end of the femur like breast cancer.

Past History

- Medical for Similar disease in other LL or other parts of the body and treatments that may disclose some diseases forgotten by the patient specially in the first medical visit not recorded in the file or the patient is trying to hide like TB, HIV, Syphilis "though rare" Sexually transmitted disease.
- Allergies.

Family History

Of Similar disease and other diseases of medical importance.

General Examination

As in the general sheet is very important to for 3 reasons:

- General assessment of the patient which may uncover another serious or general disease which should be taken in consideration while requesting investigations and/or during planning for treatment of the patients such as associated vital organ dysfunction or failure "Cardiac, respiratory, Liver, Kidney".
- May uncover the stage of the disease in cases of Lymphoma and Malignant tumors such as node metastases from SCC or Melanoma or in cases of osteosarcoma and Ewing's tumor in the liver, lung, brain or other sites.
- May be the only clue for diagnosis of the mass in the Popliteal fossa as in:
  - Systemic inflammation "Fever and rigors in cases of Acute Cellulitis/abscess or acute lymphadenitis.
  - Similar tumor "DD of multiple tumors" due to Pyaemic abscesses, multiple papillomas, sebaceous cysts, Lipomas or Lipomatosis if painful it is Dercum's disease, Multiple Exostosis, Generalized Lymphadenopathy, Multiple neurofibromatosis "associated with cafe-au-lait patches
  - Aneurysms or ischemias affecting other site of the body "Peripheral, CVS, Intestinal or Renal".

Local Examination

Swelling:

- Inspection: Position, Gait, Color, Contour, Localized swelling, trophic changes, dilated Tortious veins "Varicose Veins VV", Ulcerations, Masses. Gangrene.
- Palpation: Temperature, Tenderness, Site, Size, shape, Surface, Edge, Consistency, Mobility, Surrounding structures, Other Swellings.
- Special signs: Pulsations "Expansile or transmitted" Trans-illumination test
- Percussion: Resonant in case of femoral hernia containing bowel "not common"
- Auscultation: Bruit "Aneurysm or Machinery Murmur "Traumatic A.V. fistula".

Limb distal: for:

- Pressure effects on veins, nerves, or associated Ischemia.
- For a primary malignant Lesion "Carcinoma or Melanoma" or for a primary inflammatory lesion.

Limb Proximal: for:

- Other Similar masses.
- Arteries, Veins and Nerves.
- Associated affected inflammatory or Malignant Lymph node in the Inguino-iliac Group of LNs "The Vertical croup of the superficial inguinal LNs and the Internal iliac group are draining the LL, While the transverse group are draining the Perineum, Anal canal and Vagina into the medial half and the buttocks

and back below a line at the Level of the Umbilicus is draining into its Lateral Half".

<u>Other Lower Limb</u>: for:

- Comparison.
- A similar "Bilateral condition".

<u>Abdominal examination</u>:
For:

- Lymphadenopathy.
- Hepatosplenomegaly in cases of Lymphoma/Leukemia or Liver mets in cases of Melanoma, Osteosarcoma or other malignant tumors in the LL or in the popliteal fossa.
- Abdominal Aortic or Iliac artery aneurysms.
- Other masses such as retroperitoneal Sarcoma.
- The cause of an Ileopsoas abscess "TB spine or Crohn's d".

Chapter 6
Swelling in the Popliteal Fossa

Ahmed Farag

Abstract Anatomical background:
Boundaries:

1. The Biceps Femoris tendon (superolateral).
2. Semimembranosus reinforced by Semitendinosus (superomedial).
3. The medial and lateral heads of Gastrocnemius form the inferomedial and inferolateral boundaries, respectively.
4. Floor is made by the back of the knee Joint, Lower part of the Femur or upper part of the Tibia.
5. The Roof made by the skin and subcutaneous tissue.

Keywords Popliteal · Fossa · Mass · Examination · Anatomy · Pathology · Boundaries · Content

Anatomical Background

- Boundaries:
  1. The Biceps Femoris tendon (superolateral).
  2. Semimembranosus reinforced by Semitendinosus (superomedial).
  3. The medial and lateral heads of Gastrocnemius form the inferomedial and inferolateral boundaries, respectively.
  4. Floor is made by the back of the knee Joint, Lower part of the Femur or upper part of the Tibia.
  5. The Roof made by the skin and subcutaneous tissue.
- Contents:
  1. Popliteal artery.

A. Farag (✉)
Kasr Alainy Hospital, Cairo University, Cairo, Egypt

A. Farag et al. (eds.), *Clinical Surgical Skills Made Easy*,
https://doi.org/10.1007/978-3-031-69158-4_6

2. Popliteal vein.
3. Tibial nerve.
4. Common peroneal nerve.
5. Short Saphenous vein and Sapheno-femoral Junction.
6. Popliteal LN.

Popliteal fossa Swelling is part of the Sheet of examination of A Swelling including general and local examination, examination of a Limb namely examination of the Limb distal and Limb Proximal "See related chapter" and Areas to be examined namely both LLs, Abdomen and minimum the Virchow LN in a short as OSPE sheet "in the General examination sheet" in our daily practice it is always recommended to do a thorough though swift general examination as the clue for diagnosis may be in the General examination e.g. other aneurysms, LNs or metastases from the lesion. Or it may disclose another disease of importance like Heart failure, arrhythmias, Liver failure ….etc.

DD of a Mass in the Popliteal Fossa

1. Semimembranosus Bursa: From the ST tendon.
2. Baker's Cyst: Herniation of the Synovial Fluid through a defect in the capsule of the knee joint associated with Osteoarthritis.
3. Varicose veins: affecting the short Saphenous vein with incompetent Sapheno-popliteal Junction.
4. Popliteal artery aneurysm: from the P.A.
5. Neurofibroma: from the Tibial or Common Peroneal nerve.
6. Sebaceous cyst, abscess, Cellulitis, Lipomas …etc. from the skin and subcutaneous tissue.
7. Boney swelling: from the Lower end of the Femur or upper end of the tibia: Exostosis, benign tumors such as cysts, benign Osteoma or Chondroma or Malignant tumors such as Osteosarcoma and Ewing's tumor.
8. Acute Swelling: Rupture P.A. Aneurysm, Ruptured Baker's cyst or Semimembranosus bursa or a subcutaneous cellulitis/abscess or Acute Popliteal Lymphadenitis "Less Common"

Personal History

- Age is important to differentiate between the Baker's cyst "Old age" and Semimembranosus bursa "Younger" and between the etiologies of P.A. aneurysm due to arteritis and atherosclerosis "Old age".
- Occupation: Varicose veins are more common among teachers, Surgeons and Sellers.

- Habits of Medical importance: Such as smoking in aneurysms.
- Contraceptive pills: Are contraindication to use injection sclerotherapy to treat Varicose veins for dear of spreading thrombosis into the deep system of veins.

- **Complaint:**

- Swelling in the back of the knee which may be:
  - Painless.
  - Painful:
    1. In acute or associated with pain such as Baker's Cyst which is associate with Osteo arthritis.
    2. Pain not related to the swelling may be:
       - Due to Varicose Veins in cases of affected Short saphenous System.
       - Due to distal ischemia associated with P.A. aneurysm
       - Due to Nerve pain in cases of Neurofibrosarcoma.
       - Due to a primary inflammatory or painful malignant lesion in the limb distally metastasizing into the Popliteal LN.
       - Pain may be in the proximal LNs at the Groin affected by the pathology in the Popliteal fossa or the limb distally.

Present History

- Onset:
  1. Trauma?
  2. Inflammation?
  3. Mode of Onset?
     - Immediate in Ruptured Baker's Cyst or ruptured P.A. Aneurysm.
     - Acute "Hours" in Acute abscess, Cellulitis or Acute Popliteal LN.
     - Gradual or accidentally identified in the rest of swellings.
- Course: Progressive "Rapid or Slow progression", Regressive "spontaneous or on treatment such as in cases of inflammation".
- Duration: Very short "Rupture PPA or Baker's cyst", short "Inflammation" Weeks, months or years in the rest of pathologies"
- Associated Symptoms:
  - Osteoarthritis in Baker's Cyst but absent in Semimembranosus bursa.
  - Acute Limitation of the movement of the knee in Acute situation "Rupture PA Aneurysm or SM Bursa and in acute inflammation" associated with fever and rigors in the acute cellulitis abscess or acute Lymphadenitis.
  - Distal edema in cases of Varicose veins with skin pigmentation and ulcerations in secondary varicose veins.

- Claudication pains if PA aneurysm is associated with distal arterial disease or Blue toe Syndrome from repeated distal embolization in cases of mural thrombosis in PA aneurysm.
- Acute distal critical ischemia "Pain, Pallor, pulseless distal limb with acute loss of function which may show later mottling, Cyanosis and acute wet gangrene from simultaneous compression on the Popliteal vein" with edema in cases of acute rupture of PAA.
- Multiple similar Swellings in the same limb "Groin" incases of inflammatory or neoplastic "Secondaries from squamous cell carcinoma or primary neoplastic cause such as Lymphoma or Leukemia" enlargement of the Popliteal LN.
- Multiple lipomas.
- Boney swellings like exostosis or metastases.

Past History

- Medical for Similar disease in other LL or other parts of the body and treatments that may disclose some diseases forgotten by the patient specially in the first medical visit not recorded in the file or the patient is trying to hide like TB, HIV, Syphilis "though rare" Sexually transmitted disease.
- Allergies.

Family History

Of Similar disease and other diseases of medical importance.

General Examination

As in the general sheet is very important to for 3 reasons:

- General assessment of the patient which may uncover another serious or general disease which should be taken in consideration while requesting investigations and/or during planning for treatment of the patients such as associated vital organ dysfunction or failure "Cardiac, respiratory, Liver, Kidney".
- May uncover the stage of the disease in cases of Lymphoma and Malignant tumors such as popliteal node metastases from SCC or Melanoma or in cases of osteosarcoma and Ewing's tumor in the liver, lung, brain or other sites.
- May be the only clue for diagnosis of the mass in the Popliteal fossa as in:

- Systemic inflammation "Fever and rigors in cases of Acute Cellulitis/ abscess or acute lymphadenitis.
- Similar tumor "DD of multiple tumors" due to Pyaemic abscesses, multiple papillomas, sebaceous cysts, Lipomas or Lipomatosis if painful it is Dercum's disease, Multiple Exostosis, Generalized Lymphadenopathy, Multiple neurofibromatosis "associated with cafe-au-lait patches.
- Aneurysms or ischemias affecting other site of the body "Peripheral, CVS, Intestinal or Renal".

Local Examination

Swelling:

- Inspection: Position, Gait, Color, Contour, Localized swelling, trophic changes, dilated Tortious veins "Varicose Veins VV", Ulcerations, Masses. Gangrene.
- Palpation: Temperature, Tenderness, Site, Size, shape, Surface, Edge, Consistency, Mobility, Surrounding structures, Other Swellings.
- Special signs: Pulsations "Expansile or transmitted" Trans-illumination test
- Percussion: Not applicable here.
- Auscultation: Bruit "Aneurysm or Machinery Murmur "Traumatic A.V. fistula".

  - ***Semimembranosus Bursa***: Cystic "Positive fluctuation test in two directions", Translucent swelling in the medial aspect of the popliteal fossa at the lateral aspect of the semi- membranous tendon which increases in size during extension and deceases in size or disappears during flexion. It happens in young patients with normal knee joint.
  - DD. ***Baker's cyst*** which occurs as herniation of the Synovial membrane in older patients with osteoarthritis. The important point in clinical DD is that removal of the Bakers cyst is not recommended because the cause of pain is due to osteoarthritis.
  - ***Popliteal Lymphadenopathy***: A well-defined rounded tender hot mass if draining an acute septic focus in the heel or back of the leg.
  - ***Varicose veins*** affecting the short saphenous system and Incompetent Sapheno-popliteal Junction: soft, cystic, compressible and Blush swelling which is tortuous and shows incompetent saphenofemoral Junction on Multiple Tourniquet test. "See Venous sheet"
  - ***Neurofibroma or neurofibromatosis*** of the Tibial nerve "In the Middle of the fossa" or Common Peroneal nerve "at the lateral aspect of the Fossa": Oblong in shape in the line of the nerve which can be moved side to side but not vertically, firm in consistency may show tenderness which may radiate as tingling or pain distally on palpation. It may be a part of neurofibromatosis.

- ***Aneurysm of the Popliteal artery***: may be traumatic "False aneurysm" after penetrating trauma or rarely blunt trauma with fracture of the Lower end femur or upper end tibia in the popliteal fossa with fractured bone causing a side tear in the artery "DD. Traumatic AV fistula with its associated distal edema, Pulsating VVs and Branham's bradycardia sign". Or due to atherosclerosis or arteritis. A Cystic Pulsating swelling "Expansile pulsations as explained in the Chapter on swellings or chapter on vascular examination" which is in the line of the popliteal artery. Proximal pressure on the artery over the lower end of the femur, decreases or stops pulsations which is regained on removal of the pressure in one heartbeat. It shows thrill on palpation and bruit on auscultation. If thrombosed and totally occluded it may be difficult to diagnose except with its associated Acute or Chronic Ischemia, based on the speed of its thrombosis.
- A Bony tumor from The Lower end of femur or upper end of Tibia: Hard in consistency and fixed to the bone at the base of the swelling and usually extends outside the limits of the Popliteal fossa.
- Skin Papillomas, Sebaceous cysts, Haemangioma, Hematomas, Subcutaneous Lipoma and subcutaneous abscess as in the Chapter on examination of swellings.

Limb distal: for:

- Pressure effects on veins, nerves, or associated Ischemia.
- For a primary malignant Lesion "Carcinoma or Melanoma" or for a primary inflammatory lesion.

Limb Proximal: For:

- Other Similar masses.
- Arteries, Veins and Nerves.
- Associated affected inflammatory or Malignant Lymph node in the Inguino-iliac Group of LNs "The Vertical croup of the superficial inguinal LNs and the Internal iliac group are draining the LL, While the transverse group are draining the Perineum, Anal canal and Vagina into the medial half and the buttocks and back below a line at the Level of the Umbilicus is draining into its Lateral Half".
- In transit metastases "Black in color" in the medial aspect or the thigh incases of Melanoma due to metastases in the Lymph vessels in its way to the inguinal LNs.

Other Lower Limb: for:

- Comparison.
- A similar "Bilateral condition".

Abdominal examination:
For:

- Lymphadenopathy.

- Hepatosplenomegaly in cases of Lymphoma/Leukemia or Liver mets in cases of Melanoma, Osteosarcoma or other malignant tumors in the LL or in the popliteal fossa.
- Abdominal Aortic or Iliac artery aneurysms.
- Other masses such as retroperitoneal Sarcoma.

Chapter 7
Examination of an Ulcer

Mohamed Yehia Elbarmelgi and Mahmoud Mostafa

Abstract Personal History It is important for the Pathology—epidemiology|| of the ulcer. E.g. Smoking, alcoholism, Spicy food in tongue ulcer.

Complaint: Loss of continuity of surface epithelium. The site of the Ulcer is of paramount importance to suggest its pathology "Etiology". At this point it is important to ask for number in the same area or in other body areas e.g. Genito-oral ulcers in Behcit's disease.

Keywords History · Personal · Ulcer · Pathology · Etiology · Number · Anatomy · Examination

Personal History (Table 7.1): It is important for the Pathology "epidemiology" of the ulcer. E.g. Smoking, alcoholism, Spicy food in tongue ulcer.

Complaint: Loss of continuity of surface epithelium. The **site** of the Ulcer is of paramount importance to suggest its **pathology "Etiology**", "Table" At this point it is important to ask for **number** in the same area or in other body areas e.g. Genito-oral ulcers in Behcit's disease. Also in the oral cavity malignant ulcers are usually single while multiple ulcers may suggest aphthous ulcers. **Pain** is also of paramount importance since Neuropathic ulcers are painless while aphthous ulcers and ulcers of Behcit's disease are very painful.

Present History

Onset: Mode of onset may be diagnostic from the pathologic point of view e.g. acute ulcers are mostly benign. While chronic ulcers may be malignant like Marjolin ulcer on top of an old unstable scar "e.g. an old burn".

M. Y. Elbarmelgi (✉)
Cairo University, Cairo, Egypt

M. Mostafa
Arab Contractors Medical Centre ACMC, Cairo, Egypt

A. Farag et al. (eds.), *Clinical Surgical Skills Made Easy*, https://doi.org/10.1007/978-3-031-69158-4_7

Table 7.1 D.D. of a lower limb ulcer

	Traumatic	Inflammatory	Venous	arterial	Trophic	SQ CC and melanoma
Personal history	Any age, sex but may be a hard work or a sports injury	Over an acute abscess like carbuncle	Usually after a secondary varicose veins	Old age if due to atherosclerosis or middle or young age if due to arteritis. Males are more affected in Burger's disease with smoking	At any age or sex	Usually middle or old age in male or female
Complaint	Painful Ulcer usually over the shin of the tibia	Signs of swelling which ulcerates accompanied by signs suggestive of local and systemic sepsis	An Ulcer over the medial aspect of the lower Leg	Ulcer over the most distal part of the Limb "Toes" associated with rest pain	A Painless Ulcer at the pressure points of the LL including the heel or the sole of the foot over the metatarsal heads	A mass or as an ulcer
Present history	Long history which may suggest an underlying Periosteitis	Short history usually in immune-compromised patient or diabetic patient with multiple septic foci on the top before ulceration or surgical drainage	History of DVT some months or years ago without wearing a protective Elastic stocking	Preceded by manifestations of Chronic ischemia or neglected acute ischemia	Painless and associated with loss of sensations in the surrounding skin	Rapidly increasing in size Melanoma may present under the toe nail
Past history	Of direct trauma to the shin bone	Similar condition or DM or immunosuppressive treatment	Of DVT	Similar condition in the other LL or other ischemias	Of loss of sensation due to congenital "Spina Bifida", traumatic, Inflammatory or Neoplastic causes	

	Traumatic	Inflammatory	Venous	arterial	Trophic	SQ CC and melanoma
Family history	Of DM or diseases of Medical importance	Similar condition in the family	Venous disease	Similar condition in the family	Similar condition	
G. Examination	For DM or diseases of Medical importance	Signs of sepsis "Fever, rigors and malaise	NAD	Other manifestations of ischemia	Specially nerves for stigmata of Syphilis, leprosy, DM and Back examination	For metastases including the Inguinal LNs and in transit mets
Local examination	Over the shin of the tibia, irregular, infected "Yellowish red floor, oozing serum or pus. Floor usually fixed to the underlying Periosteum. Sloping edge, with hyperemic margin	Slough containing base over an elevated infected tissue of the carbuncle and angry margin. When treated by removal of the slough medically or surgically the base becomes Red clean granulation tissue	Secondary varicose veins with incompetent valves. The surrounding skin is edematous, eczematous and pigmentation it is painful and covered scanty granulation even in the absence of Varicose veins "Gravitational ulcer	Gangrenous floor or edges, trophic changes in the surrounding skin such as loss of hair tapered toes, and dusky red skin, Loss of distal pulsations and level of Coldness in the distal part of the Limb	Punched out edges, the skin around it is hyper-keratotic and elevated over the pressure areas and characteristic-cally painless with loss of sensation	Melona is usually black or dark in color Squamous cell carcinoma has a raised everted edge

N.B. A Marjolin ulcer is a cutaneous malignancy usually Squamous Cell Carcinoma that arises in the setting of previously injured skin, longstanding unstable scars, and chronic wounds. It does not spread to the draining LNs due to lack of Lymphatics in the scar tissue

N.B. Rodent ulcers are a type of skin cancer. Also known as basal cell carcinoma, rodent ulcers occur in the lower most layer of your skin. They usually develop in skin areas exposed to the sun. Rodent ulcers are a very slow growing cancer that usually does not spread to other parts of your body

N.B. Ulceration is a breakdown of the skin on top of the melanoma. Melanomas with ulceration are more serious because they have a greater risk of spreading, so they are staged higher than tumors without ulceration

N.B. Tuberculous ulcers are ulcers which are usually formed by breakdown of tubercles and usually has an undermined edge

N.B. Bed Sores develop when blood supply to the skin is cut off for more than 2 to 3 hours. As the skin dies, the bedsore first starts as a red, painful area, which eventually turns purple. Left untreated, the skin can break open and the area can become infected. A bedsore can become deep

At this point we have to ask about history of trauma and/or inflammation. If we fail or forget to ask about them at this point we may miss 2 important categories in the Etiology namely traumatic ulcers or ulcers following an inflammation such as ulcers after treatment of a Carbuncle.

N.B. Venous ulcers and Ischemic ulcers may start after a minor trauma such as itching in venous ulcer or minor trauma to the big toe in Ischemic ulcers.

Course: A regressive ulcer is not usually a malignant ulcer.

Duration: A long history for years usually excludes malignant ulcers except for Marjolin ulcer.

Screening of the Body Systems: It is important from the pathology point of view such as History of Neurologic disorder can suggest Neuropathic ulcer, History of arterial disease such as Lower Limb ischemia can suggest an Ischemic ulcer. History of severe and uncontrolled Hypertension can suggest Martorell's ulcer is an uncommon ischemic and extremely painful lesion located in the distal portion of the lower limb, resulting from severe systemic and poorly controlled hypertension. It is common in women between 50 and 70 years of age. The diagnosis is clinical and mostly belated, following exclusion of other causes.

Past History of:

Medical past History: can suggest TB ulcer, Syphilis ulcer, Martorell's ulcer …etc.

Surgical Past History: Spine surgery may suggest Neuropathic ulcer and history of Burn may suggest Marjolin ulcer.

Family History:

General Examination

May suggest the Etiology such as Neurologic examination, stigmata of Syphilis, Leprosy or TB.

Local Examination

Inspection of the Ulcer

- Floor of the ulcer: the part of the ulcer which is seen by the eye without touch.
- Discharge:
- Edge: it is the Junction of the intact skin though abnormal and the floor of the ulcer. It's the most diagnostic of the pathology of the ulcer.
- Margin: the abnormal but intact skin between the edge of the ulcer and normal skin.
- Limb distal: for evidence of arterial, Venous, Nerve, or lymphatic pathology as well as deformity and musculoskeletal and/or Joint abnormality.

- Limb proximally: For draining Lymph nodes and/or other swellings or for LNs in other areas.

Palpation of the Ulcer

- Base of the ulcer: It is the tissue upon which the ulcer rests. Indurated or soft. Fixity to underlying structures special bone.
- Limb distal: for evidence of arterial, Venous, Nerve, or lymphatic pathology as well as deformity and musculoskeletal and/or Joint abnormality.
- Limb proximally: For draining Lymph nodes and/or other swellings or for LNs in other areas.

Chapter 8
Lymphadenopathy Sheet and D.D. of Multiple Swellings

Ahmed Farag

Abstract A Simple revision of the Pathology and Anatomy of the Lymphadenopathy is essential before proceeding to Clinical Sheet in order to ask relevant questions. Lymph nodes amenable for Clinical examination have known Sites in the human Body such as the Neck and face, Axillae, Groins, Intra-abdominally around the aorta——Para-Aortic and Peri-aortic|| and Iliac Lymph nodes around the Common and External iliac arteries.

Keywords Lymph · Node · Pathology · Anatomy · Examination · Sheet · Diagnosis · General

A Simple revision of the Pathology and Anatomy of the Lymphadenopathy is essential before proceeding to Clinical Sheet in order to ask relevant questions:

Box 8.1 Causes of Lymphadenopathy

- **Inflammatory**: Acute or Chronic. Specific or Non-specific.

  Acute Non-Specific: LNs draining an abscess or acute inflammation.

  Chronic Non-specific: draining a Chronic septic focus like Carious tooth.

- **Acute or Chronic Specific**: includes
  - Bacterial infections: lyme disease, tuberculosis, and cat scratch disease.
  - Viral infections: Examples include measles, infectious mononucleosis, HIV/AIDS, and cytomegalovirus (CMV).
  - Parasitic infections: Examples include toxoplasmosis and Chagas disease.

A. Farag (✉)
Kasr Alainy Hospital, Cairo University, Cairo, Egypt

A. Farag et al. (eds.), *Clinical Surgical Skills Made Easy*,
https://doi.org/10.1007/978-3-031-69158-4_8

- Fungal infections: Examples include histoplasmosis and coccidioidomycosis.
  - **Neoplastic**: Primary such as Lymphoma or Leukemia or secondary from a primary focus such as breast cancer.
  - **Autoimmune diseases**: For Examples rheumatoid arthritis, lupus, and Sjögren's syndrome.
  - **Other causes**: These include drug reactions, sarcoidosis, Castleman disease and allergies.

Lymph nodes amenable for Clinical examination have known Sites in the human Body such as the Neck and face, Axillae, Groins, Intra-abdominally around the aorta "Para-Aortic and Peri-aortic" and Iliac Lymph nodes around the Common and External iliac arteries. Other Lymph nodes like Epitrochlear Lymph nodes and Popliteal Lymph nodes are amenable to clinical examination.

Personal History (Box 8.1 and Box 8.2)

The most specific to the **Pathologic** diagnosis is:

Age: T.B., Lymphoma and Leukemia are more common in young age. Metastatic Lymph nodes from cancer are common in old age and metastatic axillary Lymph nodes from breast cancer is more common in the middle age.

Residence: Past and Present such as T.B or Filariasis from endemic areas.

Pet animals: Such as Cats for the cat scratch disease or Toxoplasmosis and Birds for Psittacosis.

Complaint: Single or Multiple Swellings at the **anatomical site of the Lymph nodes** is Lymphadenopathy till prove otherwise. "DD: Multiple lipomas, multiple neurofibromatosis, Multiple Pyaemic abscesses, multiple malignant metastases, multiple exostosis. All are not at the anatomical site of Lymph nodes".

Box 8.2 Causes of Localized and Generalized Lymphadenopathy

• **Localized**: **Inflammatory**: Non Specific: Acute or chronic Specific: Acute "e.g. measles" or Chronic "e.g. T.B." **Neoplastic**: Primary "e.g. Lymphoma" Secondary "from e.g. carcinoma of the oral cavity"	• **Generalized**: **Inflammatory**: Infectious Mononucleosis or HIV **Neoplastic**: Lymphoma or Leukemia

Site: Hodgkin's disease and tuberculosis usually starts in the cervical Lymph nodes while Filariasis and Syphilis usually starts in the inguinal Lymph nodes. Epitrochlear LNs are enlarged in the second stage of Syphilis "Rare nowadays".

Fever, Loss of weight and Loss of appetite: Low grade night sweat and night fever with loss of weight and loss of appetite is more common with TB, an intermittent fever with Filariasis and fever and Pruritis may be associated with Lymphomas "in Hodgkin's disease, intermittent bouts of remittent fever (Pel-Ebstain fever). Acute High grade fever can be due to an Acute Non-Specific inflammation or due to Acute Specific inflammation like Infectious Mononucleosis.

Primary Focus: is important for localized Lymph node enlargement, Breast and chest wall in axillary LN enlargement while Anal, Vaginal or Perineal or LL lesion "Inflammatory or Neoplastic" is asked for in Inguinal LN enlargement.

N.B. Axillary LN enlargement "Posterior group" and Inguinal L.N. enlargement "Lateral half of the transverse superficial inguinal LNs" can be due to a lesion in the back of the patient above and below the level of the Umbilicus respectively.

N.B. Don't forget to examine the 4 backs:

- Back of the Breast.
- Back of the scrotum.
- Back of the knee.
- Back of the patient.

Painful or Painless

N.B. Authors prefer to include this in the complaint so as not to be missed and will help to suggest a possible **pathology** at this early phase of the clinical sheet.

Pain in the involvement of the lymph nodes painful? The nodes are painful in both acute and chronic inflamed LNs, but are painless in lymphomas and secondary carcinoma.

Present History

Onset: including **mode of Onset** was it associated with Local or Systemic Symptoms **of Inflammation** and **the First Group of Lymph node affected** if there is a generalized lymphadenopathy.

Course: Regressive or stationary are suggestive of benign nature of the disease.

Duration: The Longer the duration "Years" suggests the benign nature of the disease.

Analysis of the Complaint

Pain: Type of pain and its relation to Alcohol intake "Half of the patients having Hodgkin's Lymphoma have pain in their enlarged LNs on drinking alcohol". While inflammatory Lymph nodes are painful except in T.B.

Fever: Type, grade and course of fever as mentioned in the Complaint.

Primary Focus: inflammatory or Neoplastic in localized LN enlargement.

Loss of appetite and Loss of Weight: as mentioned above.

Pressure effects: on nerves, vessels or nearby structures.

Screening of Body System: CNS, PNS, Cardiac, Respiratory, Eyes,
GIT, Urinary, Hepatobiliary, Gynecologic, Skin and Musclo-skeletal.

N.B. Sarcoidosis which is a non-caseating granulomatous disease affecting the LNs can affect the eyes, lungs, Skin and Joints.

Past History: TB, Syphilis, HIV and Malignancy, allergy to Medications.

Family History: Such as T.B and, Malignancy.

General Examination

General Look of the patient: for Malnutrition, cachexia, a anemia and loss of weight.

Other Lymph nodes:

Abdominal Examination: Liver, Spleen, including para-Aortic LNs, Mesenteric LNs, Iliac LNs. Or a Primary Malignancy in cases of enlargement of the Virchow's Lymph node in the Neck.

Chest Examination F for Pulmonary TB and Despine Sign for enlarged Tracheo-Bronchial "Mediastinal" LNs.

Limb Examination: For Primary Pathology e.g. Melanoma or for pressure effect "Lymphedema", Secondary Varicose Veins, Pressure on Nerves as well as ischemia.

Catchment area: Looking for the cause of enlargement, Primary Cancer as well as inspection of waldeyer's ring in Cervical Lymphadenopathy.

Local Examination (Box 8.3)

Box 8.3 Tips During Local Examination of Lymphadenopathy

- Always remember in Local examination the Head, Neck and Mouth rather than the traditional Head and Neck.
- Also remember the Examination of the Chest is "Chest Front, Back and Breast" rather that chest and breast separately.
- Remember Examination of the Abdomen is Examination of the Abdomen Front and Back, Perineum, Gluteal region and Upper thighs.

Inspection

- Number: in the same area or in the other areas of the LN.
- Site: Neck, Axilla, Intra-abdominal "Aortic or Common Iliac LNs" or Inguino-iliac LNs. The group affected in each of those areas are of diagnostic importance if they are inflammatory or secondary Neoplastic LNs.
- Size: in Centimeters or Inches. A Lymph node less than 2 CMs, oval in shape and firm inconsistency is usually non-specific LN.
- Shape: rounded or irregular LNs are mostly pathologic LNs especially when large.
- Surface: usually smooth except when amalgamated LNs which feels as undulating surface.
- Surrounding structure "Skin, Muscle and other structures": Scar, Fistula, Deep or superficial to the muscle, Pushing, compressing or infiltrating surrounding structures like Trachea, arteries, veins .....etc.
- Special signs: Fluctuation Test.
- Other swellings "Catchment area and other groups of LNs": Catchment area: Looking for the cause of enlargement, Primary Cancer as well as inspection of waldeyer's ring in Cervical Lymphadenopathy.

Palpation

Number: in the same area or in the other areas of the LN.

- Temperature: Warm in Chronic inflammations and hot in Acute Lymphadenitis.
- Tenderness: Inflammatory.
- Site: as in Inspection.
- Size: as in inspection.
- Shape: as in inspection.
- Surface: usually smooth except when amalgamated LNs which feels as undulating surface.
- Surrounding structure "Skin, Muscle and other structures": Skin may be normal and un-attached to the Lymph node, acutely inflamed in Acute Lymphadenitis with abscess formation, dusky red but not hot if attached to a tuberculous LN but later on may become ulcerated or having a sinus discharging caseous material. Relation to the nearby muscle is essential for DD. E.g. DD between enlarged upper deep cervical LN "under the sternomastoid from a swelling from the cervical part of the Parotid gland "Superficial to the sternomastoid" after contraction of the muscle by active flexion of the head while counteracting this movement by pressure upwards by the hand of the examiner under the chin of the patient.
- Edge: Usually well-defined edge in most of the cases irrespective to pathology except in acute non-specific lymphadenitis with large abscess formation.

- Consistency: Cystic in acute inflammation with acute abscess formation "Red, Hot Tender" or due to Cold abscess formation due to TB "Cold abscess i.e. not hot".
- Mobility: Over the surrounding structures and in Relation to each other "as detected by moving any 2 lymph nodes simultaneously in opposite directions" they may be discrete "Separable and move freely over each other, Matted where each LN can felt separate but cannot be moved in opposite direction as if glued to each other "Due to Periadenitis in TB and arranged like a rosary beads", or amalgamated where a group of LNs form a mass with a wavy surface where no LNs keeps its shape such as in highly malignant variants forms of Non-Hodgkin's Lymphoma known in the past as Lymphosarcoma.
- Special signs: mainly Fluctuation test or transmitted Pulsations from underlying artery.
- Other swellings "Catchment area and other groups of

LNs": Including the spleen which is considered as a Group of LNs below the diaphragm.

Auscultation: d'Espine sign is a bronchial breathing heard over the vertebral spines (on the back) below the level of tracheal bifurcation; below the fourth thoracic spine in adults if there is subcarinal (Mediastinal) lymphadenopathy.

Investigations

Laboratory: C.B.C., Liver Function tests, ESR, CRP, Tumor markers for Lymphoma "e.g. LDH and Beta 2 microglobulin" and markers for a primary tumor causing LN metastases, Viral markers for Epstein Barr Virus, CMV, HIV …etc.

Radiologic: Plain X-ray Neck and Chest may show Displacement of the trachea, an enlarged Tracheo-bronchial LN. And LN calcification in Tabes Mesenterica "tubercular degeneration of the mesenteric glands with emaciation and derangement of nutrition". Ultrasonography for the LN breaking down and other structures such as involvement of the other groups of LN or other organs like Liver, Spleen, thyroid, Breast....Etc. It can also determine the size, shape and internal structure of the LNs "Hilar/Cortex ratio, preserved Hilum or other internal abnormality in the LN. Ct, MRI and PET-CT are more sophisticated and more expensive but can give a lot of information concerning the Site, cause and size of the affected LNs and should be requested by a specialized doctor.

Instrumental: Laryngoscopy "direct or indirect, Upper and lower GI endoscopies. Laryngoscopy and even diagnostic laparoscopy may be requested to determine the diagnosis and management of Lymphadenopathy.

Pathologic diagnosis:

- Needle biopsies:
  - Fine needle for cytology "or aspiration of fluids for cytology, to study the characters of the cells including the mitotic figures and the nuclear-cytoplasmic ratio suggestive of malignancy.
  - Tru-Cut needle biopsy for Histopathology
  - Endoscopic biopsies.
- Surgical Biopsies:
  - Incisional: a Small wedge of the lesion.
  - Excisional: the lesion is removed totally and sent for pathology.

The Histopathology can be examined as:

- Frozen section "Immediate"
- Paraffin blocks.

Sections from Paraffin blocks are examined with Haematoxyline and Eosin or specific stains.

Chapter 9
General Limb Sheet

Ahmed Farag

Abstract By Limb in this sheet we mean both Upper and Lower Limb with some differences due to different functions. Limb complaints such as varicose Veins, Ischemia, and Joints vs. edema, Swellings and ulcers had been dealt with in the other Clinical books as different sheets which ignores the fact that the limb is a body area which contains many structures similar to the head and neck, Chest and Abdomen.

Keywords Limb · Examination · Sheet · Diagnosis · Clinical · Mass · Ulcer · Pain · Edema

By Limb in this sheet we mean both Upper and Lower Limb with some differences due to different functions. Limb complaints such as varicose Veins, Ischemia, and Joints vs. edema, Swellings and ulcers had been dealt with in the other Clinical books as different sheets which ignores the fact that the limb is a body area which contains many structures similar to the head and neck, Chest and Abdomen. The Diagnosis like any other area in the body should be based on Anatomical and a pathologic diagnosis. And that the Clinician should fulfill the rule that he has to remember other areas which should be examined namely Abdomen, Back, perineum and left lower neck for Lymph nodes in short cases and using the Marsh of examination mentioned in the general sheet in Long cases.

Personal History

Helps to determine the probable anatomic and pathologic diagnosis e.g. leg complaints in a patient above 70 years of age are most commonly to be due to ischemia, osteoarthritis and venous compression at the iliac vessels due to metastatic malignant lymph nodes, leg complaints in females in the childbearing period is most probably of venous origin e.g. DVT or Varicose veins, while leg complaints in a

A. Farag (✉)
Kasr Alainy Hospital, Cairo University, Cairo, Egypt

A. Farag et al. (eds.), *Clinical Surgical Skills Made Easy*, https://doi.org/10.1007/978-3-031-69158-4_9

teenager male patient may raise the suspicion of osteomyelitis, bone tumors or traumatic lesions specially in the knee Joint …etc.

Handedness i.e., right or left handed are essential in the upper limb and occupation is important in both upper and lower limbs.

Complaint: localized swellings (painful or painless), Ulcers, Generalized swelling (edema), leg pain "What Brings and what relieves" helps to refer to *Anatomical diagnosis* such as Joint pain including intra-articular or extra-articular causes "at the site of a joint and increases by movement" or *pathologic diagnosis* such as Venous pain, varicose veins "increases by standing and relived by elevation", Ischemic pain "which increases by exercise and decreases by rest" or neurogenic pain, together with.

Onset, Course and Duration Help in determining the provisional anatomic and pathologic diagnosis which will help the Clinician to proceed in the rest of the present History as:

- Sheet of Varicose Veins (Primary or Secondary).
- Ischemia (Acute, Chronic, severity, etiology, Risk Factors and other ischemia).
- Swelling (specific areas such as femoral triangle or popliteal fossa or otherwise).
- Edema (Unilateral or Bilateral, pitting or non-pitting, Localized or part of generalized edema).
- Leg Ulcer (DD).
- Leg Pain (DD).
- Gangrene (Types)
- A combination of the above.

Past History and Family History Such as DM which is a risk factor for failure of treatment of ischemic, cardiac disease e.g. AF or previous myocardial infarction which may suggest an embolic origin of acute ischemia, Hypertension which may precipitate a dissecting aortic aneurysm (Typically not presenting as a lower limb complaint) or intake of certain medications such as Ergot products for treatment of migraine as a cause of peripheral gangrene specially in the upper Limb.

General Examination

As mentioned in the Marsh of examination including examination of the pulses all over the body to rule out associated ischemias and aneurysms, Signs of systemic metastases in malignant lesions in the limbs, cardiac condition as a source of ischemia in the limbs …etc.

Reserving the Abdominal examination to the stage after the examination of the lower limbs

March of Examination in a Limb (Upper or Lower)

- Inspection
- Gait (applicable only in the lower limb e.g. limping, and specific gaits in neurology).
- Position (e.g. elevation in inflammations and DVT, Dependency hanging the limb from the side of the bed close to a fan in severe ischemia).
- Deformity such as the position of rest in the hand infections, Volkmann's ischemic contraction, Duputryn's contracture, Nerve, joint and boney deformities and Gigantism in congenital A-V fistulae for DD), Shortening, gigantism, joint and boney deformities).
- Color (pale, Cyanotic, Mottled, Fixed color changes or gangrene in Acute ischemia or dusky red coloration and or gangrene in Chronic ischemia).
- Contour: Normal, Unilateral or Bilateral Symmetrical change in the contour (Wasting or edema) or Unilateral or Bilateral non symmetrical change such as localized swellings (diagnosed as anatomic and pathologic diagnosis) or varicose veins.
- Skin: Trophic changes (Skin atrophy, loss of hair, hyperkeratosis, unhealthy nails and tapering of the Toes), Ulcers (describe) or gangrene (describe).
- Active Movement.
- Palpation
- Temperature.
- Distal Pulses.
- Special examination and special tests for varicose veins, Swellings, Ulcers, ischemia.
- Limb distal: for veins, arteries active movements and sensations.
- Limb Proximal: for inguinal and Iliac Lymph nodes, examination of the abdomen, perineum, back and buttocks for the lower limbs and for Axillary Lymph nodes, H&N, mouth, chest and breasts for the upper limb lesions.
- (E.g. secondary varicose veins due to enlarged inguinal lymph nodes secondary to a squamous cell carcinoma of the buttock or a malignant lesion in the anal canal, Scrotum or Vulva. Or pain in the upper limb due to Pancoast tumor at the apex of the lung infiltrating the lower brachial plexus or due to malignant supraclavicular lymph nodes due to advanced breast cancer or malignant tumor in the mouth.

Percussion: Not applicable.

Auscultation for arterial bruits.

Chapter 10
DD. of Limb Edema

Ahmed Farag

Abstract Edema of a Limb can be part of General cause of edema due to:

- Cardiac causes Such as in Heart failure.
- Renal Causes: Due to renal failure and Nephrotic Syndrome —Nephrotic syndrome is the combination of nephrotic-range proteinuria with a low serum albumin level and edema.||
- Liver Cell failure: Usually due to decrease Liver Synthesis of Albumin||
- Nutritional Edema: due to decreased intake of Proteins especially essential Amino acids.
- Angioneurotic edema.

Keywords Limb · Edema · Examination · Diagnosis · General · Local · Cause · Pitting · Non-pitting

Edema of a Limb can be part of **General cause of edema** due to:

- Cardiac causes Such as in Heart failure.
- Renal Causes: Due to renal failure and Nephrotic Syndrome "Nephrotic syndrome is the combination of nephrotic-range proteinuria with a low serum albumin level and edema."
- Liver Cell failure: Usually due to decrease Liver Synthesis of Albumin.
- Nutritional Edema: due to decreased intake of Proteins especially essential Amino acids.
- Angioneurotic edema:

Edema in a Limb may be due to a Local **cause of edema** "Isolated Limb edema" Which may be:

1. **A Localized edema**: Not involving the whole limb and is over a specific pathology like inflammatory due to cellulitis, a deep abscess or over an osteomyelitis or due to a tumor Such as a sarcoma.
2. **A Generalized edema** of a Limb due to:

A. Farag (✉)
Kasr Alainy Hospital, Cairo University, Cairo, Egypt

A. Farag et al. (eds.), *Clinical Surgical Skills Made Easy*,
https://doi.org/10.1007/978-3-031-69158-4_10

- Venous obstruction: due to a DVT or Proximal compression on a vein by pressure from an enlarged malignant LN or malignant tumor in the Groin or axilla.
- Lymphatic due to Lymph vessel "congenital absence or hypoplasia, or infiltration by a malignant tumor "in-transit" Mets or LN obstruction by a tumor or inflammation" or its removal by Block dissection "Prophylactic or therapeutic" treatment of a malignant tumor in Breast "Axillary radical LN dissection" or Malignant tumor in the Anal Canal Vulva, Perineum, Lower Limbs or Abdominal wall below the level of the umbilicus "Front and back including buttocks". Filariasis should be suspected in the Endemic areas of the disease. ": Filariasis due to a parasite called Wuchereria bancrofti or other species transmitted by Mosquito which is endemic in some tropical countries like Africa and India."

Personal History

Age is important in cases of Lymphatic cause of edema which may appear early due to congenital absence or hypoplasia of the Lymphatic vessels Lymphedema Precox or later on in Life known as Lymphedema tarda. "Lymphedema praecox: This is the most common type of primary lymphedema. It generally develops in females at puberty. On the opposite hand Lymphedema tarda is a hereditary lymphedema occurs in adulthood, typically in the middle age."

Residence: Residing or coming from some tropical countries like Africa and India where Filariasis is endemic..

Complaint: Swelling of the upper or Lower Limb. The Later may be Unilateral or bilateral. It may be Painful or Painless which may or may not be associated with Fever.

Time-Out: Generalized or Local cause of edema.

Present History

Onset: Mode of onset, which may be acute in acute inflammation "abscess which is usually associated with pain and Fever" Acute Filariasis "Fever, Rigors, painful swollen Limb", DVT "tender calf muscle and mild distal edema".

Trauma: Surgical dissection in Axillary or Inguino-iliac LN dissection.

Inflammation: Fever +/− Rigors, redness, hotness and pain in cases of acute non-specific inflammation "Cellulitis and abscess".

Course

Progressive: in Venous causes of edema if left untreated.

Regressive: in Acute non-specific inflammation “Cellulitis or abscess with treatment.

Stationary: in congenital Lymphatic aplasia and hypoplasia if there is no recurrent cellulitis.

Remittent: in cases of recurrent cellulitis on top of Lymphedema which leaves the limb after subsidence of inflammation in a worse condition “more increase in girth and size due to obstruction of more Lymphatics”.

Associated Symptoms

- Anorexia “Malnutrition edema” or Low Protein diet “Kwashiorkor” which is Kwashiorkor is a disease marked by severe protein malnutrition and bilateral extremity swelling. It usually affects infants and children, most often around the age of weaning. The disease is seen in very severe cases of starvation.
- Symptoms suggestive of Heart failure “Dyspnea, orthopnea, Paroxysmal nocturnal Dyspnea with edema of the dependent parts of the body but not the face or eyes”, Renal Failure “Edema of the face and eyes with puffiness of the lower eye lid” or Advanced Liver disease “associated with Jaundice, ascites …etc.”
- Angioneurotic edema after exposure to allergen with wheezes and respiratory embarrassment, swollen face and lips and Urticaria “Itching”.

Past History: of a similar condition or allergies to certain medications, food or allergens and seasonal recurrence,

Family History: of Similar condition or allergies.

General examination: For:

- Cause of Generalized edema “Anasarca, when massive” Such as: Heart failure, Liver Failure, Kidney failure, Nutritional edema “Kwashiorkor”, Angioneurotic edema and Generalized Lymphadenopathy.
- An Effect of the pathology causing LL edema “e.g. Pulmonary embolism which may be massive “an Emergency life threatening” Moderate or minor repeated with Dyspnea, Tachycardia, Chest pain due to Pleurisy over a Pulmonary infarction which gives the sound of pleural rub during auscultation”
- A cause of edema such as Distant Mets from a tumor causing venous obstruction in the Abdomen such as Hypernephroma “Renal Cell Carcinoma” extending as a tumor thrombus into the IVC or Generalized Lymphadenopathy causing a Groin mass of LNs compressing the vein or Filariasis “Elephantiasis of the Skin of the Scrotum “Rare and may or may not be associated with LL elephantiasis”**Local examination:**

- **Inspection**:

Distribution of Edema

- Localized such as over an abscess or at the site of trauma "+/– Hematoma".
- Diffuse Below the Knee: DVT "during or after decumbency including P.O., Rupture Plantaris Tendon "after an acute sudden exercise. It may be due to Filarial Lymphedema or after acute block in the superficial or Acute "traumatic" A.V. Fistula femoral and/or Popliteal artery "Thrombotic i.e. Acute or embolic i.e. sudden" or after acute rupture of PA aneurysm, Baker's cyst or SM bursa.
- Diffuse Above the knee: Proximal Ileo-femoral DVT with or without impending Venous gangrene "Phlegmasia cerulea dolens (PCD)". A traumatic AV Fistula affecting the Femoral artery and Vein "Bucher's Thigh", or proximal Lymphatic obstruction "mainly congenital Lymphedema".

N.B. Phlegmasia cerulea dolens (PCD) is a potentially life-threatening complication of acute DVT characterized by marked swelling of the extremities with pain and cyanosis, which in turn may lead to arterial ischemia and ultimately gangrene with high amputation and mortality rates.

Palpation: Pitting "a pressing finger can leave an indentation mark which lasts for some time after removal of the pressing finger" of the Non- Pitting. Temperature "Cold in Ischemia or warm due to repeated attacks of cellulitis", Pulsations and Sensations.

Auscultation: Machinery Murmur "Systolic and Diastolic in traumatic A.V. fistula.

DD. Localized Gigantism due to"

1. Klippel–Trénaunay syndrome: A rare condition present from birth where blood and/or lymphatic vessels aren't formed correctly, and there are abnormal connections between arteries and veins (A-V fistulae). "No Bruit DD. Traumatic A-V Fistula"
2. Maffucci syndrome: a rare skeletal disorder characterized by the development of multiple, benign enchondromas within the bones, predominantly affecting the hands, feet, and limbs. These enchondromatous formations often lead to skeletal deformities and limb shortening.
3. Macrodystrophia lipomatosa: is a rare congenital disorder characterized by the localized overgrowth of a portion of an extremity, with the foot being the most commonly affected site. The overgrowth primarily consists of adipose tissue, though other mesenchymal components can also be involved.
4. Neurofibromatosis:
5. Lipoatrophic diabetes: is a rare skin condition that appears during childhood or adolescence, characterized by fat loss affecting large areas of the body, particularly the face, arms, and legs.

Chapter 11
Limb Pain Sheet

Ahmed Farag

Abstract General plan:

- Like other areas in the body studied in this book: diagnosis rests on two pillars namely anatomical diagnosis—Which organ or structure causes this pain|| and pathologic diagnosis—The disease affecting the organ or structure in the Limb||.
- Pain may arise in the limb or referred from a pathology in another area proximal to the Limb.

Keywords Limb · Pain · Examination · Organ · Structure · Anatomy · Pathology · Pillars

General Plan

- Like other areas in the body studied in this book: diagnosis rests on two pillars namely anatomical diagnosis "Which organ or structure causes this pain" and pathologic diagnosis "The disease affecting the organ or structure in the Limb".
- Pain may arise in the limb or referred from a pathology in another area proximal to the Limb e.g. a pathology in the Nek, Axilla or chest may cause pain in the upper limb and a pathology in the Abdomen or Lumbar Spine can cause pain in the Lower Limb.
- Accordingly in case of a pain in the Upper Limb, the areas to be examined are "Both Upper Limbs, Head and Neck and mouth, Chest Front, Back and breast "i.e. the upper half of the body above the diaphragm" and at least the Liver from the lower half of the body. While in pain of the Lower Limbs areas to be examined are both Lower limbs, Abdomen front, back including the spine and perineum "i.e. the lower half of the body below the diaphragm" and a minimum

A. Farag (✉)
Kasr Alainy Hospital, Cairo University, Cairo, Egypt

A. Farag et al. (eds.), *Clinical Surgical Skills Made Easy*,
https://doi.org/10.1007/978-3-031-69158-4_11

to be examined is Virchow LNs in the Lt Supraclavicular area in the Short case Examination.

N.B. In our Clinics It is always recommended by the authors of this book to do a complete though swift General examination in the Marsh of General examination mention in the Chapter of General examination because of the following reasons mentioned before namely:

- We have to assess the general condition of the patient which may have an impact on his/her management "We are treating the patient not only the disease.
- We may discover a more serious disease in the patient.
- To assess the effect of the patient complaint or disease on the general condition of the patient "Stage of the disease in case of malignancy or Systemic manifestations of Sepsis or T.B for example.
- The Only Clue for diagnosis may be in the General examination e.g. Ischemia in other parts of the body or Polyneuritis.

Causes of Pain in a Limb

It is Important to Bear in mind the causes of Pain in the Limb at the First Time out after Hearing the Personal History and the Complaint of the patient. This will guide us as Clinicians through the rest of our examination namely history taking and Examination.

- **Lower Limb:**
  - Nerves: Neuritis, Pressure on Nerves by Disc Prolapse or Spondylitis, Mets in the Spine, Direct infiltration by Pelvic malignancy.
  - Arteries: Ischemic pains.
  - Venous: Varicose veins and venous thrombosis.
  - Musculoskeletal: Arthralgia, Arthritis, Osteomyelitis, Fractures after direct or indirect trauma "Marsh fracture", Muscle hematomas from direct or indirect trauma "e.g. Rupture of Plantaris tendon".
  - Skin and Subcutaneous tissue: from trauma or Inflammation including Skin "e.g. Erythema", Subcutaneous tissues "Cellulitis" or deep Fascia "Fasciitis".
  - Pain may be referred from the abdomen like pain on extension of the hip or pain in the thigh and hip during walking in cases of acute retrocaecal appendicitis or acute Psoas abscess. Or renal pain referred to the inner aspect of the thigh in females. N.B. Pain in the knee may be referral from a pathology in the Hip.
- **Upper Limb:**
  - Nerves: Neuritis, Pressure on Nerves by Disc Prolapse or Spondylitis, Mets in the Spine, Direct infiltration by Pancoast Tumor.
  - Arteries: Ischemic pains. "Including Vasospastic disorders".

- Venous: e.g. axillary or Subclavian vein thrombosis.
- Musculoskeletal: Arthralgia, Arthritis, Osteomyelitis, Fractures after direct or indirect trauma Muscle hematomas from direct or indirect trauma".
- Skin and Subcutaneous tissue: from trauma or Inflammation including Skin "e.g. Erythema", Subcutaneous tissues "Cellulitis" or deep Fascia "Fasciitis".
- Pain referred from angina Pectoris, causing pain in the inner aspect of the Left arm, Mastitis or Mastalgia "due to Hormone changes" which may be Cyclic or non-cyclic according to its relation to menstruation. Biliary pain may radiate into the right shoulder.

Personal History

Age and sex: Vasospastic disorders Such as Raynaud's disease "such as fingers and toes—to feel numb and cold in response to cold temperatures or stress" is more common in Young Females. While Burger's disease (also known as thromboangiitis obliterans affects blood vessels in the body, most commonly in the arms and legs.) is more common in middle aged males.

Occupation: Prolonged standing increases the incidence of varicose veins while prolonged sitting can lead to DVT.

Habits of medical importance: e.g. Cigarette Smoking worsens the arterial ischemia.

Complaint:

- The exact site of pain in the Limb "Distribution" and Pain in one or more Limbs. Pain in a glove a stoke distribution is pathognomonic of Peripheral neuritis and Pain in the four limbs suggests a Systemic disease Such as Peripheral neuritis.
- Pain in the distribution of a nerve or dermatome suggests a compression on a nerve or a nerve root "The later has a distribution of a dermatome". Similarly arterial, venous or local site of pain have a special Distribution as will be mentioned later in the present history and examination section.

Present History

Onset

- Mode of Onset:
  - Sudden after direct or indirect trauma such as hematomas, Fracture and in March fractures are metatarsal fractures caused by repetitive stress i.e. after a vigorous waking for a prolonged Period of Time. Rupture Plantaris tendon can happen after similar exercise DD. DVT which takes hours to manifest

itself. Also Arterial Embolism causes immediate and sudden pain DD. Thrombotic cause of Ischemia. Acute disc prolapse presents by sudden shooting pain after an indirect trauma such as lifting a heavy weight in a faulty position.

  - Acute: i.e. within hours in inflammation e.g. 'Cellulitis and abscess" and in venous thrombosis.
  - Chronic such as Chronic Osteoarthritis, Pain due to varicose veins or Chronic Ischemia.

- Was the Onset associated with trauma or inflammation?:
- Trauma may be direct or indirect, Inflammation may be acute non-specific "Fever, Rigors, malaise, Redness hotness and acute loss of function" or Chronic Specific like T.B Hip with generalized malaise, loss of weight, night sweat and Night fever.

Course: Progressive in Chronic Ischemia, Osteoarthritis, Peripheral neuritis. And Intermittent in pain from arterial, Venous "VV.", Nerve or Joint origin.

Duration: If long history of pain i.e. Years it usually excludes Malignant cause of pain.

Analysis of Pain (Table 11.1)

After Excluding Skin and subcutaneous tissue bones, fascia "Flat feet" and masses as a cause for pain: Pain can be due to Veins, arteries and Nerves.

Past History

Of Disease of medical importance or treatment: mainly DM, Anticoagulation for DVT, Surgery or stents for vascular disease, Heart disease "A source of arterial embolization", Previous Decumbency in bed for DVT, Vigorous exercise for rupture Plantaris tendon or March Fracture. T.B. Back or Spine pain or disc prolapse.

Family History

For D.M.

Table 11.1 DD. of analysis of pain in the limb

Analysis of pain	Venous "Varicose Veins"	Arterial Ischemia	Nerve	Joint pain Osteo-arthritis
Type	Bursting or distending pain	Claudication" muscle spasm" or Rest pain in severe cases	Electric or lancinating shooting pain	Boring pain
Site	Ankles	Claudication in one level below the Obstructed vessel. And rest pain in the toes, feet or higher	In a distribution of a nerve "e.g. Sciatica" or in a dermatome distribution	At the joint
Referral	–	–	Nerve or dermatome distribution	–
What brings pain?	Prolonged standing	Walking in Claudication and elevation in rest pain	Positional	Worse in the morning
What relieves pain?	Walking and Elevation "absent in the morning"	Dependency and cooling of the limb by a fan "A Characteristic position in vascular words"	Positional	Improves by walking
Associated Symptoms	Dilated Tortious Veins	Absent distal pulsations at the ankle or at the Wrist "except in small vessel disease "micro-angiopathy or in Reynaud's Disease No trophic changes in Claudication but with trophic changes in Rest pain	Paresthesia (e.g. Tingling and numbness)" or Anesthesia with or without muscle wasting in the muscles supplied by the affected nerve or root value	Crepitus sounds during movement +?- Locked joint "Sudden failure of movement due to entrapped loose bodies

N.B. pain due to DVT though improves by elevation like varicose veins it is also increased by walking which should be forbidden for fear of pulmonary embolism PE for the first few weeks after Thrombosis till the thrombus is fixed to the vessel wall. DD. Rupture Plantaris tendon which usually happens after vigorous exercise. Duplex examination is needed for DD in most cases

N.B. Osteoarthritis is a degeneration in a Joint while Arthritis is an inflammation in the Joint which may be infective "Non-Specific" or Specific infection e.g. T.B., Metabolic like Gout or an autoimmune like Rheumatoid arthritis

In arthritis Systemic manifestation of sepsis or TB as mentioned before. Gouty arthritis which is due to increased Level of Uric acid in the blood with deposition in any joint including big joints but characteristically appears in the big toe with inflammatory signs "Redness, swelling and hotness. In attacks exacerbated but red meat other types of foods rich in Purines

N.B. Flat foot is a part of congenitally weak mesenchyme such as inguinal hernias, hemorrhoids and varicose veins. Pain is in the sole of the foot increases by prolonged standing relieved by sitting but not essentially by elevation of the legs

N.B. Morton metatarsalgia: The etiology and pathogenesis of Morton's Neuroma remain controversial chronic trauma, ischemia, bursitis and entrapment neuropathy have been proposed as possible etiologic factors. Careful history and clinical examination is essential to establish the diagnosis. However, if the clinical picture is doubtful, radiological investigation is recommended

General Examination

- Manifestations of chronic ischemia or associated ischemia "Cardiac, CVS, intestinal or renal ischemia". Associated upper Limb Ischemia in Vasospastic disorders "Reynaud's disease, ergot poisoning, or Chilblains".
- Streptococcal throat infection as a cause of rheumatic Fever.
- Pulmonary embolism in DVT.
- Glove and Stock anesthesia in D.M. or nerve nodules in Leprosy.
- Heart failure or AF as a Source of embolic acute ischemia.
- Musculoskeletal pains in other areas of the Body due to Rheumatoid arthritis, Fibromyalgia, or Gouty arthritis.

Local Examination

Inspection: Compare Both Limbs

- Position of the Limb: in the Joints; flexion Rotation deformities are common in pain due to intra-articular or extra-articular pathologies "Trauma which is either direct or indirect, inflammations specific or non-specific and neoplastic causes as primary bone tumors or Secondaries". An acute osteoarthritis will be in the position of rest.
- Gait: in the Lower limb.
- Deformity: In both the upper and lower limbs which may be the cause or the result of pain.
- Color:
  - Pale in acute Ischemia which later on becomes mottled with fixed color changes and finally gangrene.
  - Color may be dusky red discoloration in Chronic Ischemia, due to excessive extraction of Oxygen from the RBCs during its slow movement in the ischemic Limb.
  - Color may be Cyanotic in Phlegmasia Cerulea dolens due to severe Iliofemoral thrombosis or may be swollen in.
  - Pale in Phlegmasia Alba Dolens "the patient with swollen and white leg because of early compromise of arterial flow secondary to extensive DVT".
  - Abnormal pigmentation with ankle flare of Spider varicosities in varicose veins.
- Contour: as Compared to the other Limb which may be due to:
  - Normal contour.
  - Increased Contour "Localized or generalized".
  - Wasting which may be localized due to nerve compression or a nerve root compression affecting the muscles supplied by the diseased nerve or nerve root or generalized muscle wasting as in ischemia.

- Trophic changes: is Chronic Ischemia.
  - Skin: atrophy.
  - Hair: Loss of hair compare to the other LL.
  - Nails: Loss of Luster.
  - Tip of the toes: Tapered due to loss of subcutaneous fat.
- Active Movements: generalized absence in acute embolic Ischemia but may be maintained in chronic ischemia by the tendons of the muscles proximal to the level of Ischemia or gangrene: Active movement of a gangrenous toe in dry gangrene. A limited movement after trauma or inflammation.
- Ulcers:
  - Neuropathic ulcers will be mainly at the pressure point at the heel or over the heads of the metatarsal bones.
  - Ischemic ulcers will be at the tip of the toes "the most distant from blood supply".
  - Venous ulcers will be at the inner aspect of the lower Leg where the skin perforators drain directly into the deep venous system "Direct perforators at the ankle.
- Gangrene:
  - Dry gangrene in Chronis ischemia.
  - Wet gangrene "Life threatening from Generalized Toxemia" due to sudden traumatic simultaneous occlusion of the arteries and veins or Acute arterial ischemia.
  - Infective gangrene such as Diabetic foot due to Microangiopathy or accelerated atherosclerosis or in Gas gangrene from a Gas forming organism affecting a damaged muscle e.g. after Crush injuries "A hospital emergency".
- Limb Proximal: For LNs and masses.

Palpation

- Pulsations: In Ischemic pain starting from distal to proximal "The Level of Vessel obstruction is one level higher than the lost pulsation".
- Sensations: Superficial and deep sensations.
- Temperature: as compared to the other limb:
  - Localized hotness over inflammations and trauma.
  - Coldness in Ischemia with a level as felt by the back of the fingers "The Level of the arterial occlusion is one level higher than the level of the Level of Temperature change ".
  - N.B. an acute or Chronic ischemic limb may be warm due being wormed by an overlying Blanket i.e. Poikilothermic which means that it takes the temperature of the surrounding atmosphere due to the loss of the heat regulating mechanism brought to the Limb by blood. A Chronically ischemic limb may be warmer than the normal limb due to subclinical bacterial infection.

- Passive movements: Helps to detect Joint disease from other causes of pain.
- Swellings; may be the cause of pain such as Saphena Varix, a tumor or an arterial aneurysm showering emboli to the distal limb.
- Ulcers: See Above in the skin.
- Limb Proximal: For Groin swelling as a cause of pain "e.g. due to nerve compression", LN mets from a tumor causing pain in the Lower Limb.
- Abdominal and Pelvic examination: To detect a primary tumor or inflammation causing enlarged LNs causing pain in the Lower Limb or sending metastases in the vertebrae causing radiating pains in the LL or even direct mets in the bones of the lower limbs causing pain or even a pathologic fracture.

Investigations

- Laboratory: for D.M., leprosy, Tumor markers.
- Radiologic:
  - Plain X-ray for the osteomyelitis, Peri-osteitis, bone cysts, mets or Primary tumors, Joint space, capsule and articular surface during rest or in stress position for subluxation of joints.
  - Ultrasonography and Duplex: For venous and arterial disease. Recently US is used for Joint and Peri-articular pathology.
  - CT, MRI and Angiography: For tumors, soft tissue masses and arterial disease.
- Instrumental: EMG and nerve conduction studies.
- Pathologic: biopsies: are examined in paraffin sections or as an immediate frozen section. The Paraffin sections are examined using H&E stain or special stains:
  - Needle "Fine Needle Aspiration Biopsy and Cytology FNABC or Tru Cut Needle Biopsy.
  - Surgical: Excisional or Incisional.

Chapter 12
Examination of the Thyroid

Alexandra M. Zaborowski and Ruth S. Prichard

Abstract Basic anatomy of the thyroid: The thyroid gland is located in the anterior neck. It lies inferior to the laryngeal prominence of the thyroid cartilage and anterior to the larynx and trachea. It is composed of two lobes measuring approximately 4 cm that are joined together by a narrow isthmus in the midline at the level of the 2nd to 4th tracheal rings. The function of the thyroid gland is to produce triiodothyronine (T3), thyroxine (T4) and calcitonin which play an important role in regulating metabolism.

Keywords Thyroid · Sheet · Examination · Gland · Sheet · Neck · General · Local · Hyperthyroidism

Basic Anatomy of the Thyroid

The thyroid gland is located in the anterior neck. It lies inferior to the laryngeal prominence of the thyroid cartilage and anterior to the larynx and trachea. It is composed of two lobes measuring approximately 4 cm that are joined together by a narrow isthmus in the midline at the level of the 2nd to 4th tracheal rings. The function of the thyroid gland is to produce triiodothyronine (T3), thyroxine (T4) and calcitonin which play an important role in regulating metabolism.

A. M. Zaborowski (✉)
Breast/General Surgery RCSI, Dublin, Ireland
e-mail: zaborowa@tcd.ie

R. S. Prichard
Department of Breast & Endocrine Surgery, St Vincent's University Hospital, Dublin 4, Ireland
e-mail: Ruthprichard@rcsi.ie

A. Farag et al. (eds.), *Clinical Surgical Skills Made Easy*,
https://doi.org/10.1007/978-3-031-69158-4_12

Embryology

The thyroid is the first endocrine organ to develop, beginning around the 4th week of gestation. It arises as an endodermal invagination of the tongue at the foramen caecum and descends through the tongue to its final location anterior to trachea and larynx by week 7, developing into two lobes joined by an isthmus. It begins to secrete thyroid hormone by the 12th week. The descent of the developing thyroid gland gives rise to the epithelialized tract called the thyroglossal duct which usually degenerates by the 10th week of gestation. In some individuals the thyroglossal duct persists giving rise to a thyroglossal cyst which presents as a midline neck lump that rises on protrusion of the tongue. If left untreated a thyroglossal cyst can become infected or and form a fistula to the skin. The surgical procedure to excise a thyroglossal duct cyst is known as the Sistrunk procedure and involves excision of the entire duct, cyst and a portion of the hyoid bone.

Blood Supply

The thyroid gland is supplied by two main arteries; the superior thyroid artery and the inferior thyroid artery. The superior thyroid artery arises from the external carotid artery and lies in close proximity to the superior laryngeal nerve. The inferior thyroid artery arises from the thyrocervical trunk which is a branch of the subclavian artery and lies in close proximity to the recurrent laryngeal nerve. In approximately 3% of individuals, an anatomical variant known as the thyroidea ima artery or artery of Neubauer exists. It most commonly arises from the brachiocephalic trunk, left common carotid artery, or arch of the aorta. Venous drainage of the thyroid is via the superior, middle and inferior thyroid veins. The former two drain into the internal jugular vein whilst the latter drains into the brachiocephalic vein.

Examination of the Thyroid

1. Inspection
   - Ask the patient to sit upright on the examination table.
   - Assess for any obvious midline neck swelling.
   - Is there localised or generalised swelling of the gland?
   - Ask the patient to swallow sips of water and observe whether the swelling moves as the patient swallows. The thyroid gland or a thyroglossal cyst will move upwards on swallowing. In rare cases of advanced thyroid malignancy, the gland may not rise if it is fixed to surrounding structures.
   - Ask the patient to protrude their tongue and observe whether the swelling rises. A thyroglossal cyst will move upwards on tongue protrusion.

- Inspect the skin for scars from previous surgery. A thyroidectomy scar is typically found at the base of the neck.
- Inspect the neck for dilated veins which may occur in the setting of thoracic inlet obstruction caused by retrosternal extension of a goitre.

2. Palpation

- Stand behind the patient and ask them to gently flex their neck. Neck flexion relaxes the muscles and facilitates examination of the thyroid.
- Palpate the thyroid cartilage and cricoid cartilage. The thyroid gland lies inferiorly.
- Using the pulps of the fingers of both hands, palpate both thyroid lobes and the isthmus systematically. Examine each lobe at a time.
- Consider the following features:
  - Size.
  - Is it possible to palpate the lower border? Inability to define the lower border suggests retrosternal extension.
  - Is there localised vs generalised enlargement?
  - Is there a discrete nodule palpable?
  - Consistency: a hard gland suggests malignancy or fibrosis/Riedel's thyroiditis whilst a rubbery gland suggests autoimmune thyroiditis (Hashimoto's).
  - Tenderness: the gland may be tender in subacute thyroiditis (de Quervain's thyroiditis).
  - Fixation/tethering to surrounding structures is suggestive of malignancy.
  - Is there a palpable thrill? A thrill may occur in the setting of thyrotoxicosis.
  - Is there palpable cervical lymphadenopathy?

3. Percussion

- Percuss over the manubrium and sternum to assess for retrosternal extension.

4. Auscultation

- Auscultate over both lobes to assess for a bruit. A bruit reflects hypervascularisation of the thyroid gland and may occur in hyperthyroidism.

5. Pemberton's sign

- Ask the patient to raise both arms above their head so that their upper arms are touching the sides of their face. Keep the arms raised for 1 minute or until signs of venous congestion appear.
- A positive Pemberton's sign is when bilateral arm elevation causes facial plethora/cyanosis or distension of the neck veins which indicates thoracic inlet obstruction due to retrosternal extension of a goitre.
- Listen for stridor.

Assessment of Thyroid Status

Thyroid disease may result in hyper- or hypothyroidism. Both states are associated with different clinical findings affecting multiple systems. These clinical features should be considered as part of the thyroid exam. The main findings are summarised below.

Clinical Features of Hyperthyroidism

1. General inspection

   Inspect for low BMI, signs of weight loss and anxiety.
2. Eyes

   - Examine for exophthalmos (eye protrusion) which can occur in Grave's disease. In exophthalmos the sclerae are not covered by the lower eyelid and the eye will be visible anterior to the superior eyelid.
   - Inspect for complications associated with proptosis such as chemosis, corneal ulceration, and ophthalmoplegia.
   - Assess for Dalrymple's sign: lid retraction causing the upper and lower sclera to be visible.
   - Assess for von Graefe's sign: lagging of the eyelid on downward movement of the eye.

3. Hands

   Look for signs of sympathetic overactivity:

   - Ask the patient to stretch out their arms and look for a fine tremor.
   - Inspect the nails for onycholysis (separation of the nail plate from the nail bed). Onycholysis in hyperthyroidism is known as Plummer's nails.
   - Inspect the palms for erythema and perspiration.
   - Look for thyroid acropachy: clubbing and soft tissue swelling associated with Grave's disease.
   - Measure and characterise the pulse: sinus tachycardia or atrial fibrillation.

4. Upper limb

   - Assess for proximal myopathy by asking the patient to raise their arms above their head.
   - Examine upper limb reflexes: hyperreflexia may be seen in hyperthyroidism.

5. Neck

   Assess for enlargement of the thyroid gland. In Grave's disease or a multinodular goitre, the thyroid may be diffusely enlarged. In the case of a solitary toxic nodule, it may be possible to palpate the individual nodule. In de Quervain's thyroiditis, the thyroid may be enlarged and tender.

6. Chest
    - Assess for evidence of a systolic murmur or congestive cardiac failure which may be precipitated by thyrotoxicosis.
    - Look for gynaecomastia.
7. Lower limb
    - Assess for proximal myopathy of the lower limb by asking the patient to stand up from the chair.
    - Assess for hyperreflexia.
    - Inspect the lower limbs for pretibial myxoedema (plaques and nodules in the skin caused by accumulation of mucopolysaccharides) which is a manifestation of Grave's disease.

Clinical Features of Hypothyroidism

1. General inspection
    Assess body habitus, look for apathy/lethargy and signs of cold intolerance.
2. Face
    - Inspect the skin: coarse, dry, yellow discoloration due to hypercarotenaemia (secondary to reduced hepatic metabolism of carotene). Vitiligo may be present in autoimmune conditions.
    - Look for evidence of alopecia.
    - Periorbital oedema may occur in severe hypothyroidism.
    - Inspect for xanthelasma palpebrarum (cholesterol deposits on the eyelids) occasionally seen in hypothyroidism.
3. Neck
    - Examine the thyroid gland which may be enlarged if there is a goitre or late in Hashimoto's thyroiditis.
    - Look for a scar from a previous thyroidectomy.
4. Hands
    - Look for peripheral cyanosis due to reduced cardiac output.
    - Measure and characterise the pulse: bradycardia.
5. Upper limb
    - Assess for proximal myopathy as described previously.
    - Assess for hyporeflexia.
    - Look for signs of carpel tunnel syndrome which may occur with hypothyroidism. Tinnel's test—tapping over the carpal tunnel elicits paraesthesia in the distribution of the median nerve distally. Phalen's manoeuvre—dorsiflexion

of the wrist (by placing the dorsal surfaces of both wrists together) for >30 s elicits paraesthesia in the distribution of the median nerve.

6. Chest
    - Assess for evidence of a pleural effusion.
7. Lower limb
    - Assess for hung-up Achille's reflex (also known as Woltman's sign) which is caused by myxoedema. A positive Woltman's sign is delayed relaxation of the foot after eliciting the Achille's reflex.

Differential Diagnosis of Thyroid Swelling

The thyroid may be enlarged due to a solitary thyroid nodule or may be diffusely enlarged (i.e. goitre).

Solitary Thyroid Nodule

1. Benign
    - Simple cyst
    - Colloid cyst/nodule
    - Follicular adenoma
    - Dominant nodule in multinodular goitre
2. Malignant
    - Primary thyroid carcinoma (papillary, follicular, medullary or anaplastic)
    - Secondary carcinoma (rare)

Causes of a Goitre

The most common cause of a goitre globally is iodine deficiency. In the developed world, the majority are idiopathic. Other relatively common causes include thyroiditis (Hashimoto's, subacute granulomatous, postpartum), Grave's disease, sporadic or familial multinodular goitre (toxic or non-toxic). Examples of rarer causes include inborn errors of metabolism or drugs such as lithium.

Radiological Assessment of the Thyroid

Ultrasound (US) is the first line imaging modality to evaluate the thyroid. The most common indication for US evaluation is thyroid nodules identified on clinical examination or incidentally. US is widely available, does not involve the use of ionising radiation, and can guide decision-making about which nodules require a fine needle aspiration (FNA) for cytology. Benign nodules are typically hyper-echoic and cystic with peripheral vascularity on colour flow or Doppler. US features of malignant nodules include predominantly solid components, eggshell type calcifications, irregular margins, nodular vascularity and associated lymphadenopathy. The size of a thyroid nodule correlates poorly with risk of malignancy. The ultrasound 'U' classification of thyroid nodules allows stratification of nodules as normal (U1), benign (U2), indeterminate (U3), suspicious (U4) or malignant (U5), and guides further investigation (e.g. FNA). U2 nodules do not require FNA in the absence of risk factors for malignancy whilst U3–5 nodules should have an US guided FNA.

Follow Up of Thyroid Nodules

The follow up of thyroid nodules depends on the US appearances and the result of the FNA. Nodules with benign US features (U2) and benign cytology (Thy2) do not require follow up imaging. Nodules with indeterminate/suspicious features and insufficient cytology (Thy1) or benign cytology (Thy2) should have a repeat FNA.

Chapter 13
Abdominal Examination Sheet

Ahmed Farag and Reem Awad Alharbi

Abstract Personal History: Besides starting the patient-doctor relationship and filling the file document, it determines which disease can be responsible for the patient complaint (Epidemiology). Name, Sex, Age, religion, Race, Occupation, Residency, marital status, Number of Children and their age and Sex, Menstrual History in Females and History of intake of contraceptive Pills, Special habits of Medical importance.

Keywords Abdomen · Pelvis · PR · Gynecologic · Examination · Mass · Pain · Areas · Sheet

Personal History

Besides starting the patient-doctor relationship and filling the file document, it determines which disease can be responsible for the patient complaint "Epidemiology".

Name, Sex, Age, religion, Race, Occupation, Residency, marital status, Number of Children and their age and Sex, Menstrual History in Females and History of intake of contraceptive Pills, Special habits of Medical importance. **It should interpreted after the Complaint**.

A. Farag (✉)
Kasr Alainy Hospital, Cairo University, Cairo, Egypt

R. A. Alharbi
Surgery Department, College of Medicine, Princess Nourah Bint Abdulrahman University, King Abdullah University Hospital, Riyadh, Saudi Arabia

A. Farag et al. (eds.), *Clinical Surgical Skills Made Easy*,
https://doi.org/10.1007/978-3-031-69158-4_13

Complaint

Mass (Figs. 13.1, 13.2 and 13.3): **"Site"**: in which quadrant of the abdomen? they are divided into 4 quadrants and 9 anatomical areas. Each involves certain organs i.e. anatomical diagnosis, **"Painful or Painless"** which indicates a possible Pathology.

Abdominal Pain: "Site" may be from an anatomical organ in this site **or referred** from another site:

The abdomen is anatomically divided into 9 areas using 4 lines.

2 vertical lines called the mid-clavicular lines and 2 transverse lines the inter-spinous line between the two Anterior Superior Iliac spines ASIS and the subcostal line connecting the tip of the 9th costal cartilage it is also known as the trans-pyloric plane.

Right hypochondrium: The organs found in this region include the gallbladder, the right lobe of the liver, the upper part of the right kidney, and part of the large bowel (right hepatic flexure). Distal stomach and first part of the duodenum and the right suprarenal gland.

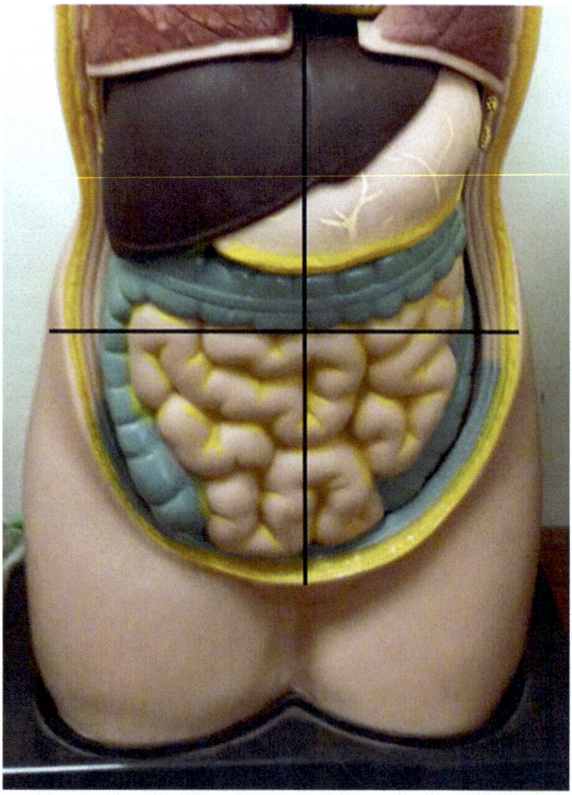

Fig. 13.1 Swelling in the left upper quadrant may be from the organs anatomically residing in this area such as stomach, liver, left side of the transverse colin, spleen, left kidney, suprarenal, tail of the pancreas, para-aortic lymph nodes, aorta, as well as the anterior and posterior abdominal wall

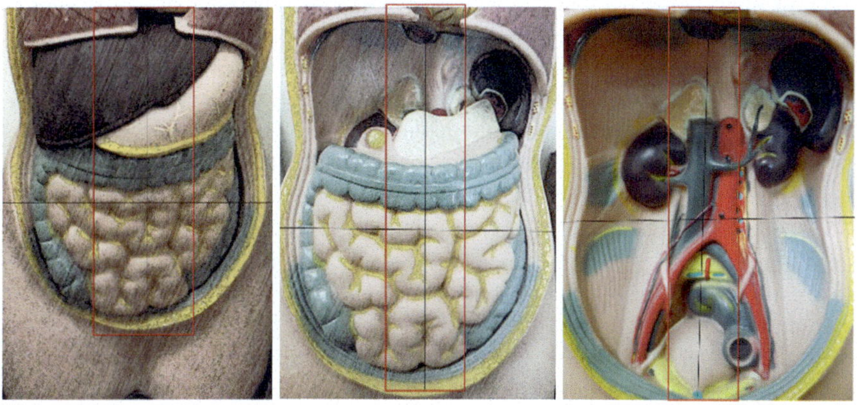

Fig. 13.2 Swelling in the left upper quadrant may be from the organs anatomically residing in this area such as stomach, liver, left side of the transverse colin, spleen, left kidney, suprarenal, tail of the pancreas, para-aortic lymph nodes, aorta, as well as the anterior and posterior abdominal wall

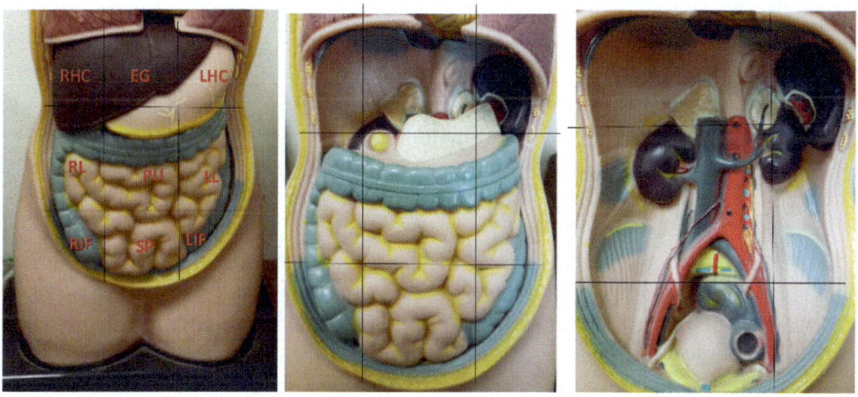

Fig. 13.3 9 Areas of the abdomen where masses or pain is referred to: Right Hypochondrium "RHC", Epigastrium "EG", Left Hypochondrium "LHC", Right Lumbar "RL", Peri-Umbilical "PU", Left Lumbar "LL", Right Iliac Fossa "RIF", Supra-Pubic "SP" and Left Iliac Fossa "LIF". They are divided by lines: 2 mid-clavicular lines "Nipple Lines in males" and s transverse lines: trans-pyloric plane and the inter-spinous plane between the 2 anterior superior iliac spines"

Epigastric region: this region include the esophagus, stomach, aorta, inferior vena cava, the adrenal glands, the central area of the liver and the left lobe of the liver, part of the pancreas, part of the large bowel (transverse colon), and part of the small bowel (third part of duodenum).

Left hypochondrium: The organs found in this region include the spleen, tail of the pancreas, part of the stomach, the upper part of the left kidney, and parts of the large bowel (left splenic flexure and part of the transverse and descending colon).

Right lumbar region: The organs in this region include the right kidney, part of the small bowel (second part of duodenum), and part of the large bowel (ascending colon).

Umbilical region: The organs in this region include the aorta, inferior vena cava, iliac arteries and veins, and part of the large bowel (transverse colon). This is also the abdominal region that holds most of the small bowel (third part of duodenum, jejunum, and ileum).

Left lumbar region: The organs in this region include part of the left kidney, part of the pancreas, part of the small bowel (jejunum), and part of the large bowel (descending colon).

Right iliac fossa: The organs in this region include the lower part of the large bowel (cecum, appendix), and part of the small intestine (ileum). In the female reproductive system, the right ovary and right fallopian tube when enlarged are also in this region. Abnormally situated organs such as Ectopic kidney, a transplanted Kidney or an undescended testis.

Hypogastric "Supra-Pubic" region: The organs in this region include the bladder, part of the large bowel (sigmoid colon, rectum), and the small bowel (mostly the ileum). In the female a large ovarian cyst grow in the midline up-to the umbilicus or higher, the uterus is in this region. A Horse shoe kidney may be present in this area.

Left iliac fossa: The organs in this region include part of the large bowel (sigmoid colon), and part of the small bowel (mostly the ileum). In the female reproductive system, the left ovary and left fallopian tube are also in this region. Or abnormally located organs like an ectopic kidney or undescended testis may be palpable in this region.

N.B. Abdominal wall masses, masses from the iliac bones or back muscles, Lymph nodes around the major arteries and retroperitoneal masses such as lipomas or sarcomas should be integral part of the DD of a mass in the abdomen.

N.B. A wandering spleen may be palpated in any quadrant of the abdomen "A rare case of abnormally mobile spleen" but it can be identified by its sharp anterior border and the splenic notch along this border.

Time-Out

- At this point we think of a differential diagnosis for the first time. E.g. A painful swelling in the left Lower quadrant in a 70 years old male is indicative of Diverticular disease (DD). If the swelling is painless, it may be indicative of Colon Cancer "CA" in the left Colon. If it is painless it is CA left Colon.
- A painful mass in the right Lower Quadrant in a teenage patient indicates the possibility of an appendicular mass with a Differential Diagnoses including Crohn's disease and Ileo-caecal Tuberculosis (T.B.) if the patient resides in Africa or India. Additionally while Ileo-Psoas abscess can be caused by T.B. or Crohn's D.

If this mass is in a 60 years old male it is.

Important to consider the differential diagnosis of Caecal cancer, in order to exclude it as a Possibility.

Present History: It is used in the pathology Section of the diagnosis.

Onset:

It involves the Mode of onset "The pattern in which the disease symptoms initially appear in a person" and was it associated with trauma or inflammation?

Mode of onset where instantaneous onset "Seconds or minutes" occurs with trauma such as Acute abdomen after violent cough may be due to rectus sheath hematoma due to rupture of the inferior epigastric artery at the arcuate ligament "Indirect trauma due to violent contraction of the Rectus abdominis muscle", Acute onset over hours which happens in acute inflammation, Slow onset over days or weeks such as malignant tumors such as Intestinal obstruction in Cancer left Colon, Insidious onset over years such as benign tumors or Accidentally discovered "Like breast mass discovered during shower or while having a check-up or investigation for another complaint" such as benign and malignant tumors. Putting in mind that accidental discovery may be preceded by trauma which draws the attention to the lesion.

Course:

Types of the course are Fig. 13.4:

Rapidly or recently rapid progression in weeks or months e.g. malignant till prove otherwise. Slowly Progressive such as Benign tumors, Regressive usually inflammatory and rarely if ever Neoplastic except in malignant obstructive Jaundice like Peri-ampullary Carcinoma of the duodenum which can undergo one remission due to sloughing of the growth once before regrowth.

Intermittent Course which characterized by remissions and exacerbations with return to the base line before the attacks such as autoimmune diseases or Cellulitis in a normal limb due to repeated traumata or in DM.

Remittent Course "i.e. symptoms disappear or lessen on the passage of time" Like repeated Cellulitis in a limb suffering from Lymphedema which leaves the limb in a worse condition than before the attack.

Duration:

Long duration over years indicates a rather benign pathology.

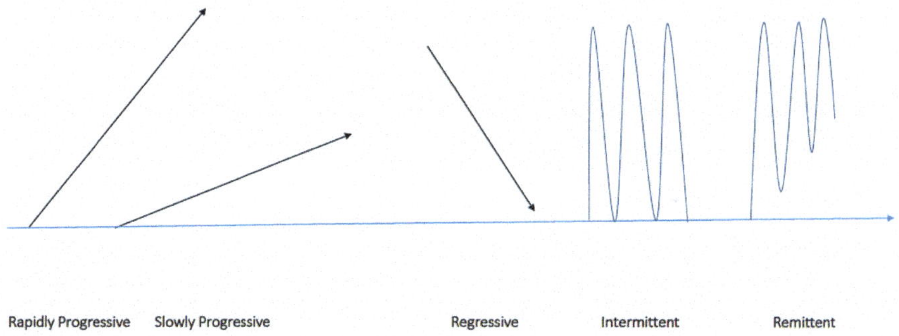

Fig. 13.4 Types of the course

Analysis of the Complaint

1. **Pain**: Site of pain, Type of Pain, referral of pain, what brings pain, what relieves pain and associated Symptoms.
   - Site of pain "Anatomy": Unlike masses, Pain may be from the organs in the anatomical site or referred from another site. E.g. testicular pain can be due to testicular pathology like Epidydmo-orchitis or referred from a ureteric stone causing renal Colic.
   - Type of pain "Anatomy and sometimes pathology": pain may be Colicky or Non Colicky. The later may be burning, stitching, and lancinating, deep boring pain … etc.
   - Colicky pain comes from a hollow organ like Bowel, ureter, Uterus and Fallopian tubes. Or biliary pain in the presence of Gall bladder. N.B. the biliary ducts itself have scanty smooth muscle to cause pain when obstructed after removal of the Gall bladder "Cholecystectomy".
   - In cases of appendicitis when there is Colic it indicates an obstruction of its lumen and the tendency to perforate early which indicates the need for urgent surgery specially when associated by repeated vomiting due to reflex pylorospasm as opposed to inflammatory cause of appendicitis where the pain is Non colicky and may be associated with just nausea or vomiting once.
   - Referral of pain "Anatomy": e.g. Pain in the right upper quadrant of the abdomen which refers to the right shoulder or to the right lower ribs, is Gall bladder pain till prove otherwise. Supra-pubic pain which refer to the tip of the penis is from the Urinary bladder pathology e.g. U B stone.
   - What brings pain "Anatomy and Pathology": Acid food dyspepsia refers to gastric origin, Fatty dyspepsia refer to Biliary and Gall bladder disease, while intolerance to dairy products or wheat refer to Small bowel origin. Dyspepsia to all types of food refers to Colonic origin. N.B. CA caecum may present as Dyspepsia group of patients.
   - What relieves pain or discomfort "Anatomy": if relieved by Vomiting or intake of alkalis both refers to gastric origin. If pain is relieved by passage of stools or Gases it refers to Colonic origin.
   - Associated Symptoms "Anatomy": Nausea, vomiting or Hematemesis and Melena "soft black stools" refer to Gastric or duodenal origin, Distension and bloating refers to GB or Small Bowel origin and exaggerated Gastro-Colic reflex, Diarrhea, Constipation, alternating bowel habits, red blood per rectum, Tenismus or Mucous per rectum are suggestive of Colonic or rectal origin.

2. **Vomiting:**
   - **Type of Vomiting**: Projectile vomiting "A Noisy Vomiting with Throwing of food for some distance indicates A Mechanical obstruction, while regurgitated vomiting "Silent with no Force" indicates Ileus. DD. Regurgitation of food due to esophageal obstruction which doesn't contain gastric contents "The food is regurgitated as it is swallowed".

- **Content**: Acid Vomiting is a Character of peptic ulceration, Vomiting of food without bilious content indicates pyloric obstruction due to gastric or duodenal ulcer or Cancer stomach at the Pylorus. Bilious vomiting in early Intestinal obstruction, Feculent Vomiting indicates a Late Intestinal obstruction or a rare Gastro-colic Fistula due to penetrating Gastric Ulcer or Cancer.
- **Relation to pain or discomfort**: If pain is relieved by Vomiting a gastric pathology is suspected, otherwise a Lower pathology in the GIT is suggested or an Extra-intestinal pathology is the cause e.g. a peritoneal or CNS cause of Vomiting.

3. **Jaundice:** or Yellow discoloration of the Sclera and body. We have to ask for the Depth of Jaundice, the color of Urine. Color of stools and Itching, age, Course of the disease and association with Chills or Fever and Splenomegaly. Age of the patient, Mode of Onset and associated symptoms as Color of Urine and stools, Itching, abdominal pain, fever and Splenomegaly are essential in DD of Type of Jaundice.

   - **Hemolytic Jaundice is characterized by:** Intermittent course with fever, Chills, Normal colored urine and stools, No itching. When it happens in Children it is a congenital Hemolytic anemia, which usually is associated with splenomegaly except in Sickle Cell anemia which causes autosplenectomy from repeated splenic infarctions associated with pain in the left hypochondrium associated with Peritoneal rub sounds on auscultation. Acquired Hemolytic anemias can happen at any age.
   - **Hepatocellular Jaundice:** is associated with enlarged tender liver red colored urine and normal colored stools, No Itching and usually it can happen at any age.
   - **Obstructive Jaundice:** which may be Intrahepatic obstructive Jaundice "Medical obstructive jaundice" associated with hepatocellular Jaundice due to hepatitis due to viral or auto-immune causes or Surgical obstructive Jaundice "Caused by a Blockage that requires Surgical intervention", can be due to Calcular, malignant or due to benign stricture e.g. due to surgical trauma. The Calcular obstructive Jaundice is characterized by being intermittent, light jaundice, dark colored urine, normal colored stools, No itching may be associated with fevers and chills "Charcot's Tirade" while Malignant obstructive Jaundice is Characterized by Progressive course except in Periampullary Carcinoma which may have one remission, deep Jaundice may be olive green discoloration, Dark colored urine, Pale colored stools and itching with Glazed nails in the dominant hand from itching.

4. **Hematemesis and Melena**. Hematemesis is the vomiting of blood, which may be obviously red or have an appearance similar to coffee grounds. Melena is the passage of black, tarry stools. DD. peptic ulcer, cirrhosis with esophageal or gastric varices, gastritis, esophagitis, Mallory–Weiss tears, and malignancy.
5. **Bleeding per rectum**. Hematochezia is the passage of fresh blood per anus, usually in or with stools. "Differential diagnosis of rectal bleeding includes com-

mon etiologies such as anal fissures, constipation, and hemorrhoids. Less frequently encountered causes include anal cancer, angiodysplasia, colonic neoplasia, inflammatory bowel disease, and ischemic colitis."

6. **Change of the bowel habits.**

   Recent change in the bowel habits "weeks, months or one year" i.e. Constipation, diarrhea or alternating bowel habits.

Screening of Body Systems

- **GIT:**
- **General** such as appetite and recent change in body weight.
- **Upper GI Symptoms:** Dysphagia, regurgitation, Heart-burn, hyperacidity, Dyspepsia, nausea, Vomiting, satiety, Colics, Hematemesis and or Melena.
- **Lower GI: Colonic** distension, Colonic pain, Diarrhea, Constipation, Bleeding or Mucous per rectum.
- **Anal and rectum**: Tenismus, bleeding, mucous or discharge per anus, swelling, prolapse or pain and its relation to defecation.
- **Hepato-Biliary:** Pain and/or swelling in the upper right quadrant of the abdomen. Jaundice.
- **Spleen:** Pain and/or swelling in the Left upper quadrant of the abdomen. +/− Manifestations of hypersplenism.
- **Urinary Symptoms:**
- **Upper Urinary:** Loin pain, Renal Colics, Mass or Symptoms suggestive of Uremia.
- **Lower Urinary which includes:**
- Urine Color: Amber or normal, red due to blood jaundice or dye, white due to phosphaturia or Chyluria or Prune Colored due to vitamin A or B12", abnormal contents "Air or Pneumaturia, crystals or Crystaluria, Stones or Necrotic tissue or Necroturia" and act of micturition: Frequency, urgency, precipitancy, urge incontinence, Start of the act, stream of urine, Termination of the act, post-operative dripping, and double micturition.
- **Chest symptoms:** Cough, wheezes, Expectoration and hemoptysis.
- **Cardiac Symptoms**: Palpitation, chest pain during exercise or during rest may present as pain in the upper abdomen, Left shoulder, inside the left arm or left sided neck or signs of heart failure such as Dyspnea, orthopnea or Paroxysmal nocturnal Dyspnea.
- **Neurologic Symptoms:**
- Central or peripheral.
- **Musculoskeletal:** Pain, deformity, weakness.

Past History

- Diseases such as infective hepatitis, Cirrhosis, cancer, Inflammations especially IBD, operations, blood disease such as hemolytic anemias …etc. and diseases of medical importance such as TB, DM, HTN, Cardiac disease, chest disease like Bronchial asthma renal or liver failure.
- Medications which may affect the surgical decision such as anticoagulation, Corticosteroids, Statins, or other medications which may uncover an associated medical condition forgotten by the patient during history taking "Not uncommon event in our clinics".
- History of allergy to medications: if omitted this can subject the doctor to a serious medico-legal and can subject the patient to a major health care error "An avoidable one".
- N.B. We usually don't forget the indications of a medication but it is a major health care problem to forget the contraindication, the most common of them is allergy to a certain medication or group of Medications". "The authors".
- Dietary habits and supplements: such as Garlic and Ginseng can cause an intra-operative or P.O. increased bleeding. They should be stopped before surgery.

Family History

- Medical Diseases of medical importance.
- Cancer and its site in the first and second degree relatives.
- Allergies.
- Problems during anesthesia.

General Examination

In Long Cases a recommended sequence of examination (Marsh of Examination) is needed to achieve the 3 goals of General examination:

1. General assessment of the patients to exclude other associated Systemic or local disease not presented by the patient in the history. For example: During general examination of a 36 years female with post Cesarean section incisional hernia and general an unexplained tachycardia was discovered and diagnosed as Primary thyrotoxicosis. If it had not been detected, she could die from Thyrotoxic Crisis during Anesthesia.
2. Stage of the disease: Not only in cancer but in organ failure or dysfunction e.g. Liver, Kidney, Pulmonary, Cardiac or Neurologic dysfunction.
3. The only clue for diagnosis may be in the General examination. E.g. Cervical or Lymphadenopathy in a patient with obscure epigastric mass or Surgical obstruc-

tive Jaundice may suggest Lymphoma. Another example Café au-lait patches in an obscure multiple subcutaneous swelling which would suggest Multiple neurofibromatosis.

N.B. The items mentioned in general examination are for screening of the patient in general examination but never enough for local examination.

- **General look**: Normal or Abnormal "e.g. Toxic, earthy, anxious, Apathetic look ...etc.
- **Decubitus in Bed**: Elevated leg in DVT, hanging limb beside the bed near a fan in critical ischemia, folded on himself in pancreatic pains and aortic aneurysm.
- **Upper Limb** in the following sequence: Fine tremors, Flapping tremors, Nails (Clubbing, vertical ridging, spooning ...etc.), Palm of the hand (warmth, color, sweating), Pulse on both sides for equality in volume and arrival) delayed pulse in one side compared to the other is pathognomonic of a proximal aneurysm. Then sampling of pulse on one of them for rate and rhythm if they are equal on both sides. Water Hummer Pulse and Blood pressure.
- **Vital Signs** namely Temperature and Respiratory rate.
- **Head and Neck**: Jaundice, Pallor, Central cyanosis, Supraclavicular and Virchow Lymph node +/− thyroid gland and the main group of the deep cervical lymph nodes deep to the sternomastoid on both sides.
- **Chest**: front and back including the heart and lungs and both breasts in males and females.
- **Lower Limbs**: for pedal pulse, edema "Unilateral or bilateral, Pitting or Non-pitting" and tender calf muscles.

Abdominal Examination

General plan (Box 13.1):

Box 13.1 Abdominal Examination: General Plan

• **Inspection**: • **Contour**: 1. Symmetrical: Flat, Distended or Scaphoid 2. Asymmetric: Masses, Central distension or distended Flanks • **Subcostal angle**: Acute, Obtuse or flared Costal margins • **Epigastrium**: for masses, Divarication of the recti and Epigastric hernias • **Umbilicus**: Position, hernias, discharge, Sinuses or nodules • **Suprapubic**: Hair, Masses, Fistulae and Scars • **Inguinal regions and upper thighs "Femoral triangles"**: for Hernias, Masses, Scars and sinuses • **Lateral Abdominal wall**: Color, Striae "alba, Nigra or Rubra", Scars, Dilated Veins, or masses • **Back and buttocks**: For Swellings, Sinuses, Hernias • **Perineum**: for Masses, Sinuses and orifices "Urinary, Anal and Vaginal orifice	• **Palpation:** 1. Superficial: "By the flat of the hands" for Masses tenderness and Rigidity. 2. Deep: For Organs, Masses related to organs and Masses not related to Organs. • **Percussion:** For Organs, Masses and Ascites. • **Auscultation:** For Bowel sounds, Bruits, Venous Hum, Rub "friction sounds" and Breath sounds "In dead Silent abdomen due to severe Ileus" **Investigations:** Laboratory, Radiology, Instrumental and Pathology

Inspection:

- **Contour:**

1. **Symmetrical:** Flat, Distended or Scaphoid.
2. **Asymmetric:** Masses, Central distension or distended Flanks.

- **Subcostal angle**: Acute, Obtuse or flared Costal margins.
- **Epigastrium:** for masses, Divarication of the recti and Epigastric hernias.
- **Umbilicus:** Position, hernias, discharge, Sinuses or nodules.
- **Suprapubic:** Hair, Masses, Fistulae and Scars.
- **Inguinal regions and upper thighs "Femoral triangles":** for Hernias, Masses, Scars and sinuses.
- **Lateral Abdominal wall:** Color, Striae "alba, Nigra or Rubra", Scars, Dilated Veins, or masses.
- **Back and buttocks:** For Swellings, Sinuses, Hernias.
- **Perineum:** for Masses, Sinuses and orifices "Urinary, Anal and Vaginal orifice.

Palpation:

1. **Superficial: "By the flat of the hands"** for Masses tenderness and Rigidity.
2. **Deep:** For Organs, Masses related to organs and Masses not related to Organs.

Percussion: For Organs, Masses and Ascites.

Auscultation: For Bowel sounds, Bruits, Venous Hum, Rub "friction sounds" and Breath sounds "In dead Silent abdomen due to severe Ileus".

Investigations:

1. Laboratory.
2. Radiology.
3. Instrumental.
4. Pathology.

Examination for Organs

Examination for the Liver

General Examination may reveal:

Earthy look, Fetor hepaticus "occurs when your breath has a strong, musty smell", Jaundice, malnourishment "due to loss of appetite or very strict restriction of proteins" with or without disturbed level of consciousness "Hepatic Coma or pre-coma".

Hands may show Flapping tremors of the hands on sudden dorsiflexion of the wrist or spontaneously where there is Rhythmic repeated flexion-extension repetition like a flapping wing of a bird. Nails show":

Clubbing: Lovibond angle sign: When you view your fingernail from the side, it should have a slight dent at the base. This dent, known as the Lovibond angle, makes a slight upward curve as your nail grows toward your fingertip. In the early stages of nail clubbing, the nail and nail bed look flat from the side".

Stages of Clubbing

1. Increased fluctuance & bogginess of nail bed
2. Loss of normal $<165°$ angle between nail and cuticle
3. Increased curvature of nail
4. 'Drum sticking' of distal digit
5. Hypertrophic osteoarthropathy: Shiny, striated appearance,

Leuconychia "is a White discoloration due to hypoalbuminaemia", and/or Koilonychia "which is Spooning of nails due to iron-deficiency anemia".

Palmar erythema: affecting the thenar and Hypothenar eminences "Compare with your hand in order to nullify the effect of ambient temperature".

Water-Hammer pulse or increased pulse pressure "Elevated Systole and decreased diastole" due to increased intrahepatic A-V shunts in advanced liver disease. Scratch marks due to itching in obstructive Jaundice and ecchymosis due to hypo-Prothrombinaemia.

Head, Neck and mouth: Jaundice, Fetor Hepaticus, Anemia, Lymphadenopathy as part of generalized lymphadenopathy including Hepatomegaly and/or Splenomegaly, or Isolated left supraclavicular (Virchow's node, metastatic invasion from intra-abdominal malignancy metastatic also to the liver.

Congested external Jugular vein in heart failure which may cause congestive Hepatomegaly and may be Pulsating in severe tricuspid regurge.

Chest examination: Gynaecomastia "A disc like enlargement of the male breast due to relative increase in estrogen hormone due to failure of its inactivation in the failing liver" and Spider nevi which is dilation of preexisting central arterioles from which numerous thin- walled capillary branches radiate like spider legs, carrying away freely flowing blood.

Lower Limb: For pitting edema "usually pitting and bilateral due to hypoalbuminemia or due to associated Renal failure "Hepato-renal Syndrome or due to heart failure as cause for hepatomegaly. And clubbing of the toe nails. Scratch marks due to itching in obstructive Jaundice and ecchymosis due to hypo-Prothrombinaemia.

Inspection: stand at the foot of the patient and see the contour of the abdomen with the light coming from the opposite side in order to exaggerate any shadows of a localized mass.

Generalized distension or distended flanks, may be due to ascites and Localized swelling due to the liver is in the right hypochondrium and may reach down to the RI Fossa.

Other findings include Flared up costal margin "Due to hepatosplenomegaly", Obtuse subcostal angle specially in males "Normally it is an acute angle in males and obtuse in normal females", Divarication of the Recti "is a stretching of the linea alba with abnormal widening of the gap between the two medial sides of the rectus abdominis muscle (increased inter-recti distance), It becomes apparent when we ask the patient to raise his upper art of the body like what we do in abdominal wall exercise", Downwards shift of the umbilicus, which is normally equidistant from the Xiphoid process and the Symphysis pubis "Which indicates an upper abdominal swelling". Caput Medusae "The swelling usually appears around the umbilicus, and the veins branch out from a central point" It is compressible with rapid refill and veins shows a refill from the side of the umbilicus on 2 finger emptying test. The Umbilicus may show a true Umbilical hernia "with the umbilical Scar on its summit due to increased intra-abdominal pressure DD. From para-umbilical hernia with the umbilical scar on its side. Inguinal hernias are common due to an increased intra-abdominal pressure and occasionally dilated vertical veins in the flanks "indicating an inferior vena cava obstruction due to compression of the IVC by the cirrhotic liver if there is liver tissue behind the IVC when it lies in its position very close to the liver as it receives the hepatic veins. Characteristically the blood flow in those veins are flowing from below upwards in the same direction of flow in the IVC being collaterals trying to compensate for its obstruction.

Superficial Palpation

Start with superficial palpation in the diagonal area to where is the mass "in this case start from the left iliac fossa" and move through the 9 areas of the abdomen in an S-shaped way. E.g. start from the LLQ to the LL, LHQ, EG, UA, SP, RIF, RL then to the RHQ. Or from the LIF, SP, RIF, RL, UA, LL, LHQ, EG then RHC.

Superficial palpation may give most of the needed information and increases the patient's confidence and reassure him concerning his worries about discomfort or pain during examination.

It gives very important information regarding messes and its location and if intra-abdominal or abdominal wall as well as tenderness and rigidity over the mass or in another area of the abdomen.

Deep Palpation

The patient should be lying supine with his knees flexes "in order to release tension on the deep layer of the abdominal wall fascia" Place your right hand on the patient's abdomen in the right lower quadrant (RIF). Ask and teach the patient how to take a deep but gentle breath like a sigh before putting you hand. Start from the right iliac fossa with your hand warm and gentle in order to avoid reflex guarding of the patient especially in anxious patient and reassure him that he will not feel pain as much as you can. Start from the right iliac fossa with your hand warm and gentle in order to avoid reflex guarding of the patient especially in anxious patient. Then move your hand up towards the right costal margin, staying lateral to the rectus muscle "in order to avoid mistaking the tendinous intersection of the rectus muscle with the lower edge of the Liver".

Feel for the liver edge: Ask the patient to take deep breaths in and out. Feel for the edge of the liver with the radial border of your index finger of your relaxed hand resting gently, comfortably and fully on the patient abdomen as the liver descends during inspiration. "In each position repeat make your hand steady and don't move it in order to receive the lower edge of the liver. The liver moves up and down with respiration and wait until the edge strikes or touches your hand. Repeat the respiratory cycle 2 or 3 times in each position in order to be sure that no edge had struck the radial border of your index finger.

N.B. you can use the tips of your fingers instead but some patients do guarding in response to it.

N.B. Your hand "Fingers, Knuckles and wrist", should be on the same horizontal level with the patient abdomen so it is better to do it while sitting on a comfortable stool or chair while doing this part of the examination.

Record the position of the liver edge by advancing your hand up on finger breadth at a time during expiration and note the point at which you first feel the liver edge. This represents the lower border of the liver "It can be marked with a pen on the body of the patient".

N.B. Edge may be sharp or rounded edge. In case of sharp edge like in cirrhosis You can sharply demarcates when the anterior surface of the liver ends and when it lower surface starts".

The same should be done for palpation of the left lobe of the liver starting from the umbilicus proceeding in the midline between the two recti using the tips of the fingers rather than the radial border of the index finger because of the narrow space between the 2 recti which may become larger in the presence of divarication of the Recti as detected during inspection.

Percussion

Upper border: Percuss down along the mid-clavicular line (MCL) to find the upper border of the liver. In female patients, percuss down from the axilla. Or elevate the hands of the patient above her head in order to spread the breast tissue over the chest wall and percuss from the mid-clavicular line as in male.

N.B. Don't percuss for the liver in the parasternal area which is normally dull being the area of the hilum of the right lung.

N.B. Percussion of the Chest for the Upper border of the liver should be a deep percussion because the liver is deep to the lung and the percussion for the lower border of the liver should be a light percussion because the liver is superficial to the intestine and is just below the abdominal wall and the last few intercostal spaces.

N.B. light percussion gives the consistency and character of the superficial organs while deep percussion give the tone of deeper organs. "Light knocking of the door is needed if people are just behind the door at home and heavy knocking is for people at a longer distance from the door".

Tidal percussion: Percussion is a heavy percussion for the upper border of the liver starts at the second intercostal space and is resonant due to the lung tissue full of air and moving down space by space we can notice a change of the resonance which indicates the upper border of the liver "usually the 5th Intercostal space" before it becomes dull at just one space lower to it. Asking the patient to take and hold a deep breath makes the changed note at the level of upper border of the liver becomes fully resonant, due to downwards movement of the diaphragm. Tidal percussion confirms the position of the upper border of the diaphragm.

The Lowe border of the right lobe of the liver is normally not palpable but can be located by superficial percussion 2 finger breadths below the right costal margin and the lower border of the left lobe is again not palpable between the 2 recti but can be located by light percussion half way between the Xiphoid process and the umbilicus in normal population or a hand breadth "measured by the patient's own hand" below the Xiphoid process of if the umbilicus is shifted downwards due to other reason apart from the liver.

Size: Record the size of the liver in centimeters. A normal liver span is between 6 and 12 cm.

Character: Note the character of the liver, such as smooth, craggy, or tender.

Additional notes:

This examination should be performed with the patient lying on their back (supine).
If the liver is enlarged, it may be palpable even when the patient is not inhaling.
The liver should not be tender to palpation.
The liver surface should be smooth.

Examination for the Spleen

General examination: For

1. Signs of Hypersplenism: namely anemia, Leucopoenia "increased incidence of upper respiratory tract infections" and/or Thrombocytopenia: Easley bleeding gums or Skin petechiae and/or skin bruises.

   N.B. Petechiae are pinpoint, round spots that form on the skin. They're caused by bleeding, which makes the spots look red, brown or purple. The spots often form in groups and may look like a rash. The spots are often flat to the touch and don't lose color when you press on them "DD. Mosquito bites".
2. Causes of Splenomegaly:
   - Infections "Bacterial such as Splenic abscess by embolization from Mitral valve digitation called sub-acute bacterial endocarditis, Viral such as infectious mononucleosis, Protozoal such as malaria and trypansomiasis".
   - Congestive: due to portal hypertension due to liver cirrhosis or Bilaharzial Peri-portal fibrosis or portal vein thrombosis due to e.g. umbilical sepsis in a neonate.
   - Blood disease: Hemolytic anemias.
   - Neoplastic: Lymphomas or Leukemia's and Myelofibrosis.
   - Autoimmune: Sarcoidosis, Amyloidosis, Rheumatoid arthritis (Felty's syndrome).
   - Metabolic: in lipid storage disease "Gaucher disease".
   - N.B. Causes of Massive Splenomegaly:
     - chronic myeloid leukemia,
     - visceral leishmaniasis
     - Malaria.
     - Gaucher disease.

Abdominal examination of the spleen:

- Inspection: A localized fullness in the Left hypochondrium which may be associated with generalized abdominal distension mainly in the flanks if associated with ascites in congestive splenomegaly. In Huge spleen, the mass may extend downwards and medially into the eight iliac fossa "the most common", transversely into epigastrium or directly downwards into the left iliac crest. N.B. the weight of the Spleen and the resistance of the Phreno-Colic ligament determines the direction of enlargement of the huge spleen.

- Superficial palpation: gives a lot of information on the site, Size, surface tenderness, rigidity and even the anterior sharp border and the splenic notch especially in large and huge spleen with weak abdominal wall "due to malnutrition and/or moderate ascites".
- N.B. in massive ascites the spleen may not be felt by superficial palpation and can be felt only by dipping".
- Deep palpation for the spleen:

1. From the right iliac fossa: The most common way in order to avoid missing a massive spleen if you start higher where the firmness of the spleen can be mistaken for the firmness of the abdominal wall, a mistake which can be avoided by superficial palpation". We use the tips of the fingers of the right hand "usually" lateral to the right rectus abdominis muscle and asking the patient to take a deep sigh while depressing our hand as much as we can without hurting the patient "the best time to do this is during expiration" then the examiner asks the patient to take 2 or 3 successive deep but gentle sigh. N.B. the hand should be still waiting for the tip of the spleen "which moves up and down with respiration" to hit the tips of his examining fingers. If the spleen is not felt at this position we advance our hands one inch at a time towards the tip of the 10th costal margin. Spleen is only felt below the costal margins when it is enlarged 2 or 3 times more than normal "Normal spleen is not felt" if you feel the spleen clinically it is a pathologic spleen. Characteristically the spleen have a sharp anterior border with a notch which is felt if the spleen is moderately enlarged "The most important DD. From the kidney" other clinical signs of differentiation is mentioned in the table (Table 13.1).
2. In the right lateral position with the left hand pushing the left lower rib cage to push a minimally enlarged spleen into the examining finger tips of the right hand.
3. Sitting position in order to use the gravity to pull the small splenomegaly below the costal margin to be felt by the tips of the fingers.
4. From the left iliac fossa in heavy huge spleen e.g. in Chronic Myeloid Leukemia CML".
5. From the epigastrium.
6. Dipping by rhythmic dipping of the extended fingers at the inter-phalengeal "IPJ" joints flexed rhythmically at the Knuckle joints of all fingers Like flapping of a wing of a bird" over the expected enlarged spleen through the fluid medium of a massive ascites.

Examination for the Left Colon

In the Left Iliac fossa normally felt like a soft vertical structure in the left iliac fossa by Flexing the knees of the patient and asking him to take a sigh and felling the colon by the fingers of both hands over each other moving in a direction

Table 13.1 Clinical difference between Splenomegaly and a kidney mass

	Spleen	Kidney
Site	LUQ but may extend into UA, Epigastrium and RIF. Or extends into the left lumbar and LIF	Renal angle but can reach the anterior abdominal wall if markedly enlarged
	Cannot be pushed into the renal angle	Fills the renal angle or can be pushed into the renal angle
Anterior border and notch	Sharp with a notch if large enough	Rounded
Upper border	Cannot be felt "you cannot insinuate your hand between the mass and the costal margin.	Can be felt
Ballottement	No	Yes
Repercussion	No	Yes
Percussion	Dull all through and is continuous with the Liver Dullness Resonant renal angle Traube's area: Dull	A band of resonance "of the colon" is above the anterior surface of the mass Dull renal angle Traube's area: Resonant

N.B. Ballottement. I.e. the movement of the mass between two hands one in the renal angle and one at the anterior surface of the mass "Like a ball" and Repercussion means that the mass is felt at the renal angle when pushed anteriorly like a gentle thrust by the examining fingers it moves up the drops back on the hand in the renal angle

N.B. Troube's area: surface markings are respectively the left sixth rib superiorly, the left mid axillary line laterally, and the left costal margin inferiorly and one finger breadth from the left edge of the sternum. The Traube's are is hyper-resonant on percussion due to the overlapping resonance of the Lung and fundus of the stomach. The Dullness of the Traube's area may be dullness all through the area or may be encroached upon from:

- Behind due to splenomegaly
- Below due to an enlarged left lobe of the liver, a stomach fundus mass, Massive ascites or after a meal
- Above due to a left pleural effusion
- Anterior due to a massive pericardial effusion

perpendicular to the longitudinal axis of the colon when the hand are depressed as much as possible during the expiration phase of the sigh. Better to be felt against the Iliacus muscle which is possible in most cooperative and thin patients in absence of marked tenderness and rigidity. It may be tender, spastic or has a mass which may be mobile of fixed.

Examination for the Urinary Bladder, Uterus or a Pelvi-Abdominal Mass

Usually in the Suprapubic area or the hypogastrium. They are intra-abdominal masses "their EDGE disappear on contraction of the abdominal wall" and their upper border are felt by the ulnar border of the left hand and its lower border cannot be Felt if they originate from the pelvis except in some ovarian masses or cysts with a long pedicle. They are dull on percussion DD. From mesenteric cysts and mass from the sigmoid colon.

Examination of the Abdominal Aorta and the Iliac Arteries

With its related Lymph nodes which may be felt when pathologically enlarged.

Examination of Intrabdominal Mass Not Related to Organs

In the right iliac fossa, epigastrium or umbilical area by the rolling movement of the two hands over each other during the expiration phase of a deep sigh better to reach the posterior abdominal wall or the vertebrae "Avoid the silly mistake early in your career to easily feel the vertebral column in a patient with week abdominal wall and Lumbar lordosis and mistaking it as a retroperitoneal tumor".

Examination for Ascites

History of enlargement of the abdomen usually over months which is progressive in course. The most common cause is Liver Cirrhosis. Less Common causes are Constrictive Pericarditis, T.B. peritonitis, malignant ascites "especially of G.I. or ovarian origin", Chylous ascites and Pseudomyxoma peritonei.

Acute ascites with painful and tender liver is due to Budd-Chiari syndrome (BCS) is an uncommon disorder characterized by obstruction of hepatic venous outflow. The obstruction may be thrombotic or non-thrombotic anywhere along the venous course from the hepatic venules to junction of the inferior vena cava (IVC) to the right atrium.

History can include besides the mode of onset any T.B. toxemia "Loss of weight, night sweat and night fever", History suggestive of infective hepatitis or alcoholism and history suggestive of intra-abdominal malignancy.

General examination: Stigmata of Liver failure, constrictive pericarditis "engorged neck veins and Edema LLs", metastases from intra-abdominal malignancy "e.g. enlarged and hard Virchow's LN", Left Pleural effusion may suggest a benign ovarian tumor "Meigs syndrome" which is a rare presentation.

Abdominal Examination: Contour shows distended abdomen especially in the Flank.

Percussion the patient is in a 10 degrees head up position we start percussion in the midline from the epigastrium downwards until we find dullness "D.D. Full urinary bladder so ask the patient to urinate before the examination. Then we move towards the flanks from the last point of resonance till the anterior axillary line on both sides. Normally it is resonant.

N.B. the anterior axillary line is a line between the anterior fold of the axilla till the anterior superior iliac spine ASIS where the peritoneal cavity ends".

Beyond this line there is normal dullness being in the retroperitoneal area.

If dullness is discovered we change the position of the patient and ask him to lie on his left side and re-percuss the abdomen.

Shifting dullness means that the some of the dull area in the supine position becomes resonant when it is away from the table and some of the resonant areas on the lower side becomes dull due to the shift of the peritoneal fluid by gravity.

Minimal ascites cannot be felt except by percussion of the umbilical area in the supine position which is normally resonant and re-percussion in the Knee elbow position where it becomes dull.

Massive ascites filling the whole abdominal cavity cannot be felt except by tapping the abdomen on one side with the ulnar border hand of the patient pressing firmly at the midline of the abdomen and perceiving the thrill by the other hand of the examiner put on the opposite side of the abdomen. N.B. the pressure excreted by the patient's hand in the midline prevents transmitting the impulse through the abdominal wall.

Digital Rectal Examination as Part of Abdominal Examination and for Anorectal Complaint

Abdominal examination is not complete without "Per-rectal (or Digital Rectal' Examination "PR" or "DRE" and Per-Vaginal Examination "PV".

DRE or PR as a Primary examination are indicated in:

- **A.R. Complaints** which needs PR as a primary examination are Pain, bleeding, swelling, itching "Pruritis Ani", and discomfort, Tenismus "repeated unproductive urge to defecation", Bleeding per rectum, mucous discharge, Rectal Prolapse "Complete or partial mucosal prolapse, Anal Incontinence or Constipation.
- PR "or DRE" in **Gynecologic complaints** is indicated in suspected Rectovaginal Fistula "Post-delivery or rarely Primary after an abscess Seen once by one of the authors or in a neglected hard Stool impaction in an elderly patient Seen only twice in 44 years of practice". And in uterine or Vaginal vault prolapse after hysterectomy to assess for the presence of associated Rectal Prolapse.
- DRE" or PR" is indicated in **Urinary Symptoms** in males specially for examination of the Prostate, base of the Urinary bladder, and Bulbar urethra "Chapter on Urologic examination".

Present History

- Age is essential in every complaint mentioned above for the suspected pathologies:
  - In Newborn Imperforate anus “Low or High and the later with or without a Fistula and Hirschsprung’s disease “will be covered in Chapter for Pediatric Examination”.
  - Piles, fissure, Fistula, and rectal Prolapse “Complete or mucosal DD. Prolapsed piles” are common at any age from childhood even in infancy “Though less common except in Pediatric surgical clinics”.
  - Cancer is older age usually above 40 but recently it may present with higher percentage at a younger age “The cause is not fully understood”.
  - Bleeding Per rectum in Child hood and in young adults may be due to Juvenile polyp, Polyposis Coli or Inflammatory Bowel Disease “IBD” (Crohn’s disease, Ulcerative Colitis, or their variants “Microscopic Colitis and Indeterminate Colitis”. The IBD is usually associated with diarrhea and Mucous per rectum but if affecting the A.C mucosa and Lower rectum they may be associated with Obstructed Defecation Syndrome ODS “Due to spasm of the A. Sphincter due to Pain “Anismus”, Tenismus, Bleeding and mucous per rectum and Peri-anal irritation “Pruritis ani” more frequently seen now in the Colorectal clinics at any age after adulthood.
  - Anal Incontinence “A.I.” in Childhood Usually presents after operations for Hirschsprung’s disease, high imperforate Anus or Spina Bifida, in the middle age after Anal Operations or vaginal deliveries and at any age but mainly at the Extremes of age due to fecal impaction “Retention with Overflow”. Early postoperative A.I. can be after Rectal or Colonic resections “Called Low anterior resection syndrome LARS”, or following extracolonic Major Surgeries are mainly due to fecal impaction or Pelvic Collection. The latter is associated with tenismus, Mucous and mucous per rectum.
- Sex: Pain the Prostate may present as anal pain and Vice Versa, while associated Anal Incontinence is more common in Females with repeated vaginal deliveries which is more in the form of Stress Urinary incontinence.
- Menstrual History and Deliveries.

Complaint

Pain, bleeding, swelling, itching “Pruritis Ani”, and discomfort, Tenismus “repeated unproductive urge to defecation”, Bleeding per rectum, mucous discharge, Rectal Prolapse “Complete or partial mucosal prolapse, Anal Incontinence or Constipation.

N.B. Red Flag Symptoms: warning symptoms which needs Colonoscopy or at least Sigmoidoscopy are: Tenismus “repeated unproductive urge to defecation”, bleeding per rectum, mucous discharge. They are suggestive but not pathognomonic of cancer since it resembles the symptoms of other diseases such as IBD, Complicated Hemorrhoids and other causes of pain and bleeding per rectum.

First Time Out: Provisional diagnosis based on the patient's complain and the Type of patient "Epidemiology" as interpreted as anatomy and pathology.

E.g. painless bleeding per rectum associated with defecation in a young adult "described as a Splash in the Pan of fresh blood at the end of defecation" is suggestive of Hemorrhoids for DD" while such Bleeding not related to defecation in an older patient is suggestive of cancer till prove otherwise.

Present History

Onset, Course and duration:

Onset: Mode of Onset is usually acute, recurrent acute or chronic onset in all The Anorectal pathologies. Its association with indirect trauma at the onset in the form of straining may suggest acute attack of Hemorrhoids, anal fissure and Sometimes Perianal abscess. Association with local and systemic acute inflammatory symptoms is suggestive of Perianal suppuration "=/– Fistula" or Pilonidal abscess "=/– Fistula".

Course: as an Exception from the general sheet, Intermittent or regressive course is not suggestive of the benign nature of the disease.

Duration: The longer the duration "Years" the possibility of benign nature of the pathology is suggested".

Analysis of the Complaint

Pain:

- Pain in the Anal canal "Back passage" but sometimes it presents as Anterior pain "Urinary or gynecologic". Those patients are referred to the Surgeon from Urologists and gynecologists, after negative examination and investigations are negative.
- Type of pain may suggest the pathology: in cases of anal fissure it is a Razor type of pain, while in the hemorrhoids it is burning pain or like irritation" pain in the abscess is a throbbing like pain all of them may refer anteriorly specially in males to cause pain in the urinary passage.
- Reference of pain: Anal pain may refer anteriorly with Urinary and Gynecology symptoms. N.B. Anal pain never refer to Lower limbs "A common presentation of Spine pathology "Disc or otherwise" as lower limb pain during defecation.

- What Brings pain? Anal pain increases with Constipation "Hard stools", diarrhea "more irritating than hard stools", spicy food, prolonged sitting on toilet seats and/or straining during defecation.
- What relives pain? Is it related to defecation or not is the most important question to ask the patient for it because pain due to Hemorrhoids or fissure are related to defecation. Continuous pain "Pain not related to defecation", may be due to abscess formation, IBD or even Lowe rectal cancer or anal cancer. Pain not related to defecation may be due to Chronic causes of pelvic pain such as: Coccydynia, Levator syndrome, Proctalgia Fugax "pain due to spasm in the Levator Ani which awakens the patient from sleep and is a grapping pain in the bottom which may be severe and happens in patients with anxiety or with a lot of Psychological pressure at work or in their social life", Pyriformis Syndrome "Presents with deep rectal or anal pain which refers to the Buttocks as pointed by a single finger of the patient. They need referral to a pain Clinic after exclusion of organic lesions.
- What relieves pain? Venotonics medications, Local Ointments, suppositories, Sitz baths are characteristically effective in most of the patients with hemorrhoids and anal fissure. Persistent symptoms on those treatments has to raise the possibility of other pathology associated with the 'e.g. hidden abscess, IBD or pelvic pain syndromes.
- Associated symptoms: including Bleeding, Tenismus and mucous per rectum are warning signs which may need further investigations "e.g., Laboratory, radiology or endoscopy +/− biopsies", Associated Urinary Symptoms "Dysuria, Frequency, Burning micturition, Pneumaturia or Fecaluria", associated Gynecologic conditions "Discharge, Gases or stools per vagina" or associated gynecologic prolapse and Systemic manifestations suggestive of sepsis or metastases from advanced Colorectal malignancies.

- Bleeding per rectum:

  - Duration: Long duration "Years" suggests benign pathology.
  - Fresh or altered? Fresh blood suggested an Anal pathology e.g. Hemorrhoids" except when associated with hypotension "A high GI pathology may cause massive bleeding per rectum and needs Gastroscopy at the same time of Colonoscopy. In Chronic bleeding with anemia and Normal Upper GI endoscopy and Normal colonoscopy even in the presence of Hemorrhoids, Small bowel visualization using Barium Sulphate Follow-through Studies, Multislice CT, CT entrography, MRI entrography. Enteroscopy or capsule endoscopy must be done to exclude small bowel source of Bleeding before treating the Hemorrhoids by Surgery or modern techniques.
  - Amount: Small amounts suggests anal pathology while Large amounts may suggest Higher pathology in the Colon "E.g. Angiodysplasia, diverticular disease or cancer" or higher source of bleeding from the Small bowel, Stomach or even esophagus "E.g. Esophageal varices due to portal hypertension" .
  - Relation to defecation: Bleeding not related to defecation suggest pathologies other than Hemorrhoids.

- Mixed with stools or not? Bleeding from Hemorrhoids usually at the end of stools or rarely at the start of defecation. Blood mixed with stools suggests a higher pathology in the rectum, Colon or Higher.
- Painful or painless? Pain from Hemorrhoids is usually painless but may be painful "Irritation" if severely engorged or with spices. Fissures rarely bleed except in patients on anticoagulation or with coagulopathy. Pain with fissure suggests associated internal piles and warrants endoscopy to exclude another pathology.
- Associated Symptoms: If bleeding per rectum is associated with Colics, this refers to Colonic or higher pathology. Association with mucous and tenismus raises the possibility of Malignancies, proctitis "Radiation, IBD, or infective' etiology.

- **Mass** (Table 13.2: The mass may be persistent or recurrent.
- Persistent mass may be prolapsed piles "Fourth degree", Sentinel piles "Skin tag of a fissure or acute due to anal abscess or acute perianal Hematoma.
- A mass which protrude from the anal verge during spontaneously or manually and returns **spontaneously** or by pushing "DD. Piles, Partial mucosal Prolapse or Complete rectal prolapse" Ask the patient about the length, Size and if he noticed the cooler of the Prolapse and if he has a digital photo of the Prolapse".

DD. of Acute Perianal Hematoma "Acute rupture of one of the perianal veins into the limited space of the perianal tissue under the perianal skin "Being limited by the fibrous extensions of the central tendon of the Longitudinal Muscle ani and fixed to the Perianal skin in this area. DD. from the abscess is with the associated local and systemic inflammatory sign. If the patient notices a bluish color and that it developed instantaneously after straining it suggests an acute perianal hematoma. DD. Carcinoma of the Anal Canal.

- **Discharge**: Pus "Abscess or Fistula" or Mucous "Cancer or inflammation"
- **Itching "Pruritis ani"**:
    - Associated with generalized Itching or Urticaria "Think of systemic cause mainly allergies, Urticaria and much more important it may be a sign of Lymphoma Hodgkin's, Non-Hodgkin's or cutaneous Types of Lymphoma

Table 13.2 DD. Of a Lump protruding from the Anal Canal "A.C." during straining"

	Hemorrhoids	Mucosal Prolapse	Complete rectal Prolapse
Size and shape	Grape size and shape	Finger like	Cylindrical
Distribution	Partial or Complete Circumference of the Anal canal	Partial of the Circumference of the A.C.	Complete Circumference
Length	Less than 5 Cms	Less than 5 Cms	More than 5 Cms
Color	Plum Colored	Pink	Pink

  like Sezary Lymphoma and Mycosis fungoides ", both are Types of T cell Lymphoma.
  - Localized Perianal Itching with excoriation which may be due to fecal soiling due to painful anal condition due to A. fissure, Fistula-in-Ano or an acute attack of hemorrhoids. If it occurs by night it may be due to pin worm infestation. Where the female worm lay its eggs on the perianal skin during sleep. It may be associated with vaginal irritation.
  - Other causes of Pruritis Ani involve, contact dermatitis, Cancer, fungal infections and sometimes DM.

- Incontinence and Constipation will be addressed in the Chapter of Pelvic examination.
- Recent Change in the bowel habits in an old age usually suggests a warning sign in the old age.
- Systemic manifestations suggestive an acute perianal or Pelvic suppurations, Signs of distant metastases to the Liver, Lung, Bone or brain, or Systemic manifestations associated with IBD in the eyes, Spine, skin or Jaundice due to sclerosing Cholangitis. Or other auto-immune disorders associated with the IBD especially autoimmune thyroiditis.

General Examination: For the following reasons;

- Assessment of the general Condition of the patient and discovery of any associated Systemic disease.
- Assessment of the stage of the disease in cases of cancer and if the cancer.
- Assessment of the cause of disease on the General condition of the patient e.g. anemia, Malnutrition of Cachexia.
- The Only clue for diagnosis may be in the general examination e.g. Systemic manifestation of acute Fever suggests Perianal or Pelvic suppuration as a cause of anal pain. Liver, Lung, Bone, brain or Skin metastases suggests Advanced AR malignancy, Systemic manifestations associated with IBD as Iridocyclitis "both the iris and ciliary body become inflamed", Ankylosing spondylitis, Pyoderma Gangrenosa usually suggests an IBD as a cause of anorectal Symptoms. Hyperpigmented macules, or spots, on the oral mucosa, lips, nose, hands, feet, and anogenital region.

N.B. Peutz-Jeghers syndrome (PJS) is an inherited condition that puts people at an increased risk for developing hamartomatous polyps in the digestive tract, as well as cancers of the breast, colon and rectum, pancreas, stomach, testicles, ovaries, lung, cervix, and other types of cancers.

Digital rectal Examination: is covered in the Following Chapter in details but simple important points are to be highlighted Here:

Inspection of the perianal skin for:

Signs of dermatitis "Wet inflamed perianal skin" DD. Paget's disease which is looks like eczema but dry.

Prolapsed Piles, Cancer of the Anal Canal or perianal skin, Anal Fissure, Anal Fistula "Closed or discharging pus, the number of the openings and its relation to the anal Canal described as Clock face and its distance from the anal verge, Its relation to the vagina, scrotum or Buttocks" DD. Hiradenitis suppurativa. Pilonidal area for abscesses or sinuses. Do Wink reflex at this point to assess sensation in the saddle area. Notice ulcers and/or masses in the perianal and at the anal verge "Cancer, Acute Perianal hematoma "Acute external piles', Interno-external piles including its color and shape "Uncomplicated or Acute thrombosed piles", skin tag associated with anal Fissure. Report on the color of skin "Inflamed" in association with any mass. Bright red inflamed skin suggests an anal abscess while a dusky red thick skin suggests Crohn's disease or Malignant infiltration.

Scar of previous operation. Take a note of the size of the anal verge during rest "Normal, Patulous "you can see the anal canal mucosa in some cases associated with complete rectal prolapse". Shape of the anal canal "Rounded in normal people, Keyhole, strictured or markedly deformed. Then ask the patient to squeeze to notice the muscle power and any change in the above data. Finally ask the patient to strain as he does during defecation and notice any protruding mass "DD table (Table 13.2)".

N.B. The anal wink, anal reflex, perineal reflex, or anocutaneous reflex is the reflexive contraction of the external anal sphincter upon stroking of the skin around the anus.

Palpation

- By a well lubricated Gloved finger after telling the patient the procedure and approval, reassuring him in the presence of a chaperon, we ask the patient to push down as what he does during defecation while the index finger gently pressing at the anal verge at "O'clock position while the patient is in the Left lateral position. The finger is introduced slowly which the patient is at the zenith of straining to be fully in the anal canal. The examination should be abandoned immediately if the patient feels any pain. This test should not be done in cases of anal fissure which is easily diagnosed by inspection being at the anal verge. If there is any red flag signs further examination should be done with colonoscopy or Sigmoidoscopy under anesthesia.
- As we advance the fingers in the anal canal during DRE we can have a lot of information at the index passes in the anal canal we can feel any mass, Spasm and tone of the EAS together with IAS. During rest and squeeze. As we introduce the finger to its full length we can feel:
- Anteriorly by the index finger: We can feel the rectal wall, mass Tenderness all around. We can feel the base of the Urinary bladder and the Seminal vesicles opposite the terminal Phalanx, the Prostate opposite the Second phalanx and the anal canal surrounding the proximal phalanx in males. The Terminal Phalanx can palpate the Cervix Uteri by the tip of the Phalanx, the Vagina opposite the rest of the terminal Phalanx and by the whole length of the middle Phalanx and the Anal Sphincter surrounding the proximal phalanx in Females. The Prostate, the Bulbar Urethra in males and the posterior wall of the vaginal are better felt by the termi-

nal phalanx "being most rich in touch receptors' during gradual withdrawal of the finger outside the anal canal with some flexion of the distal IP joint of the index finger, in order to assess the size, smoothness, Tenderness or any masses in the Prostate in males and assesses any abnormality in the posterior vaginal wall during rest "organic lesion "e.g. mass or rectovaginal fistula" and during straining at defecation for a rectocele. The finger is then reintroduced fully in the center of the rectum and ask him to strain in order to assess for the Presence of rectal prolapse "intussusception" as a cause of obstructed defecation.

- N.B. in both sexes the Douglas pouch can be felt anteriorly for pelvic abscesses, Masses "Plummer's Shelf in Intracoelomic spread of Intra-abdominal or breast cancer, Sarcoma botryoides or botryoid sarcoma is a subtype of embryonal rhabdomyosarcoma, that can be observed in the Douglas Pouch and many other sites.
- The ventral "Volar" aspect of the examining index finger is rotated to face the Sacrum posteriorly to feel the rectal wall for tenderness or masses or internal opening of a Fistula, extra rectal abscesses "Pelvic "pelvirectal" or cysts including Dermoid Cyst or Tailgut cysts (TGCs) are rare congenital entities arising from remnants of the embryological postanal primitive gut, tumors from the sacrum "Chordoma or Schwannoma". And Coccydynia.
- The examining finger can assess the Puborectalis muscle as the degree of Anorectal junction during rest, Squeeze and attempted defecation in normal subjects or patients presenting with Symptoms of anal incontinence or obstructed defecation syndrome.
- The Finger the feels each side of the rectum and extra-rectal tissue separately for masses, abscesses and tenderness. The levator ani can be felt by hooking the tip of the index finger to try to roll the Pubococcygeus and Iliococcygeus part of the Levator ani "L.A." muscle against the related pelvic wall for any tenderness "L.A. syndrome".
- The Examining gloved finger is then withdrawn an inspected for discharge "Blood, Mucous or Pus".

Gynecologic and Vaginal Examination for General Surgeons

Most common conditions likely to come up to the General surgeon and needs gynecological examination are:

- Acute abdomen due to:
  - Inflammatory Pelvic disease IPD.
  - Ectopic pregnancy.
  - Acute Salpingitis, Salpingo-oophoritis and/or abscess.
- Mass:
  - Uterine Fibroids.

  - Benign ovarian tumors or Cysts "Simple or Chocolate cysts".
  - Ovarian Cancer.
  - Uterine Body cancer.

- Other presentations:

  - Rectovaginal fistula.
  - Endometriosis causing Colonic, Rectal or other pathologies.

Personal History

- Age: of great importance since benign and malignant tumors are more common in the middle age or older age.
- Marital status and/or sexual activity.
- The use of contraceptives: May increase the incidence of vaginal discharge. And the Use of Intrauterine Device "IUD" may increase the incidence of ectopic pregnancy and Inflammatory Pelvic disease "IPD" and may present to the surgeon with acute abdomen.
- The Use of hormonal replacement therapies "mainly estrogen": may increase the incidence of endometrial carcinoma.
- The use of Anti estrogens like Tamoxifen: increased relative risk of developing endometrial cancer for women taking Tamoxifen mainly for treatment of breast cancer.
- Habits of medical importance: Smoking, Alcohol use or recreational drugs.

Complaint

- Abnormal Vaginal bleeding "Menorrhagia, Metrorrhagia or Postmenopausal spotting.
- Dysmenorrhea.
- Vaginal prolapse.
- Abnormal Vaginal discharge
- Urinary incontinence.
- Dyspareunia.
- Non Gynecologic presentation such as abdominal mass "Lower abdomen, Suprapubic or Pelvi-abdominal mass or as an Acute abdomen.

First Time-out: Provisional diagnosis based on which disease can do this complaint in this type of patients".

Present History

Onset, course and duration.

Detailed Menstrual History:

Use of contraception.

Enquire In detail about the nature of the presenting complaint and the history of the presenting complaint. First listen to the patient. Then ask about:

- Age at menarche and menopause.
- Regularity of the menses.
- Dysmenorrhea.
- Date of LMP "Last Missed Period'. Did the Last Period seem normal? When the last period is missed or was abnormally scanty suspect an ectopic pregnancy "disturbed "Ruptured" or Undisturbed.
- Vaginal discharge. If there is a vaginal discharge, ask about its amount, color, and smell. Is it causing the patient to itch?
- Date and result of the last cervical smear test.
- Vaginal prolapse.
- Urinary incontinence.
- Coitus, present or past. (Are you sexually active?). Coitus during the period may predispose to severe inflammatory Pelvic disease "IPD" presenting as acute Lower abdominal pain.
- Dyspareunia.
- Use of contraception.

Past Medical History

- Past gynecological history.
- Past reproductive history: previous pregnancies in chronological order, including terminations and miscarriages.
- Past medical history.
- Past and recent miscarriage
- Current, past, and childhood illnesses
- Surgery.
- Recent visits to the doctor.
- Drug history
- Prescribed medication.
- Over-the-counter medication.
- Recreational drug use.
- Allergies.
- Contact with Pet animals e.g. Cats: For Toxoplasmosis.

Family History

- About parents, siblings, and children.
- Anyone in the family had a similar problem?
- In the case or a suspected Sexually Transmitted disease "STD", ask about the partner.

General examination: For assessment of the Following:

- General condition of the patient and any associated surgical disease not reported by the patient e.g. cardiac, respiratory renal or liver dysfunction ...etc.
- Assessment of the stage of the disease e.g. in cases of Cancer.
- The Only Clue for diagnosis may be in the General examination e.g. Severe pallor with acute abdomen in a woman in the Childbearing period with history of missed or scanty last period raises the possibility of disturbed ectopic pregnancy.

Abdominal examination: Is essential for ascites, liver or peritoneal spread in Ovarian cancer.

Gynecological (Bimanual) Examination

Inspection: Inspect the vulva paying close attention to:

The pattern of hair distribution, the labia majora and clitoris.

Palpation

- Palpate the labia majora.
- Try to palpate Bartholin's gland (the structure is not normally palpable).
- Lubricate the index and middle fingers of your gloved right hand.
- Use the thumb and index finger of your left hand to separate the labia minora.
- Insert the index and middle fingers of your right hand into the vagina at an angle of 45 degrees.
- Palpate the vaginal walls.
- Use your fingertips to palpate the cervix. Assess the cervix for size, shape, consistency, and mobility. Is the cervix tender? Is it open?
- Palpate the uterus: place the palmar surface of your left hand about 5 cm above the symphysis pubis and the internal fingers of your right hand behind the cervix and gently try to oppose your fingers in an attempt to "catch" the uterus. Assess the uterus for size, position, consistency, mobility, and tenderness. Can you feel any masses?
- Palpate the right adnexa: place the palmar surface of your left hand in the right iliac fossa and the internal fingers of your right hand in the right fornix and gently try to oppose your fingers in an attempt to "catch" the ovary. Can you elicit excitation tenderness? (Look at the patient's face.)
- Use a similar technique for palpating the left adnexa.
- Feel the Urinary bladder and urethra anteriorly.

- Feel the Douglas pouch, Rectum and Anal Canal posteriorly.
- Once you have removed your internal fingers, inspect the glove for any blood or discharge.

DD. of an Abdominal Mass

Very Important Questions Should Be Answered Namely

- Intra-abdominal or an abdominal wall mass?: Does the mass disappears or does not disappear with contraction of the abdominal wall muscle. By inspection and by palpation.
- Contraction of the abdominal wall muscle can be done by asking the patient to lift his upper part of the body with his arms across his chest.
- N.B. during palpation the disappearance of the edge of the mass "rather than its surface" is more clinically reliable since the rigidity of the surface of the mass will be replaced with the rigidity of the contracted abdominal wall muscle.
- Does the swelling moves with respiration?: If the swelling moves up and down with respiration this is important anatomically since this mass is from an organ related to the diaphragm "Liver or Spleen" or from an organ related to an organ related to the diaphragm "Gall bladder (GB) mass which is intimately related to the Liver".

DD of a Mass in the Right Hypochondrium

- Abdominal wall swelling: "The swelling stationary in size and its edge remains palpable on contraction of the abdominal wall": Differential Diagnosis (DD) of an abdominal wall mass:
    1. Soft tissue tumor: "e.g. Desmoid tumor or soft tissue sarcoma"
    2. Hernia: Swelling at the site of a hernia orifice or the site of a previous scar, which increases on standing and decreases on Lying down "Disappears if not complicated" which gives an Expansile impulse on cough,
    3. Lipoma: Soft and semi-fluctuant in consistency, lobulated surface with a slippery edge:
    4. Hematoma: History of direct or indirect trauma like severe cough in cases of rectus sheath hematoma with later on bluish discoloration of the skin due diffusion of blood into the subcutaneous tissue.
    5. Abscess: Acute onset with systemic signs of inflammation id large "Fever, rigors and malaise" and Local signs of inflammation "swelling, Pain, redness,

hotness and tenderness". When fever becomes hectic and pain becomes throbbing, pus formation should be suspected "stage of suppuration".

6. Cyst: true cysts are rare and false cysts like seromas after trauma or Surgery "Not uncommon", they show positive cross fluctuation test.
7. Metastasis: Rare such as the sister Marry Joseph nodule at the umbilicus from intra-abdominal malignancy.

- Gall bladder Mass: Due to acute Cholecystitis, Mucocele of the gall bladder or rarely due to malignant tumor.
- Gall bladder masses are intra-abdominal and moves up and down with respiration, globular in shape "Pear Shape" which is continuous with the liver and its dullness in continuous with the Liver dullness. In acute Cholecystitis there is fever, rigors. Jaundice is an indication of involvement of the Common Bile duct in the pathology "Stone in the CBD, edema or tumor".
- Right upper quadrant tenderness: This is a sign of inflammation in the gallbladder.
- Murphy's sign: This is pain when the doctor palpates the right upper quadrant during deep inspiration.
- Courvoisier's sign: This is a palpable, non-tender gallbladder in a jaundiced patient which raises the possibility malignant obstructive jaundice.
- Diffuse Liver Mass: Nonalcoholic fatty liver disease (NAFLD), Alcoholic liver disease (ALD), viral hepatitis, Hepatitis caused by medications and toxins, autoimmune liver disease, Hepatic steatosis, Cirrhosis and Hepatic fibrosis.
- The symptoms of diffuse liver enlargement can vary depending on the underlying cause. However, some common symptoms include: Upper abdominal pain or discomfort, Fatigue, Loss of appetite, Nausea and vomiting, Jaundice (yellowing of the skin and eyes), Dark urine, normal color of stools, Swelling of the abdomen and legs and Itching.
- Localized Liver mass: Hepatic adenoma: Hepatic adenoma is a benign tumor of the liver. It is most common in women of reproductive age who are taking oral contraceptives. Hepatic Haemangioma which is the most common type of liver tumor. Liver metastases or a primary liver tumor. "The most common are the Hepatocellular carcinoma HCC or Cholangio-Carcinoma". Hydatid cyst of the liver. Palpable Reidel's Lobe of the liver.
- Kidney mass "Renal Swelling": By inspection from behind you can notice a full renal angle as compared to the other side" or it is visible abdominally when markedly enlarged and can be palpated by superficial palpation and deep palpation abdominally "A rounded border all through "DD. From the Liver and spleen where both usually have a sharp lower border and sharp anterior border respectively". By palpation there is a Swelling which fills the renal angle or can be pushed to the renal angle "between the last rib and the Erector spinae muscle and above the iliac crest "Normally it is empty being occupied by the flexures of the colon", you can reach its upper border "DD. Of Liver and spleen" and shows a dull renal angle when it fills the renal angle and characteristically there is a band of resonance over the selling abdominally being deep to the Colon.

- Auscultation Just above and lateral to the umbilicus may reveal a bruit "A renal artery stenosis". When markedly enlarged it touches the anterior abdominal wall.
- Supra-renal swelling: when markedly enlarged which looks like a kidney swelling but it does not fill- or can be pushed to the renal angle. I tis suspected when the patient presents with truncal obesity, hypertension, hirsurism and or precocious puberty. It may be without any systemic effects.
- Carcinoma of the Hepatic Flexure of the Colon: which shows an intra-abdominal swelling which does not move up and down with respiration and usually firm to hard in consistency.
- A tumor from the second part of the duodenum. Rare and can be diagnosed by exclusion.
- A swelling from abnormally high sub-hepatic appendix: Acute mass, abscess or tumor.

DD of a Mass in the Epigastrium

- Fatty hernia of the Linea Alba: In the midline with or without minimal shift from the midline. It feels like a Lipoma, it shows an Expansile impulse on cough and usually partially reducible and may be multiple.
- Mass from the Left Lobe of the Liver: "Vide-Supra"
- Gastric swelling: An intra-abdominal swelling which does not move with respiration, It is usually associated with gastric type of dyspepsia and firm to hard in consistency.
- Pancreatic Pseudo-cyst: An epigastric mass and when suspected a nasogastric tube may be felt over the mass. DD. A large pancreatic true cyst.
- Enlarged Para-Aortic Lymph node: Usually Primary as Lymphoma "alone or as a part of Generalized Lymphadenopathy 'An example for the importance of General examination as the only clue for clinical diagnosis' or a secondary e.g. from a malignant Testicular tumor hence the importance of examination of the scrotum as an integral part of the Abdominal examination.
- Aortic aneurysm: A mass in the epigastrium which may extend to the Umbilical region which shows an expansible pulsations synchronous with heart beats. N.B. the Aorta bifurcates into the 2 common iliac arteries one inch below and to the left of the umbilicus".
- Mass in the transverse colon: An intra-abdominal swelling which does not move with respiration which is associated with change in bowel habits, bleeding per rectum or dyspepsia few hours after meals "due to Gastro-colic reflex".

DD of a Mass in the Left Hypochondrium

- Abdominal wall mass.

- Enlarged spleen.
- Left Kidney mass.
- Left supra-renal mass.
- Mass from the tail of the pancreas.
- Gastric mass.
- Mass from the left Colon.
- Mass from an enlarged left lobe of the liver.

DD. of a Mass in the Right Lumbar Region

- Abdominal wall mass.
- Right Kidney swelling.
- Mass from the ascending Colon.
- Appendicular mass retro-caecal position.

DD of a Mass in the Umbilical Region

- Umbilical hernia, Mass or caput medusa and Metastases "Rare" from intra-abdominal Tumor "Sister Mary Joseph nodule".
- Desmoid tumor of the abdominal wall: A locally malignant tumor "Doesn't metastasize" and is related to Fibromatosis and Sarcoma.
- Mesenteric cyst: An intra-abdominal mass, which is cystic in consistency, moves freely in all directions with a band of resonance over its surface "intestine". The last three are called Tillaux's triad.
- Carcinoma of the transverse Colon "Redundant T. Colon"
- Small bowel tumors:
- Retroperitoneal Lipoma or sarcoma: may reach a large or huge size with no symptoms related to other systems e.g. GI, Urinary or others.

DD of a Mass in the Left Lumbar Region

- Abdominal wall mass:
- Left Kidney mass: enlarged Kidney due to hydronephrosis or tumor.
- Mass in the descending Colon:

DD of a Mass in the Right Iliac Fossa

- Abdominal wall mass:
- Inguinal Hernia: See the chapter of the hernia.
- Appendicular mass: Associated or shortly preceded with symptoms and signs of acute appendicitis with local and systemic signs of inflammation. N.B. due to the associated abdominal wall guarding, the mass may not be felt except after Anesthesia and examination under anesthesia was considered the first step before incision in the classic teaching.
- Mass in the Caecum: Usually Cancer but Ileo-caecal Crohn's disease, T.B and rarely Actinomycosis are seen.
- Iliac adenitis:
- Ectopic mobile kidney:
- Transplanted Kidney: History of Transplantation and the scar over the transplanted kidney help in diagnosis.
- Undescended testis: Empty Ipsilateral scrotum.
- Retroperitoneal sarcoma:
- Ileo-psoas abscess: History suggestive of T.B. or Crohn's disease. The swelling usually extends under the psoas fascia to below the inguinal ligament which is cystic with Cross fluctuation between the cyst below and above the inguinal ligament.
- Ileo-caecal T.B.: History of T.B, residence in an endemic area and T.B toxemia "Night sweat, night fever and loss of weight".
- Actinomycosis:
- Mass from the Iliacus muscle: like Psoas abscess but solid in consistency.
- Mass from the iliac bone: e.g. Chondroma or Chdorosarcoma. It is fixed at the base in all directions. Usually large, hard with lobulated surface.
- Pelvic swelling: The most common is a tubo-ovarian mass.
- Aneurysm of the iliac arteries: a swelling in the course of the iliac artery which shows expansile impulse with each heartbeat.
- Ileopsoas hematoma due to indirect trauma in over anti- coagulated patient "Marivan toxicity". Seen by the author once in his career.
- Iliac Lymphadenopathy. Which may be isolated or part of systemic lymphadenopathy. And may be <u>Inflammatory</u> i.e. Acute or Chronic and each may be specific or non-specific or <u>Neoplastic</u> "Primary or secondary".

DD. of a Mass in the Hypogastrium "Suprapubic Area"

- Abdominal wall mass:
- Bladder swelling: due to retention of urine "Acute or Chronic" the chronic retention is painless and may reach up to the umbilicus "e.g. neurogenic bladder".

Acute retention is markedly painful and smaller in size. Lower border cannot be felt.

- Uterine swelling: Such as pregnancy or large uterine fibroid. Again its lower border cannot be felt except in some fibroids.
- Ovarian mass: Usually cystic and freely mobile its lower border may be felt having a long pedicle.
- Pelvic abscess: in the Douglas pouch from a complicated tubo-ovarian abscess, perforated appendix, perforated diverticulitis or carcinoma. Fever rigors, abdominal tenderness and rigidity PR and PV examination reveals a tender and boggy swelling in the Douglas pouch.
- Sigmoid Colon mass. Diverticulitis and Peri-diverticular mass "Abscess or phlegmon" or cancer colon.

DD of a Mass in the Left Iliac Fossa

- Abdominal wall mass: Vide Supra.
- Inguinal Hernia: Vide Supra
- Mass in the Sigmoid Colon: Vide Supra
- Iliac Lymphadenopathy: Vide Supra
- Ectopic mobile kidney: Vide Supra
- Transplanted Kidney: Vide Supra
- Undescended testis: Vide Supra
- Retroperitoneal sarcoma: Vide Supra
- Ileo-psoas abscess: Vide Supra
- Mass from the Iliacus muscle: Vide Supra
- Mass from the iliac bone: Vide Supra
- Pelvic swelling: Vide Supra
- Aneurysm of the Iliac arteries: Vide Supra

Chapter 14
Digital Rectal Examination "DRE"

Shimaa Alkhaldi

Abstract Obtain a detailed history: Before conducting the examination, gather information about the patient's symptoms and medical history to guide the examination. Create a comfortable environment: Explain the procedure, establish rapport, and ensure the patient's modesty is preserved. Patient positioning: The two most common positions for anorectal examination.

Keywords PR · Rectal · Anal · Canal · Examination · History · Symptoms · Position

(a) Obtain a detailed history: Before conducting the examination, gather information about the patient's symptoms and medical history to guide the examination.
(b) Create a comfortable environment: Explain the procedure, establish rapport, and ensure the patient's modesty is preserved.
(c) Patient positioning: The two most common positions for anorectal examination:

   a. Prone jackknife position: This position requires a specialized proctoscopic table. The patient kneels on a padded ledge and leans forward, resting their chest and abdomen on the table. The table is adjusted to an appropriate height and angled forward, raising the buttocks upward.

      Avoid this position: patients with decreased mobility, recent abdominal surgery, morbid obesity, late pregnancy, or arthritic conditions affecting the knees, hips, and lower back.

   b. Left lateral (Sim's) position: The patient lies on their left side with their back close to the edge of the exam table, and their hips and knees are both flexed at 90°.

(d) Lighting and equipment: Ensure that the exam room is well lit, ideally with a sink and a nearby toilet. Prepare the necessary instruments in advance.
(e) Chaperone: will ensure patient comfort and maintain professionalism.

S. Alkhaldi (✉)
King Faisal Specialist Hospital, Riyadh, Kingdom of Saudi Arabia

A. Farag et al. (eds.), *Clinical Surgical Skills Made Easy*, https://doi.org/10.1007/978-3-031-69158-4_14

Inspection and Palpation

1. Stepwise inspection: Begin by carefully inspecting the perineum, anal margin, anal verge, and sacrococcygeal region. Have an assistant retract the buttocks if needed.
2. Visual inspection: Look for specific conditions such as pilonidal disease, anal margin or anal verge lesions, hemorrhoidal disease, skin irritation, maceration or excoriation, perianal dermatoses, erythema, ulceration, drainage sites, condyloma, scarring or evidence of prior anorectal surgery, purulence, fecal soiling, anal discharge, and prolapsing tissue.
   - Valsalva maneuver: Assess the degree of perineal descent and check for the presence of genitourinary or rectal prolapse. Evaluate the pelvic floor muscles for strength and function during voluntary contraction.
3. Anocutaneous reflex: Lightly touch the perianal skin to provoke the "anal wink" or anocutaneous reflex.
4. Palpation: Palpate the area to identify tenderness, induration, or fluctuance, which may indicate a suppurative process or a firm "cord" (suggesting an anal fistula).
5. Fissure-in-ano assessment: Gently efface the anal verge to check for a fissure-in-ano.
6. Insertion technique:
   a. Lubrication: Apply a small amount of lubricant to the index finger.
   b. Insertion: Ask the patient to take a deep breath and insert the lubricated finger into the rectum, facing downward (6 o'clock position).
   c. Assess: rectal wall, stool consistency, resting sphincter tone and ask the patient to squeeze to evaluate squeeze tone accurately.
   d. External sphincter tone: Assess the tone of the external sphincter and ask the patient to bear down to feel for tightening. In female assess the perineal body bulk.
   e. Palpation of the rectal wall: Start from the 6 o'clock position and palpate clockwise to the 12 o'clock position. Then, return to the 6 o'clock position and palpate the other half of the rectal wall, feeling for masses (Note size, mobility, firmness, and relationship to surrounding structures), nodules, and tenderness.
   f. Additional assessments: Palpate presacral/retro-rectal area posteriorly. Assess the prostate gland in males and the cervix in females. Check for rectocele anteriorly and consider bimanual examination for rectovaginal septum assessment.
7. Occult Blood Test: Check any fecal material obtained during the rectal exam for occult blood using a guaiac kit. This test helps detect hidden blood in the stool.

8. Documentation: When documenting findings, describe the location in relation to anatomic position (anterior, posterior, right, left) instead of using clockface descriptors, as they depend on the patient's position during the examination.
9. DRE may be omitted: anal fissure, thrombosed external hemorrhoids, non-reducible internal hemorrhoids, tight anal stricture, and large anorectal mass. Neutropenia is considered a relative contraindication (limited evidence)
10. Anoscope, proctoscope and Rigid Sigmoidoscopy can be done as part of anal examination.

Chapter 15
Pelvic and Rectal Clinical Examination

Ilario Froehner Junior and Peter Petros

Abstract Through the pelvis, the urinary, gynecological, and gastrointestinal tracts have their respective outlets, associated with an elaborated complexity of muscles, circulatory and neurological systems.

All three compartments (urological or anterior, gynecological or middle and intestinal or posterior) work together in integrated physiology. Symptoms that occur in the pelvis can therefore involve more than one medical specialty.

Keywords Examination · Pelvic · Urinary · Gynecologic · Gastrointestinal · PR · PV · Integrated

Introduction

Through the pelvis, the urinary, gynecological, and gastrointestinal tracts have their respective outlets, associated with an elaborated complexity of muscles, circulatory and neurological systems.

All three compartments (urological or anterior, gynecological or middle and intestinal or posterior) work together in integrated physiology. Symptoms that occur in the pelvis can therefore involve more than one medical specialty.

Posterior compartment evaluation consists of anatomical and functional parameters analysis, prior and current anal continence status determination, intestinal transit and defecatory disorders detection, and the search for symptoms originating from the anterior and middle compartments (urinary and gynecological, respectively).

I. F. Junior (✉)
PELVIA Gastrointestinal Motility and Continence and at Nossa Senhora das Graças Hospital Gastrointestinal Motility Department, Pelvic and Rectal Examination, Curitiba, Brazil

P. Petros
Sydney, NSW, Australia
e-mail: pp@kvinno.com

A. Farag et al. (eds.), *Clinical Surgical Skills Made Easy*,
https://doi.org/10.1007/978-3-031-69158-4_15

Anamnesis is the paramount starting point and must be thoroughly accomplished. It is followed by physical examination that must be complete and focused on the information gathered during the anamnesis. A precise clinical examination will lead to the correct complementary test to be requested, for instance, anorectal manometry, endoanal ultrasound and Defecography studies.

Pelvic region is made up of several dynamic organ systems perfectly organized into a small space. Through the pelvis, the urinary, gynecological, and gastrointestinal tracts have their respective outlets, associated with an elaborated complexity of the muscles, circulatory and neurological systems (Fig. 15.1). Added to this, the bone framework and its joints need to maintain the necessary space for all these structures, to support them, to accommodate them and distribute the weight of the upper abdomen, chest, neck and head, to the lower limbs, articulated in the pelvis.

Symptoms that occur in the pelvis can therefore involve several medical specialties such as general practitioners, gastroenterologists, general surgeons, digestive system surgeons, oncological surgeons, coloproctologists, urologists, gynecologists, obstetricians, rheumatologists, vascular surgeons, neurologists, neurosurgeons, and dermatologists.

The difficulty in interpreting the signs and symptoms can lead to delay in the definitive diagnosis, to postponement in the initiation of the appropriate treatment, and to worsening of the clinical picture and quality of life parameters of the patients. Adequate clinical examination is essential in the orientation of the most suitable specialty, for example, coloproctology, urology and gynecology, or combined, as frequently is necessary.

In this chapter, we will discuss the pelvic examination concerning the posterior compartment of the pelvis, related to the gastrointestinal tract.

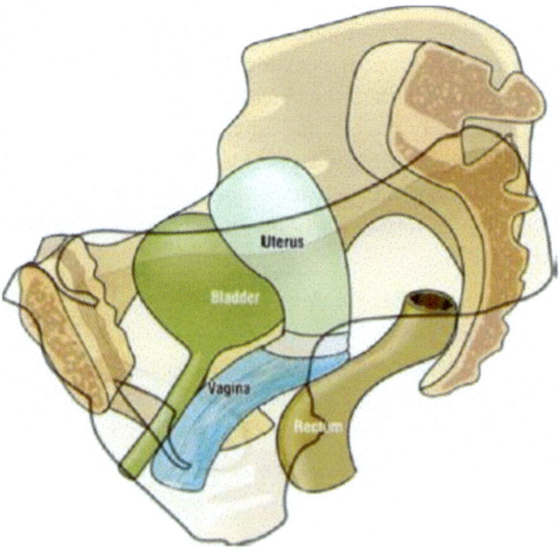

Fig. 15.1 Pelvis with organs. Anterior (urinary) compartment is in green. Middle (gynecological) compartment is in blue. Posterior (intestinal) compartment is in brown. (Adapted from: Petros P. Overview. In: Petros P. The Female Pelvic Floor. Function, Dysfunction and Management According to the Integral Theory. 2nd ed. Heidelberg: Springer Medizin Verlag; 2007. p. 3 [1])

Anatomical and Functional Aspects

The main component of the pelvic floor is made up of the levator ani muscles or the pelvic diaphragm. These muscles represent a pair of broad, symmetrical muscle leaflets composed mainly of three muscles: iliococcygeus, pubococcygeus and puborectalis (the latter two also called pubovisceral muscle).

The rectum corresponds to the last portion of the large intestine and is located in the posterior compartment of the pelvis. Following the concavity of the sacrum, and supported by the coccyx, the rectum angles sharply backwards to cross the levator ani muscle and give rise to the anal canal, an area called the anorectal ring. Surgically, this corresponds to the proximal limit of the anal canal.

Although representing a relatively small segment of the digestive tract, the anal canal is characterized by a unique anatomy and complex physiology. Like the rectum, the anal canal is also defined differently according to anatomists and surgeons. The surgical anal canal is compatible with anorectal digital examination and imaging tests such as endoanal ultrasound and magnetic resonance imaging. However, it does not correspond to the histological structure present. The anal canal is made up of the following layers: mucosa and submucosa, followed by the internal sphincter, intersphincteric space, and the external sphincter of the anus. This muscle is in close contact with the puborectalis muscle, which is the medial portion of the levator ani muscles. At rest, the anus or anal orifice is closed due to the tonic action of the sphincters and the presence of internal and external hemorrhoids (Fig. 15.2).

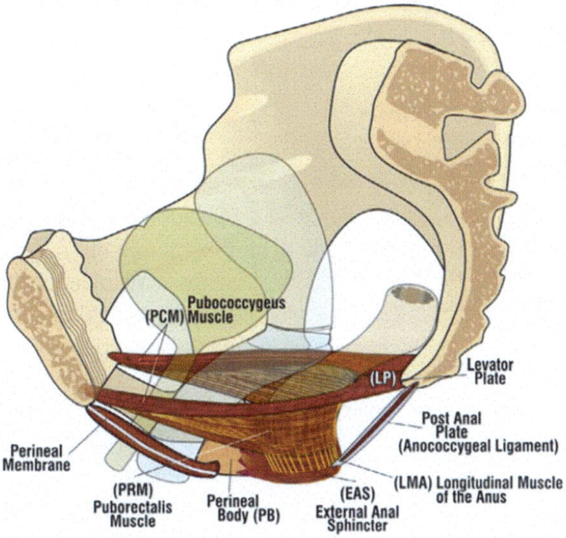

Fig. 15.2 Pelvic with organs and muscles. (Adapted from: Petros P. Overview. In: Petros P. The Female Pelvic Floor. Function, Dysfunction and Management According to the Integral Theory. 2nd ed. Heidelberg: Springer Medizin Verlag; 2007. p. 4 [2])

The Integral Theory of the Pelvic Floor

From the 1980's, a concept based on pelvic anatomy began, in which all support structures would participate decisively in physiology. The Integral Theory has initiated, grouping the pelvic structures into three anatomical-functional compartments: anterior, middle and posterior.

According to the Integral Theory, pelvic disorders are due to a complex interaction between the ligamentous structures that support it. This interaction is controlled by the sympathetic autonomic nervous system through the hypogastric nerves and parasympathetic autonomic nervous system and voluntary control by the pudendal nerve (Fig. 15.3).

The first studies demonstrated that patients undergoing urethral sling surgery at the Royal Perth Hospital had a favorable response to urinary disorders due to the action on the skeletal muscles and not the elevation of the bladder as was the surgical principle. In 1993, "posterior fornix syndrome" was described as resulting from laxity of the sacral uterine ligament. More than its description, its correction resulted in the improvement of symptoms of urgency, nocturia and pelvic pain.

The comprehensive understanding of the anatomical and functional aspects association of the three compartments highlights a remarkable interaction of the pelvic contents, commonly eliciting urinary, gynecological and evacuatory repercussions (Fig. 15.3).

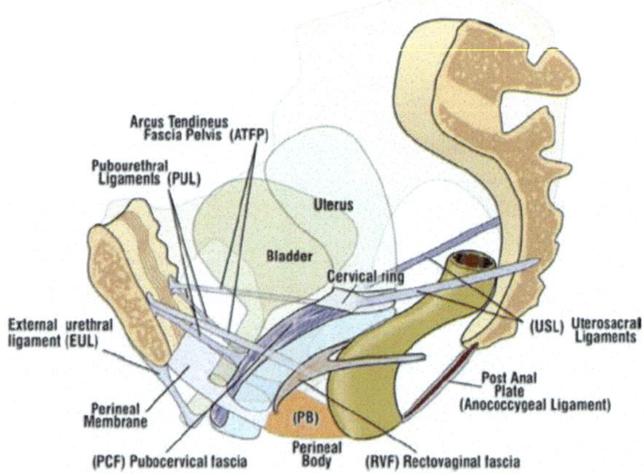

Fig. 15.3 Pelvis with organs and connective tissue. Ligamentous and membranous structures are in grey and Fascial thickening of vagina, pubocervical fascia and rectovaginal fascia are in darker color. (Adapted from: Petros P. Overview. In: Petros P. The Female Pelvic Floor. Function, Dysfunction and Management According to the Integral Theory. 2nd ed. Heidelberg: Springer Medizin Verlag; 2007. p. 3 [1])

Pelvic and Rectal Clinical Examination

Pelvic and rectal clinical evaluation consists of anatomical and functional aspects association and the determination of the current anal continence status, the detection of intestinal transit and defecatory disorders, and the existence of symptoms originating from the anterior and middle compartments (urinary and gynecological, respectively).

The evaluation is based on anamnesis, abdominal and perineal physical examination, as well as the adequate complementary tests request.

First Step: The Anamnesis "History Taking as Said by the Patient"

Anamnesis is essential. The determination of the current bowel habit allows it to be compared with the oscillations that exist throughout the patient's life and during specific conditions, such as, for example, menstrual cycles, pregnancies, or diseases. It is important to note that the occurrence of bowel movements, such as slow transit constipation, obstructed evacuation, irritable bowel syndrome and anal incontinence in some patients, occur only at these times.

Commonly, patients consider their bowel condition to be inherent to their age or normal for their current situation. Similarly, the embarrassment resulting from some conditions, such as anal incontinence, prevents the patient from mentioning these symptoms to the attending physician, such as the gynecologist in relation to urinary incontinence, and there is a need to routinely inquire about these respective symptoms. It is important to note that approximately one third of patients already have some degree of anal incontinence prior to anal surgeries, such as Hemorrhoidectomies or fissurectomies.

In addition, since bowel continence is multifactorial, many patients do not present loss of feces or gases due to the balance or compensation among these mechanisms, for instance, good rectal capacity and compliance in patients with obstetric occult lesion of the anal sphincter, highlighting the concept of "functional reserve". In these cases, some surgery, anal or intestinal, could affect this balance, predisposing to obstructed evacuation and/or anal incontinence.

Questions related to the gastrointestinal tract, especially about aspects of digestive motility, are useful—particularly in patients with chronic diarrhea, as it is an intense stress factor onto the anal canal.

Evaluations of comorbidities and previous morbid history (e.g., previous surgeries) are important in determining the differential diagnosis. Eventually, joint evaluations of other specialties, such as urology, gynecology, urogynecology, neurology, among others, become important.

Scores, indices, or measurement tools have become a fundamental item in the evaluation of patients. The importance of quantifying and objectifying some information is essential in the initial evaluation and follow-up. Also, the clarification to the patient, which informs the subjective information of their life experiences. As an example, the large number of patients who consider themselves constipated without being one.

The Continence Grading Scale, or currently the Cleveland Clinic Florida Continence Scale, from 1993, is the most widely used index worldwide in daily practice and in scientific studies for the clinical assessment of the severity of anal incontinence. It ranges from 0—complete continence, to 20 points—daily anal incontinence to gas, liquid, and solid feces, associated with the daily use of perineal protectors and with significant limitation of the patient's quality of life.

Fecal Incontinence Quality of Life Index, developed in 2000, allows the evaluation of the impact of anal continence alterations on patients' daily lives, evaluating four domains, namely: lifestyle, behavior, depression, and embarrassment.

Recently, the score for anterior rectal resection syndrome, LARS Score—Low Anterior Resection Syndrome Score, was developed in 2012 contemplating some characteristics associated with the respective syndrome, such as anal incontinence to gases and liquid stools, bowel movement frequency, fragmented or incomplete evacuation, and defecatory urgency. Its objective is to evaluate the clinical intensity of anterior resection of the rectum: from 0 to 20 points, without the syndrome, from 21 to 29, mild condition, and from 30 to 42, severe one. It does not present in its composition aspects related to solid stool incontinence, the use of perineal protectors and quality of life.

Regarding functional constipation, a specific Rome IV criteria allow diagnosis, while other scores stratify symptoms intensity, such as Constipation Scoring System, from 1996, validated for use in several countries. Its objective is determining and monitoring the intensity of this condition, including aspects of slow transit constipation and obstructed evacuation. There are 8 questions whose score ranges from "0" (normal intestinal transit) to "30" (greater intensity). "Frequency of bowel movements" ranges from "0"—up to 3 times a day at up to 3 days apart—to "4"—less than once a month. "Difficulty: painful evacuation effort" ranges from "0"—never—to "4"—always, as well as "Completeness: feeling incomplete evacuation" and "Pain: abdominal pain". "Time: minutes in lavatory per attempt" ranges from "0"—less than 5 min—to "4", more than 30 min. "Assistance: type of assistance", from "0"—no help—to "2", help with enemas or help with hands. "Failure: Unsuccessful attempts for evacuation per 24 hours" range from "0"—never—to "4", more than 6 times a day. "History: Duration of constipation (year)", the only invariable, ranges from "0"—zero—to "4", more than 20 years. The maximum possible score is 30, indicating marked constipation.

Also, when concerning gastrointestinal functional disorders or disorders of the brain-gut axis, there are Rome IV diagnostic criteria that address dysfunctions such as dyspepsia, functional diarrhea, bloating, and irritable bowel syndrome.

Diarrhea, if present, should be investigated with a view to its etiology and correction since it overloads the rectal reservoir and predisposes to anal incontinence.

Second Step: Physical Examination

Abdominoperineal physical examination is critical. In line with comorbidities, previous morbid history, and anamnesis information on intestinal transit and anal continence, the physical examination directs the diagnostic reasoning and indicates the need for complementary tests and evaluations. For example, pelvic floor and urogynecological dysfunctions often coexist with or precede anal continence disorders.

Physical examination, especially digital rectal examination, has reduced sensitivity in diagnosing the location and extent of anal sphincter lesions. Complementary evaluation can add diagnostic data in up to 98% of cases, assist in the choice of treatment in 75 to 84% of anal incontinent patients, and define the management in 10 to 19% when compared to clinical evaluation alone. The comparison between the clinical evaluation of primiparous women and the respective endosonographic evaluation resulted in the diagnosis of sphincter lesions in 3 and 33% of the patients, respectively. Clinical and manometric evaluation of 159 women treated at a specialized service for obstetric lesions of the anal sphincter, using endoanal ultrasonography as the gold standard, verified the sensitivity of only 26% of perineal inspection and the sensitivity of 67% and the specificity of 55% of digital rectal examination in the diagnosis of sphincter lesions.

Perineal inspection allows the evaluation of evident changes in anal tone, such as in the patulous anus, and the verification of perineal scars, such as obstetric lacerations, episiotomy, and perineoplasty. Anal surgeries may also suggest possible sphincter injuries. Areas with reduced anal skinfolds may indicate hypotonia or underlying muscle damage. Inspection of anal contraction allows the tonic evaluation of the sphincter circumference as well as evacuation, by diagnosing anorectal prolapses, perineal descent and perineal bulging, such as those resulting from episiotomies and displacements of the perineal body and posterior vaginal wall, common in rectocele. Perineal body provides an estimate of anterior sphincter thickness. Changes in anocutaneous sensitivity may be associated with pudendal nerve neuropathy. Anuscopy provides visualization of the distal rectum, internal hemorrhoids, pectineal line, and external hemorrhoids.

Third Step: Complementary Tests

Complementary exams allow an objective understanding of bowel movement, defecation, and anal continence.

Anorectal manometry allows the assessment of anal tone at rest and voluntary contraction. When all technical details of its performance are observed, it provides reliable data on anorectal function. Anorectal manometry assists in the localization of sphincter lesions, selecting patients with indication to undergo imaging methods, such as endoanal ultrasonography and magnetic resonance imaging. It assists importantly in the evaluation of obstructed defecation and can also be used during pelvic floor physiotherapy sessions by biofeedback.

Endoanal ultrasonography is the imaging method of choice in the evaluation of anal sphincter morphology in the study of anal incontinence. It is considered a minimally invasive test in relation to electroneuromyography and a low-cost test when compared to magnetic resonance imaging with an endoanal coil. It has sensitivity and specificity greater than 95% in the identification of sphincter lesions. It complements clinical history and anorectal manometric study and it is important in determining the etiology, due to the presence of clinically asymptomatic lesions, such as occult obstetric sphincter lesions, which occur in up to 35% of primiparous women.

Magnetic resonance imaging with endoanal coil has similar sensitivity and specificity to endoanal ultrasonography, allowing images with better definition, especially of the external anal sphincter muscle. It also allows a broad evaluation of the pelvic floor and pelvis. The evaluation of external sphincter atrophy is most often associated with pudendal nerve neuropathy and worse results of anal sphincteroplasty.

Defecography studies are indicated mainly in the evaluation of defecatory disorders associated or not with anal incontinence, allowing the identification of structural alterations, which are often difficult to locate and classify only by physical examination alone—as in the case of enteroceles and sigmoidoceles. It can be performed by fluoroscopic study, by magnetic resonance imaging and, more recently, by Endoanal ultrasound.

The pudendal nerve latency time helps to define sphincter dysfunction, whether due to pudendal nerve neuropathy or muscle injury or even mixed (neuromuscular) injury. Currently, according to the clinical context, its indication can be waived due to decreasing availability, discomfort and pain associated with its performance and, even adding data to the investigation, it modifies the conduct in a minority of cases. Although controversial, patients with pudendal nerve neuropathy have a worse prognosis when submitted to sphincter reconstruction surgical procedures. As with electromyographic studies, the evaluation of pudendal nerve latency time is restricted to a few selected cases.

Conclusions

Defecation and anal continence dysfunctions are generally challenging, often multifactorial conditions that associate complex pathophysiology with subjective data and variables impacts on patients' quality of life.

An adequate comprehension of its innumerable characteristics and interconnections allows the focused selection of complementary tests, their interpretation, the various possible forms of treatment, and the expected responses versus those obtained in each chosen therapy.

Acknowledgements I am very grateful for the indispensable support received by the Pelvia Gastrointestinal Motility and Continence team, especially to nurse Jocemari Noeli Buzato for the paramount assistance in the creation of this chapter.

I would also like to thank Nossa Senhora das Graças Hospital for the importance it has always shown for Gastrointestinal Motility, Anorectal Physiology and for our activity in this very important hospital.

References

1. Petros P. The female pelvic floor. Function, dysfunction and management according to the integral theory. 2nd ed. Heidelberg: Springer Medizin Verlag; 2007. p. 3.
2. Petros P. The female pelvic floor. Function, dysfunction and management according to the integral theory. 2nd ed. Heidelberg: Springer Medizin Verlag; 2007. p. 4.

Chapter 16
Acute Abdomen

Kimberley Logbochi Olivia Mvetimbo Tamb and Audrius Dulskas

Abstract Acute abdomen is a dreadful condition, which brings individuals to the emergency department. The word acute means that this condition must be treated immediately before it escalates and leads to a fatal result. The abdomen is a vast area of the body and includes many organs, which diseases/disturbances can manifest as an acute situation. Anatomically the abdomen is delimited by costal margins superiorly and inferiorly by the symphysis of the pubis plus pelvic bones.

Keywords Acute · Abdomen · Emergency · Examination · Anatomy · Causes · Areas · Surgical · Medical

Introduction

Acute abdomen is a dreadful condition, which brings individuals to the emergency department. The word acute means that this condition must be treated immediately before it escalates and leads to a fatal result. The abdomen is a vast area of the body and includes many organs, which diseases/disturbances can manifest as an acute situation. Anatomically the abdomen is delimited by costal margins superiorly and inferiorly by the symphysis of the pubis plus pelvic bones. The abdominal cavity is limited by the abdominal walls, diaphragm and pelvis, which contains the location of digestive organs, kidneys, spleen and ureters.

There exist two ways to divide the abdominal cavity: the four quadrants or the nine regions; those divisions come in handy when it comes to the locating the pain.

The perception of pain can be visceral or parietal. Visceral abdominal pain is from distention of hollow organs, mesenteric traction or excessive smooth muscle

Kimberley Logbochi Olivia Mvetimbo Tamb
Vilnius University Faculty of Medicine, Vilnius, Lithuania
e-mail: kimberley.mvetimbo@mf.stud.vu.lt

A. Dulskas (✉)
National Cancer Institute, Vilnius, Lithuania

A. Farag et al. (eds.), *Clinical Surgical Skills Made Easy*,
https://doi.org/10.1007/978-3-031-69158-4_16

contraction. Most often, it is deep and poorly localized in the midline. Parietal pain from parietal peritoneum and abdominal wall is lateralized and localized to the inflamed area, and conducted via intercostal nerves.

In Classic Teaching the cause of the acute abdominal pain can be presented as a House (Fig. 16.1), with a ground Floor "Abdomen Proper", Upper Floor "Chest causes of pain radiating to the upper abdomen", Basement "Pelvic causes of pain radiating to the Lower abdomen", Attic "Naso-pharynx, where in children swallowing of the infected secretions may cause an acute abdominal pain e.g. tonsillitis or adenoids", Front garden "Anterior abdominal wall e.g. a n acute hematoma of the rectus sheath", Hind Garden "Posterior abdominal wall" An Electric supply "Nerve supply e.g. Herpes zoster" and water Supply Arterial supply such as dissecting aortic aneurysm or a ruptured AA.

In order to describe the pain and identify its source, a physician must perform an excellent anamnesis and physical examination before resorting to instrumental tests. Regarding the clinical examination, the acronym SOCRATES is very useful for the assessment of abdominal pain and stands for: Site, Onset, Character, Radiation, Associated symptoms, Timing, Exacerbating and relieving factors, Severity. Physical examination should consist of:

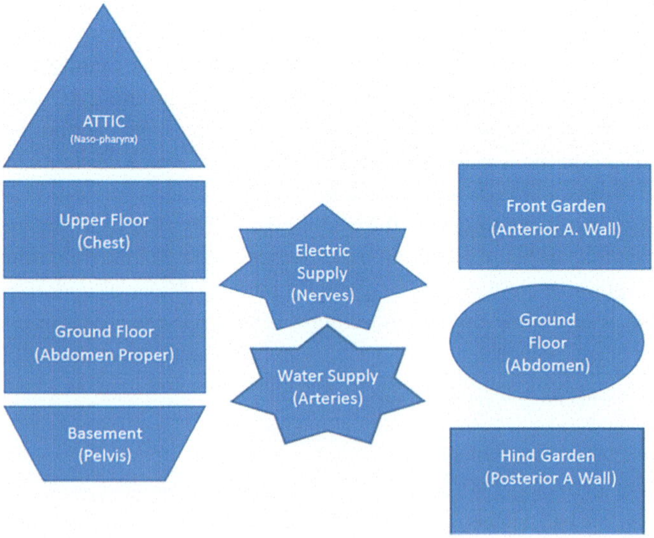

Fig. 16.1 The House model of causes of acute Abdomen

General State and Appearance Inspection/Abdominal Part Inspection

Physical examination should consist in looking at the general appearance of the patient (sharp facial expressions or so called "facies hypocraticus" means that patient is in a prolonged pain), when inspecting the abdomen, one should look at the contour, the skin, umbilicus and masses. When looking at the skin, one should notice any changes in color, ecchymosis or visible moles, scratches, bruises and Striae. If the prominence of veins is visible, this could suggest portal hypertension or vena cava obstruction. The 6F rule can explain the causes for a distending abdomen: fat, fetus, feces, flatus, fluid or full sized.

Auscultation of the Abdomen

Auscultating the abdomen, by using the stethoscope and listening to bowel sounds in each of the four quadrants, normal bowel sounds should be 5–35 bowel sounds per minute. When bowel sounds are lacking this could indicate paralytic ileus, which is when the motor function of the digestive tract is paralyzed due to a neuronal misfiring. Absence of bowel sounds may be a sign of peritonitis. Now when the opposite happens, and bowel sounds are increased this is a sign of bowel obstruction.

Palpation and Percussion of the Abdomen

Palpating the abdomen should also be held in a systematic manner using the four quadrants, light palpation first and then deeper palpation. The physician might feel tenderness, which may or may not be an indication of a disease or again voluntary guarding which is the voluntary contraction of the abdominal muscles when palpation provokes pain. Rigidity and rebound tenderness are the other clinical signs that can indicate a specific pathology. Specific sites of tenderness are important, when located in the epigastrium this implies the presence of peptic ulcer, in the right hypochondrium—Cholecystitis, in the left iliac fossa suggest diverticulitis and in the right iliac fossa could manifests as appendicitis or Crohn's ileitis. Deep and bimanual palpations can be used to assess the size of organs such as the liver, gallbladder, spleen and the kidneys. The spleen can only be palpable if it is enlarged. Murphy's sign, which is indicated by right upper quadrant pain, is often the result of acute Cholecystitis as the gallbladder can be palpated.

We will now be discussing the different situations where acute abdomen manifest itself, in a systemic manner.

Differential Diagnosis of Abdominal Pain in the Right Upper Quadrant

- Acute Cholecystitis: Acute abdomen pain is felt in right upper quadrant (RUQ), and presents itself with fever, nausea and vomiting, with cachexia appearance. The pain is characterized as constricting and radiates to the scapula. The pain seems to be exacerbated after consuming food. Tenderness is expressed in the right hypochondrium, and Murphy's sign will manifest itself during palpation as the patient will feel pain when the physician palpates the gallbladder. In confirmation of the diagnosis, laboratory bloods tests and ultrasounds will be ordered. The complete blood cell count will display an increase in C-reactive protein (CPR) and leukocytosis which is an indication of inflammation. On ultrasounds, one may encounter the gallstones and the thickening of the gallbladder wall and the enlargement of the bladder—all showing signs of acute Cholecystitis [1].
- Calcular Obstructive Jaundice: Another differential diagnosis of acute RUQ pain, can present itself with prolonged abdominal pain, nausea and vomiting. The pain usually follows a meal and may radiate to the epigastrium or right shoulder or the back. The patient may appear with jaundice and pruritus, his feces may appear pale and his urine dark; those signs suggest cholestasis. On abdominal palpation tenderness and abdominal guarding are present. Initial diagnostic evaluation includes a complete blood cell count which shows elevated total bilirubin and direct bilirubin, elevated alkaline phosphatase (ALP) and gamma glutamyltransferase (GGT). The ultrasound may show the presence of gallstones in the common bile duct and the enlargement of ducts. These may be indicative for choledocholithiasis. Painless elevation of liver function test and jaundice may be the sign of pancreatic cancer.
- Acute Hepatitis: An additional differential diagnosis of RUQ pain, can present itself with nausea, vomiting, small appetite and a fever plus minor flu symptom. The pain does not radiate. The patient appears with jaundice, stool is pale, and urine is dark. On palpation the abdomen displays voluntary guarding, and the liver is enlarged and tender during deep palpation. Then follows the laboratory tests, which shows elevated AST, ALT, total bilirubin, a prothrombin time (PT) and international normalized ratio (INR) and a comprehensive hepatitis panel which includes Hepatitis A, IgM antibody, Hepatitis B surface antigen, Hepatitis B core antibody, Hepatitis B surface antibody and Hepatitis C antibody. Based on the evaluation of the comprehensive hepatitis panel, one can determine if it is an acute or chronic hepatitis [2].
- Acute Budd-Chiari Syndrome or acute Veno-occlusive Disease: Budd-Chiari syndrome (BCS) is an uncommon disorder defined as hepatic venous outflow tract obstruction, which is independent of the level or mechanism of obstruction, given the obstruction is not due to pericardial disease, cardiac disease, or sinusoidal obstruction syndrome (veno-occlusive disease). When acute, Clinical manifestations develop rapidly over a few weeks, with intractable ascites and hepatic necrosis. Venous collaterals are not seen.

Differential Diagnosis in Epigastric Region Pain

- Acute Pancreatitis: Epigastric pain can present itself with fever, tachycardia and the pain is sudden and dull with radiation to the back. The patient will present with nausea and vomiting, and his skin may present with the Grey Turner sign, which is a flank ecchymosis with discoloration. On palpation abdominal tenderness, guarding and distention is present. A follow up with laboratory diagnosis, will display an increase in lipase, amylase, CRP and an increase in white blood cell count. Ultrasound is used as a first line diagnostic, but computed tomography (CT) scan is more specific and sensitive for the diagnosis of acute pancreatitis. The CT abdomen will show an enlargement of pancreatic parenchyma with edema.
- Complicated or active gastric or duodenal ulcer: The most common epigastric pain can characterize itself by a burning sensation. The patient presents with dysphagia, nausea, vomiting and weight loss or weight gain. Exacerbating factors are linked to food consumption, pain is increased shortly after eating or pain is relieved by eating food, depending on which one it is one can differentiate between gastric ulcer or duodenal ulcer. On palpation tenderness is present. In this case laboratory tests are not very conclusive; an upper gastrointestinal (GI) endoscopy is the preferred diagnostic tool as it will allow to examine the ulcer and take a biopsy to test it for H. pylori as it is one of the main risk factors for peptic ulcers. One of the most common complications of peptic ulcers is bleeding, which will then manifest as hematemesis which is the vomiting of blood or melena the discharge of black tarry stool or again anemia. The second most common complication is the perforation, which will lead to the leakage of bowel contents, and can lead to the presentation of shock with hypotension and tachycardia. Peptic ulcer perforation will present with pain at the shoulder and on the abdominal X-ray radiolucent air will be present below the diaphragm (Cope Zachary, Abdominal pain).
- Gastric paresis: Another form of epigastric pain presents itself with nausea, vomiting and bloating. The patient may be anorexic and present with weight loss, paleness of the skin, feeling tired. On physical examination mild epigastric tenderness and abdominal distention is expressed. Laboratory blood tests and urine, looking for signs of dehydration, one may encounter an increased HbA1c. The gold standard for gastroparesis is the gastric emptying scintigraphy to evaluate gastric motility by tracking how long it takes for a meal with a radioactive tracer to move through your stomach and empty from it.
- Gastritis: An additional form of epigastric pain can present itself with nausea, vomiting, loss of appetite, belching and bloating. The patient may present with a fever, which is indicative of an inflammation. Physical examination displayed mild epigastric tenderness. Proceeding with laboratory diagnostic, an increase in CRP and white blood cell count. The next diagnostic for a definitive diagnostic, is an upper endoscopy which may reveal a thickened and prominent rugae in the gastric fundus and reveal gastritis. The most common infection of the stomach is

by H. pylori, so additional tests such as with noninvasive tests like urea breath test to confirm the presence of the bacteria. The most common noninfectious causes could be the use of NSAIDS, which increases the risk of mucosal injury.
- DD: Acute inferior Myocardial infarction, Acute dissecting aortic aneurysm and Leaking Aortic aneurysm "See Below"

Differential Diagnosis of the Pain in the Left Upper Quadrant

- Splenic cause of Pain: Left upper quadrant pain can present itself accompanied with discomfort; the pain may radiate to the left shoulder. Sign of early satiety may be present. On physical examination, bi manual palpation on deep inspiration where the enlargement of the spleen is sensed. If percussion is used by the physician, dullness is heard when it normally should be tympanitic, called Castell's sign. Follow up with laboratory diagnostics, will display signs of anemia with low red blood cell count, a decrease in white blood cell and low platelets. The CT scan is the best diagnostic tool to determine the cause of splenomegaly.
- Supra-renal hemorrhage "Apoplexy": Acute Bleeding in the suprarenal Gland Adrenal hemorrhage is an uncommon disorder characterized by bleeding into the suprarenal glands. The hematoma may be unilateral or bilateral, and the clinical presentation can range from nonspecific abdominal pain to catastrophic cardiovascular collapse. The etiologies for this unusual disorder are diverse. Potential causes include blunt abdominal trauma, septicemia, coagulopathies, anticoagulant use, pregnancy or stress.
- DD: Supradiphragmatic cause of pain e.g. pleurisy. "See Below"

Differential Diagnostic of Right Lower Quadrant Pain

- Acute appendicitis: Right lower quadrant pain can manifest as a history of nausea and vomiting. The patient may present as anorexic and with fever due to an inflammation. Pain will be acute over the McBurney's point which is indicative of an acute appendicitis (first it may appear in the epigastric region or whole abdomen and later localize specifically in the right lower quadrant -. On physical examination the patient may present with the obturator or Rovsing signs. Psoas sign is assessed by having the patient lie supine and placing your hand just above the knee. Ask the patient to lift the right leg against resistance of your hand. This motion causes friction of the psoas muscle over the inflamed appendix, causing pain. To assess for the obturator sign, position the patient supine with their right knee bent and leg bent at the hip. Rotate the leg internally at the hip, causing the internal obturator muscle to stretch providing indirect pressure over the appendix. Rosenstein's sign, also known as Sitkovskiy sign, is another sign of acute appendicitis. It is observed when tenderness in the right lower quadrant increases when the patient moves from the supine position to a recumbent posture on the left side. There may also be a Blumberg sign (or rebound tenderness). Pain felt upon sudden release of steadily applied pressure on the abdomen indicative of peritonitis. Dunphy sign (cough test; coughing test) increased abdominal pain, localized to the right lower quadrant, with coughing. There are some more signs, but here we discussed only the most known. The laboratory diagnosis will reveal an increase in CRP, increase in white blood cell, a pregnancy test is recommended for woman of childbearing age. The ultrasound is the preferred test as it is safer choice, compared to the CT scan. A severe complication of acute appendicitis is the perforation of the appendix.

Right Lower Quadrant Pain Can also Manifest with a History of Nausea and Vomiting

- Disturbed Ectopic pregnancy: The patient is pregnant in the first trimester, has vaginal bleeding and frequent urination. Abdominal rebound tenderness and guarding is also expressed. The laboratory findings will show an increase in beta human chorionic gonadotropin (β hCG) the pregnancy hormone and an antenatal cardiotocography (CTG) to verify the viability of the fetus using an ultrasound transducer placed on the pregnant women. The best diagnostic tool is the Transvaginal ultrasound and will display an empty uterine cavity which is an indication for ectopic pregnancy.
- Necrotizing enterocolitis: Right lower quadrant pain, with a history of vomiting and the patient appears pale due to poor skin perfusion plus lethargic. Present with melena which is bloody stool and abdominal distention. On abdominal examination symptoms will mimic acute appendicitis, with tenderness and guarding on palpation. On laboratory tests will have an increase in CRP and arterial blood gases will reveal metabolic acidosis and low platelets. The best diagnostic for necrotizing enterocolitis is chest x-ray which will show the presence of gas in the bowel wall.

Inflammatory bowel diseases (IBD) can elicit pain in the right lower quadrant. Two very important IBD: Ulcerative colitis and Crohn's disease (Table 16.1).

Table 16.1 DD between Ulcerative colitis "UC" and Crohn's disease "CD"

Test	Ulcerative colitis	Crohn's disease
General assessment	Bloody diarrhea, tenismus, fatigue	Fever, weight loss, fatigue, diarrhea, anemia
Physical examination	Abdominal tenderness	Palpable abdominal mass
Laboratory test and instrumental tests	Elevated ESR and CRP, leukocytosis, thrombocytosis Ileocolonoscopy: friable, mucosa	Ileocolonoscopy best diagnostic tool for the disease: cobblestone

Differential Diagnosis of the Left Lower Quadrant Pain

- Acute Diverticulitis: Left lower quadrant pain can manifest with nausea, vomiting, constipation and bloating. The patient may present with fever due to an inflammation and abdominal distention. On physical examination rebound and localized tenderness plus guarding is present. Due to the inflammation the laboratory results display an increase in white blood cells and CRP. The most ideal diagnostic test is a CT scan of the abdomen and pelvis with intravenous (IV) contrast is used to diagnose diverticulitis: colonic outpouching and bowel wall thickening. Weakness of the muscular layer of the colon, leads to the formation of pouches in the wall of the colon, take place in the descending and sigmoid colon which would explain the left lower quadrant pain. Perforation can lead to the complication of diverticulitis [3].
- Sigmoid Volvulus: One of the most common causes of intestinal obstruction is sigmoid volvulus, when the colon twists on itself which results in obstruction. The patient shows features such as severe constipation and asymmetrical abdominal distention. On physical examination tenderness is present and on auscultation abnormal bowel sounds displayed as tympani are heard. Abdominal x-ray, for sigmoid volvulus has a specific appearance 'coffee bean' shaped.
- Colonic obstruction (Table 16.2): The interruption of the normal passage of bowel is referred to as bowel obstruction. The patient will present with abdominal pain that is gradual and can also be diffuse. It will present itself with progressive, continuous vomiting and constipation. On examination abdominal distention is present due to excessive gas. In early auscultation increased high pitched sounds are heard and percussion tympany is observed. Bowel obstruction can be classified as either small bowel obstruction or large bowel obstruction.

Table 16.2 DD between small bowel obstruction and large bowel obstruction

	Small bowel obstruction	Large bowel obstruction
Definition	Mechanical blockage of the small intestines	Mechanical blockage of the large intestines
Common causes	Intra-abdominal lesions, hernias, Crohn's disease, malignancy and volvulus	Colon carcinoma, volvulus and diverticulitis
Physical assessment	Nausea, vomiting, abdominal pain described as cramping Abdominal pain	Abdominal pain, distention and constipation Pain may be acute or chronic when malignancy is involved
Laboratory diagnosis	CBC, electrolytes, acid base…etc.	CBC, electrolytes, acid base, lactic acid, CEA tumor marker
Instrumental tests	Plain abdominal x-ray to see proximal bowel dilatation and the multiple fluid air level. Multi detector computed tomography (MDCT), oral or IV contrast optimize the CT scan data	Plain abdominal x-ray to see proximal bowel dilatation and the multiple fluid air level. CT scans are the golden standard. Contrast enema is also a useful clinical tool

Diffuse Abdominal Pain

- The most common form of diffuse abdominal pain, suggest peritonitis which is any inflammation of peritoneal layers. The pain can present as diffuse or localized. There are two types of peritonitis, primary involves the contamination of the peritoneal layers and secondary is direct contamination of the peritoneal cavity by an organ that is covered with peritoneum. The secondary is the most common and often presents as a perforation of the GI tract into the peritoneal cavity. The patient may express symptoms of nausea, vomiting and fever. On physical examination, abdominal guarding and rebound tenderness is present. Laboratory tests with a complete blood cell count, leukocytosis is present due to the inflammation. The best diagnostic tool is the use of contrast CT, and it displays the presence of free air in the peritoneal cavity 'pneumoperitoneum'.

Extra-Abdominal Causes of Acute Abdomen

- Pelvic inflammation, an inflammation caused by a bacterium migrating from the cervix to the female reproductive organs. The pain can manifest in the lower abdomen. The patient may present with fever, nausea, vomiting and abnormal vaginal discharge. Diagnosis is based on clinical symptoms, and can be supported by vaginal examination, ultrasound, cervical/urethral swab and vaginal culture. The most common pathogen that cause the inflammation are Chlamydia trachomatis and Neisseria gonorrhea (Cope Zachary, Abdominal pain).
- Torsion (Table 16.3): Ovarian or Testicular torsion.

Table 16.3 Genital torsion comparison in males and females

	Ovarian torsion	Testicular torsion
Definition	Twisting of the ovary around adnexal ligaments	Twisting of the spermatic cord structures, with loss of blood supply to the testicle affected
Onset of Pain	Sudden onset in the right lower quadrant	Sudden onset of severe unilateral scrotal pain followed by inguinal/scrotal swelling, may radiate to lower abdomen
Symptoms	Nausea and vomiting	Nausea and vomiting
Physical examination	On palpation a mass may be present	Abnormal positioning of the testes, presence of a negative Prehn sign where the elevation of the scrotal does not relieve pain
Laboratory tests	Urinalysis and inflammatory markers	Urinalysis, inflammatory markers
Diagnostic tools	Pelvic Ultrasound with Doppler	Ultrasound with Doppler
Complications	Surgical emergency as it may lead to necrosis and infertility	Emergency must be corrected as soon as possible, as saving the testicle is key to preserving fertility function

- Urinary tract infection UTI) is when one of the most common bacteria E. coli migrates and colonizes the bladder, urethra, ureters or kidneys. The infection may manifest as flank pain or abdominal pain. The patient will present with fever, chills and pyuria. Regarding laboratory test, urine culture is sufficient with the clinical findings for the diagnosis. Women tend to be prone to UTI due to the length of their urethra which is shorter than the urethra in men. Many risk factors such as sexual intercourse, urinary catheter, pregnancy contribute to the infection (Cope Zachary, Abdominal pain.
- Nephrolithiasis encompasses the passage of kidney stones that can lodge itself anywhere in the urinary tract. The condition presents itself with flank pain and the pain may radiate in the groin. The patient may present with nausea, vomiting and hematuria. On physical examination, the Murphy's kidney's punch is performed, striking the costovertebral angle which manifest as pain when it is punched. A positive sign may indicate a disease involving the kidney. In the laboratory results, one should pay attention to the parameters indicating the status of the kidney such as BUN and creatinine. Diagnostic tools include ultrasound or CT without contrast to detect the stones.
- Acute pyelonephritis, is the inflammation of the renal pelvis and parenchyma caused by an ascending bacterial infection from the bladder. The patient may present with fever, nausea, vomiting flank pain and dysuria. Clinical diagnosis is optimal for determining the condition. Laboratory results, with a focus on urinalysis, and urine culture to determine the bacteria which causes the inflammation. Inflammatory markers are increased. A diagnostic tool of choice is the CT of the abdomen and pelvis with and without contrast: infected parenchyma may be visible as striated nephogram.
- **Intra-thoracic Cause of Pain**: Inferior Infarction "Upper epigastric pain and may be associated with Nausea and Vomiting" an ECG and troponin test helps in DD. Pleurisy may cause pain in the ipsilateral side of the upper abdomen. "Chest symptoms like cough, expectation, Hemoptysis and a pleural rub may help in DD in addition to Chest x-ray".
- **Arterial Cause of Pain**: Dissecting or Leaking abdominal aneurysm or Intestinal ischemia in cases of Mesenteric vascular occlusion "arterial or venous'.
- **Nerve cause of pain** due to e.g. Herpes Zosters "pain the distribution of a dermatome and vesicles may appear later on in the same dermatome. Tabes Dorsalis due to Syphilis was common cause in the past.
- **Abdominal wall cause of pain** due to Rectus sheath hematoma: after an acute attack of spasmodic irritative cough like whooping cough will lead to injury of the inferior mesenteric vessels at its entrances to the rectus sheath at the arcuate line. The condition is suspected clinically and with later overlying bluish discoloration from the escape of the hematoma to the subcutaneous tissue of the abdominal wall after few days. Ultrasonography will help to avoid unnecessary exploration.
- **Medical cause of acute abdomen**: especially Diabetic Ketoacidosis "Smell of acetone" with DD. Of starvation ketosis, Familial Mediterranean fever FMV, Cytomegalovirus CMV and Porphyria.

Acute Abdomen in Pediatrics

- Pyloric stenosis is the hypertrophy and hyperplasia of the pyloric sphincter (part of the stomach) present in new born. The new born may appear more cranky and not seem to be able to keep food down in the stomach, after each feeding the new born projectile vomits. On physical examination, a firm, mobile nontender 'olive' mass is detected in the right upper quadrant. Due to the constant vomiting the child is dehydrated, his laboratory tests display unbalanced electrolyte and acid base dysfunctions. The gold standard diagnostic tool is the ultrasound, which shows an elongated and thickened pylorus (Cope, Zachary. 'Abdominal Pain').
- Intussusception is one of the most common causes of bowel obstruction in new born. Described as when the proximal part of the bowel invaginates in the distal part of the bowel. The new born may present with abdominal pain, expressed with sudden crying and screaming; vomiting and bloody stool. On abdominal examination tenderness is present. Routine laboratory blood tests, can be made an increase of white blood cells may be present. The most appropriate diagnostic tool is the ultrasound, due to the reduction of radiation exposure, it displays a 'pseudo kidney' or 'doughnut' sign which is indicative of intussusception. If the diagnosis is delayed this could lead to bowel ischemia, perforation and necrosis of tissues [4].
- Meckel's diverticulum one of the most common congenital abnormalities of the digestive tract, an outpouching due to the incomplete eradication of the vitelline duct in between the 7th and 8th week of gestation. The new born present with Hematochezia, passage of fresh blood through the anus. On physical examination abdominal tenderness. The most significant and non-invasive diagnostic tool is the Meckel's scan, using a radiolabeled tracer technetium pertechnetate Tc99m, which will bind to the gastric mucosa and confirm the diagnosis (Cope Zachary, 'Abdominal pain'). The condition is often characterized by a rule of 2: prevalence rate of 2% in the population, a male to ratio 2:1, incidence rate of 2% for symptomatic new born, presence of symptoms before the age of 2, a location at a distance of 2 feet to the Ileo-caecal valve, diverticular length of 2 inches and two type of ectopic tissues.
- Hirschprung disease is an inherited condition when a new born presents with an aganglionic colon segment. Characterized when the new born fails to pass meconium in its first 48 h of life, has abdominal distention and is vomiting. A rectal biopsy is key to determine the diagnosis, if not treated promptly the child could develop chronic constipation.

References

1. Strasberg SM. Clinical practice. Acute calculous cholecystitis. N Engl J Med. 2008;358(26):2804–11. https://doi.org/10.1056/NEJMcp0800929.
2. Schaefer, Timothy J., and Savio John. Acute hepatitis. (2019).

3. Wilkins T, Embry K, George R. Diagnosis and management of acute diverticulitis. Am Fam Physician. 2013;87(9):612–20.
4. Applegate KE. Intussusception in children: evidence-based diagnosis and treatment. Pediatr Radiol. 2009;39(Suppl 2):140–3.

Further Reading

Abdullah M, Adi Firmansyah M. Diagnostic approach and management of acute abdominal pain. Acta Med Indones. 2012;44(4):344–50.

Alkatout I, Honemeyer U, Strauss A, Tinelli A, Malvasi A, Jonat W, Mettler L, Schollmeyer T. Clinical diagnosis and treatment of ectopic pregnancy. Obstet Gynecol Surv. 2013;68(8):571–81.

Camilleri M, Kuo B, Nguyen L, Vaughn VM, Petrey J, Greer K, Yadlapati R, Abell TL. ACG clinical guideline: gastroparesis. Am J Gastroenterol. 2022;117(8):1197–220.

Chang HC, Bhatt S, Dogra VS. Pearls and pitfalls in diagnosis of ovarian torsion. Radiographics. 2008;28(5):1355–68.

Cope Z. Early diagnosis of acute abdominal disease. GP. 1953;7(6):35–9. PMID: 13060509.

Copelan A, Kapoor BS. Choledocholithiasis: diagnosis and management. Tech Vasc Interv Radiol. 2015;18(4):244–55.

Diamond M, Lee J, LeBedis CA. Small bowel obstruction and ischemia. Radiol Clin. 2019;57(4):689–703.

Dover AR, Alastair Innes J, Fairhurst K, editors. Macleod's clinical examination-E-Book. Amsterdam: Elsevier Health Sciences; 2023.

Epelman M, Daneman A, Navarro OM, Morag I, Moore AM, Kim JH, Faingold R, Taylor G, Ted Gerstle J. Necrotizing enterocolitis: review of state-of-the-art imaging findings with pathologic correlation. Radiographics. 2007;27(2):285–305.

Huang C-C, Lai M-W, Hwang F-M, Yeh Y-C, Chen S-Y, Kong M-S, Lai J-Y, Chen J-C, Ming Y-C. Diverse presentations in pediatric Meckel's diverticulum: a review of 100 cases. Pediatr Neonatol. 2014;55(5):369–75.

Martin RF, Rossi RL. The acute abdomen: an overview and algorithms. Surg Clin N Am. 1997;77(6):1227–43.

Singer AJ, McCracken G, Henry MC, Thode HC Jr, Cabahug CJ. Correlation among clinical, laboratory, and hepatobiliary scanning findings in patients with suspected acute cholecystitis. Ann Emerg Med. 1996;28(3):267–72.

Somwaru AS, Philips S. Imaging of uncommon causes of large-bowel obstruction. AJR Am J Roentgenol. 2017;209(5):W277–w86. https://doi.org/10.2214/ajr.16.17621.

Ta A, D'Arcy FT, Hoag N, D'Arcy JP, Lawrentschuk N. Testicular torsion and the acute scrotum: current emergency management. Eur J Emerg Med. 2016;23(3):160–5.

Toouli J, Brooke-Smith M, Bassi C, Carr-Locke D, Telford J, Freeny P, Imrie C, Tandon R. Guidelines for the management of acute pancreatitis. J Gastroenterol Hepatol. 2002;17:S15–39.

Veauthier B, Hornecker JR. Crohn's disease: diagnosis and management. Am Fam Physician. 2018;98(11):661–9.

Yeo HL, Lee SW. Colorectal emergencies: review and controversies in the management of large bowel obstruction. J Gastrointest Surg. 2013;17:2007–12.

Chapter 17
Urology Sheet

Steven Anderson, Elsayed M. Salih, and Mohammed Aboelmaged

Abstract Patients with urological complaints can be of any age, physical and mental disposition, either (or both) sex, and hail from every social background imaginable. The complaint may be of an emergency nature, in which case analgesia or other pain-relieving treatment should be available as soon as the cause of the problem is established. If the patient wishes, any interested accompanying relative or supporter should be encouraged to be present during the history-taking and final discussion.

Keywords Urologic · Examination · Sheet · History · Sexual · Pain · Colics · Urine · Micturition

Taking a Urological History

Patients with urological complaints can be of any age, physical and mental disposition, either (or both) sex, and hail from every social background imaginable. The complaint may be of an emergency nature, in which case analgesia or other pain-relieving treatment should be available as soon as the cause of the problem is established. If the patient wishes, any interested accompanying relative or supporter should be encouraged to be present during the history-taking and final discussion.

Patient data:

Name:

Age is a guide to the nature of urologic diseases. Some conditions are specific to men at certain ages e.g. BPH and prostate cancer.

Gender:

S. Anderson · M. Aboelmaged
Beaumont H, Dublin, Ireland
e-mail: stevenmarkanderson@rcsi.ie

E. M. Salih (✉)
Al-Azhar University, Cairo, Egypt
e-mail: elsayedsalih@azhar.edu.eg

A. Farag et al. (eds.), *Clinical Surgical Skills Made Easy*,
https://doi.org/10.1007/978-3-031-69158-4_17

Residence (past & present): Some diseases are common in certain ethnic groups.

Occupation (past & present): Dye and textile workers are at risk for bladder cancer.

Education

Marital status

Symptomatology

The **presenting complaint** is noted, its duration, associated symptoms and the impact it is having on the patient's life. The commonest complaints in urology are pain, lower urinary tract symptoms and hematuria.

Complaints are reported in the patient own words e.g. I have difficulty during urination. Urologic symptoms may be classified into urological, genital or systematic symptoms (Fig. 17.1).

Classification of Urological Symptoms

Pain

- Analysis of pain includes:

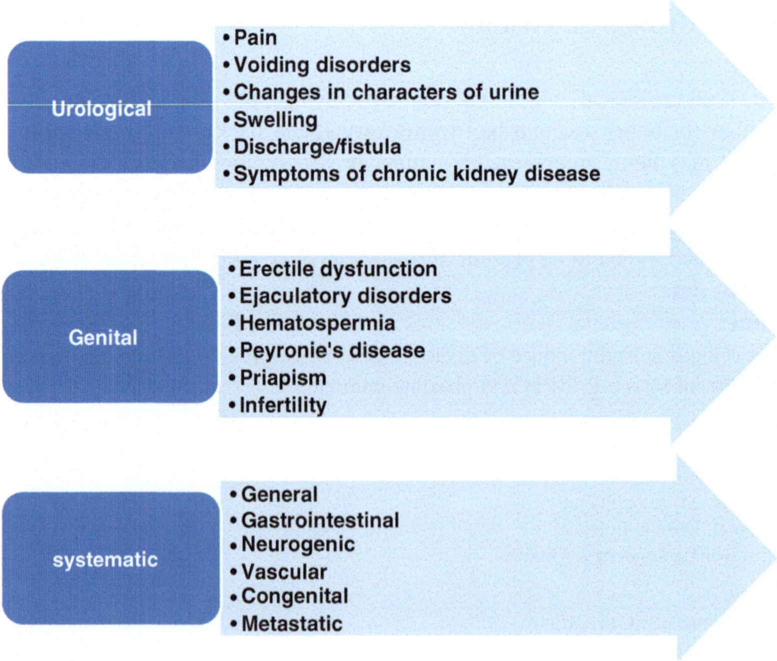

Fig. 17.1 Symptoms in urologic sheet

1. Site.
2. Severity.
3. Character.
4. Reference (Radiation).
5. What increase.
6. What decrease.
7. Associated symptoms.

Renal Pain

All types of pain can occur in kidney but the commonest are:

- Colicky pain (most common) or Dull aching pain.

  1. Dull aching pain: due to distension of renal capsule. as in:

     - Acute inflammation of the kidney.
     - Bleeding in a cyst.
     - Peripheral renal tumor.
     - Renal abscess.
     - Acute hydronephrosis.

  2. Renal colic:

     - Most common cause is stone.
     - Definition of colic: spasmodic pain which occur in hollow viscous or tubular structure lined by smooth muscle due to contraction of these muscles in an attempt to get rid of an obstructing agent.
     - Character:

     1. Colicky pain in renal angle.
     2. May radiate to epigastrium.
     3. Not related to posture.
     4. May be relieved by NSAIDs.
     5. May be associated with nausea, vomiting and diaphoresis.

Ureteric Pain

1. Upper third: (T11 – L1 sympathetic.) colicky pain similar to that of renal colic.
2. Middle third: should be differentiated from appendicitis on right side and diverticulitis on left side.
3. Lower third: (T12 - L2 symp.) (S2, 3, 4 parasympathetic.) Most common causes are stones and stricture.

Criteria: As renal colic +

- Referred to scrotal skin in male and labia major in female.
- may be referred to tip of penis.
- pain usually associated with irritative voiding symptoms (frequency, urgency).

Urinary Bladder Pain

Common causes

Full bladder (most important).
Cystitis.
Stones.

Malignancy

Criteria:

- Character: dull aching or discomfort.
- Site: supra-pubic region.
- Referred to: tip of penis.
- Relieved by: evacuation of bladder in full bladder.

Prostatic Pain

May be acute or chronic.

(a) Acute pain:

- Severe pain in the perineum.
- Associated with: dyschasia (rectal dysentery), high grade fever and urine retention.
- E.g. acute prostatitis and prostatic abscess.

(b) Chronic pain:

- Pain in perineum, lower abdomen, around anus and tip of penis.
- Due to chronic prostatitis.

Urethral Pain: Causes: stone or inflammation. Character: burning pain in urethra.
Testicular Pain.
Epididymal Pain.

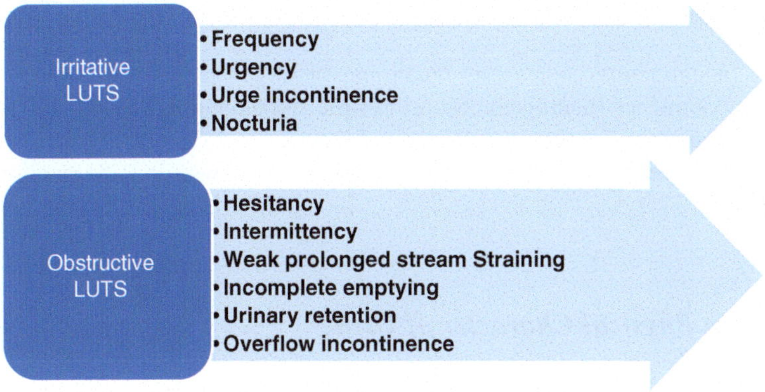

Fig. 17.2 Symptoms of lower urinary tract

Symptoms Related to act of Micturition (Voiding Disorders)

Obstructive Lower Urinary Tract (LUTs) Symptoms (Fig. 17.2)

- Causes:—infra-vesical obstruction.—The commonest cause in elderly male is BPH.
- Criteria:

  1. Weak urinary stream.
  2. Difficulty
     - To initiate (Hesitancy)
     - To maintain (Intermittency)
     - To terminate (Post-micturition dribbling)
  3. Sense of incomplete voiding.
  4. Retention of urine (acute or chronic)

Irritative Lower Urinary Tract (LUTs) Symptoms (Fig. 17.2)

- Due to bladder and urethral irritation (Malignancy, cystitis and stone)
- Criteria:

  1. Frequency: by day (Diurnal) and by night (Nocturia).
  2. Burning micturition.
  3. Urgency: strong desire to micturate which can't be postponed and can't hold urine whenever desire develops.
  4. Urge incontinence: strong desire to micturate which can't be postponed and if postponed, involuntary escape of urine drops will occur.

Day and Night Incontinence

- Stress incontinence.
- Urge incontinence (neurogenic, stone, cystitis and malignancy).
- Total incontinence as in → vesico-vaginal fistula.
- Paradoxical incontinence (false): retention with overflow as in BPH and urethral stricture.

Change in Physical Character of Urine

Volume

1. Normally—0.5–1 ml/kg/h (800–1600 ml/day).
2. Decrease in volume.
   - <400 cm^3/24 h → oliguria (least volume to excrete toxic metabolite from the body).
   - No urine/12 h (with empty bladder) → anuria.
3. **Polyuria:** Definition: urine output > 3 L/day.
   Causes:
   (a) *Renal causes: as* Nephrogenic diabetes insipidus and Diuretics.
   (b) *Endocrinal causes:* DM. and Cranial diabetes insipidus.
   (c) *Psychogenic* (compulsive water intake).

Color

- Normally → golden or amber yellow.
- Red urine → hematuria**Hematuria is the most important symptom in urology (see later).**

Aspect

- Normally → clear.
- Turbid urine → pyuria, Crystaluria, proteinuria and Chyluria.
- Chyluria: The urine looks milky due to presence of lymph. The color clears on addition of ether.
- Pneumaturia (air in urine) → UTI by gas forming organism or vesico-colonic fistula.
- Fecaluria (passage of fecal debris).
- Necroturia: The passage of pieces of tumor tissue in cases of carcinoma of the Bilaharzial bladder is described by the patient as "pieces of fat".

Urethral Discharge

Urethral purulent discharge in men due to Neisseria gonorrhea or Chlamydia trachomatis.

1. Amount
2. Color
3. Presence of blood
4. Relation of discharge to urination and ejaculation
5. Pain
6. Associated symptoms: Conjunctivitis and arthralgia
7. Relation to sexual contacts
8. Exposure to STDs

Swellings

Abdominal Swellings

Generalized (5Fs)

1. Fetus
2. Flatus
3. Feces
4. Fat
5. Fluid

Large masses

1. Renal tumor
2. Hydronephrosis
3. Pyonephrosis
4. Polycystic kidneys
5. Adrenal tumors
6. Full bladder
7. Hepatomegaly
8. Splenomegaly
9. Fibroids

Groin Swellings

1. Hernia (inguinal, femoral)
2. Enlarged inguinal lymph nodes

3. Saphena Varix
4. Hydrocele of the cord
5. Undescended testis
6. Lipoma of the cord
7. Femoral aneurysm
8. Psoas abscess

Scrotal Swelling

- Orchitis, TB epididymo-orchitis
- Testicular tumor
- Gumma of the testis
- Hydrocele: Fluid-filled cyst around the testis, which is difficult to feel.
- Epididymal cysts: A fluid-filled cyst lies behind the body of the testis.
- Varicocele
- Sebaceous cyst
- Carcinoma of scrotal skin

Cervical Lymph Node

Mass in the left supraclavicular nodes can be due to metastatic spread of testis and abdominal cancers.

The Symptoms of Chronic Renal Failure

- Lack of concentration is the earliest symptom.
- Headache
- Blurring of vision
- Epistaxis
- Dry mouth
- Tachypnea
- Palpitations
- GIT manifestations (anorexia, dyspepsia, bitter taste, constipation and bleeding)
- Genital problems (loss of libido, erectile dysfunction and infertility)
- Itching and hiccup are late.

Male Genital Symptoms

Sexual activity: Libido (interest in sex), function (ability to achieve and maintain an erection), satisfaction with sexual life and performance, condom use, problems. Testicular pain or masses, and testicular self-examination practices. History of sexually transmitted diseases (STDS), and treatments; and concerns about HIV infection.

A. **Impotence:** The consistent inability to achieve and maintain a penile erection sufficient to permit satisfactory sexual intercourse.
   1. **Organic impotence** develops gradually and is related to physical risk factors. Etiology is usually multifactorial.
   2. **Psychological impotence** has an abrupt onset secondary to marital **stress**, anxiety, insomnia, depression, and relationship difficulties. Patients will note early morning erections, and respond to different forms of sexual stimuli.

B. **Loss of libido** may indicate endocrine dysfunction e.g. Androgen deficiency.

C. **Disorders of ejaculation and orgasm:**
   1. **Premature ejaculation** is persistent occurrence of ejaculation with minimal sexual stimulation before or shortly after penetration.
   2. **Retrograde ejaculation** is backflow of semen into the bladder.
   3. **Anejaculation:** Failure to ejaculate.
   4. **Anorgasmia** is the inability to achieve the pleasurable sensation of orgasm during intercourse.

D. **Hematospermia:** The presence of blood in seminal fluid

E. **Peyronie's disease:** Curvature of the penis secondary to formation of fibrous plaques within the tunica albuginea.

F. **Priapism** is persistent or prolonged (>4 h), painful, purposeless (in the absence of sexual stimulation) penile erection.

G. **Infertility** is the inability to conceive after one year of unprotected sexual intercourse.

History of Present Illness

The chief complaint is the reason presenting the patient to the urologist.

Put the pertinent positives first, and include all the relevant negatives e.g. **no hematuria**, that help to clarify the differential diagnosis.

Symptoms are arranged in a chronological sequence. Renal colic followed by hematuria is suggestive of stones, while hematuria followed by colic may result from a tumor.

Details of the Current Symptoms (OLD CARTS)

- **O**nset: date it began, sudden or gradual, over how long?
- **L**ocation and radiation: ask the patient to point to the site with one finger and whether the pain moves anywhere else?.
- **D**uration.
- **C**haracters: nature of the symptom.
- **A**ggravating factors: What makes the symptom worse?
- **R**elieving factors: What makes the symptom better?
- **T**iming and frequency: improving or deteriorating with time

Severity

- Setting in which the symptom occurs.
- Details of previous similar episodes.
- Associated manifestations.
- Details of investigations and treatment for the current problem.
- Extent of functional disability.
- Menstrual and reproductive history for women.

Past History

The therapeutic history, whether medical or surgical.

Medical History

- Diseases as diabetes, hypertension, hepatitis, bronchial asthma, and cardiac conditions.
- **Allergies and Reactions.**
- Drugs: as hematuria with anticoagulants. Ant allergic, antihistaminic drugs precipitate LUTS, a fact that should be taken in consideration in elderly men.
- **Bilharziasis:** Bilaharzial cystitis and carcinoma.
- **Calculi:** Renal colic, passage of stones and treatment.

History of Trauma

Family History

- Polycystic kidney disease.
- Von Hippel-Lindau disease.

- Renal tubular acidosis.
- Urolithiasis.
- Prostate cancer.

Social History

Special habits to identify risk factors for particular diseases.
Smoking and alcohol.

Systematic Symptoms

1. **Gastrointestinal symptoms of urologic diseases:**
   - Acute pyelonephritis is associated with abdominal pain and distension.
   - Ureteric colic is associated with nausea, vomiting and distension.
   - Silent urologic diseases (e.g. hydronephrosis, staghorn stone, chronic pyelonephritis and cancer) may present with gastrointestinal symptoms that mislead the clinician.
2. **Neurologic disorders: may** cause urinary and sexual dysfunction:
   - **Disease:** Diabetes mellitus, Multiple sclerosis, Cerebro-vascular disease, Spinal cord injury and Parkinsonism.
   - Pelvic surgery (hysterectomy, abdomino-perineal resection).
3. **Vascular disorders: Hypertension** may be a manifestation of renal vascular disorders or adrenal masses.
4. **Congenital disorders:**
   - Adult polycystic kidney, von Hippel-Lindau and tuberous sclerosis complex are autosomal dominant diseases.
   - Undescended testis and hypospadias have hereditary tendency.
5. **Symptoms of metastases:**
   - Bones: Pain, swelling, nerve compression, spontaneous fracture.
   - Lungs: Persistent cough, hemoptysis, blood-staining, pleural effusion.
   - Liver metastases develop late symptoms.
   - Brain: Headache, vomiting, visual disturbances, convulsions.
   - Adrenal metastases are usually bilateral and primary tumors of the breast and lungs should be taken in consideration.
6. **General symptoms:**

Fever, Weight loss and cachexia in cases of malignant tumors and manifestations of uremia.

The Physical Examination

General

- The patient should be courteously invited to lie comfortably on their back with arms by their sides, on a couch in a warm private room.
- In so doing, their mobility in transferring from their chair (or wheel-chair) to the couch is assessed and any help they require is noted.
- If the patient cannot lie comfortably because of a skeletal deformity or injury, examination must be carried out in an alternative position.
- If the patient cannot straighten one of his legs, or if it causes pain to do so, he may have psoas irritation due to a retroperitoneal abscess, mass or retrocaecal appendicitis.
- If the patient is female, a male doctor may wish to request the presence of a chaperone, or vice versa.
- The patient should be asked to expose his or her abdomen, groins and genitalia.
- Inspection of the hands, face and neck and palpation of the radial pulse, cervical and supraclavicular areas are routine.
- Signs of any gross cardiovascular, respiratory, obesity or wasting disease are usually evident.

The Abdominal Examination

Inspection

- The abdomen is inspected and any asymmetry, distension or surface lesions (scars, skin lesions, sinuses) noted on a diagram together with other findings.
- The patient should be asked to point to the area of pain.

Palpation

- The abdomen is palpated in the nine anterior areas and in the two renal angles. During this, keep a close watch on the patient's face and eyes to detect tenderness, while causing the minimum of pain.
- Note any mass: assess its site, size, surface, consistency, mobility and tenderness.
- If it is in the loin, can it be palpated bimanually? Can you get above or below the lump? A renal mass is detected in the right or left upper quadrants; it may or may not be tender; only its lower margin is palpable and it may not be possible to get above it; the mass should be palpable bimanually unless it is too small; it should be slightly mobile downwards on inspiration.

- A distended bladder is palpable suprapubically as a dome-like mass this can be difficult in obese patients. The palpable.
- Bladder may or may not be tender; it is not possible to get below it.

Percussion

- A **renal mass** should be resonant to percussion (in theory) because, unlike the spleen or liver, it is a retroperitoneal structure, overlying which is gas-filled bowel.
- **A distended bladder** is dull to percussion, because it lifts the peritoneal contents away from the abdominal wall.

Auscultation

Not particularly helpful in the diagnosis of urological disease, but nevertheless. An important part of the abdominal examination.

Local Examination

The Groins and Genitalia

(a) Examination of the male groins and genitalia:

- General inspection for signs of chronic disease, abnormal body hair or Gynaecomastia.
- Examination of the external genitalia is made to assess the presence, size and
- Consistency of the testes in the scrotum. Absent testes indicate cryptorchidism and small soft testes suggest testicular failure. Bulky epididymis may indicate vasal obstruction. The presence of both vasa is confirmed by palpation of structures in each spermatic cord that feel like string.
- A careful inspection is made for the presence of a Varicocele by standing the patient up. A large Varicocele is obvious with the patient lying, while a moderate one may only be detectable with the patient standing, classically described to feel like a bag of worms.
- Examining the penis, a Phimosis or hypospadias
- The foreskin, if present, should be retracted to ensure it is not tight and to reveal the glans penis. The urethral meatus is inspected to ensure it is in the normal position and is not scarred.
- The penile urethra and the corpora cavernosa are examined if the history suggests a relevance.

(b) Examination of the female genitalia:

- it is done at the same time as a vaginal examination. This is not always necessary, but is indicated if the complaint relates to incontinence or other perineal symptoms.
- The ideal situation is with adequate light and the patient as relaxed as possible, lying in the left lateral position. A lubricated Simms speculum is inserted and the vaginal introitus is inspected for surface lesions or masses.
- The patient is asked to cough; any descent of the anterior or posterior vaginal walls or the cervix are noted; any urinary leakage is noted.
- If indicated, a bimanual vaginal examination is performed to palpate the cervix and adnexae (with the patient supine).

The Digital Rectal Examination (DRE)

- For diagnosis of prostatic lesion as BPH and cancer, bladder lesion and other pelvic lesions.
- the patient is examined in supine position, the left lateral position, or in the knee-elbow position
- Examination will be uncomfortable but quick. Patients with rectal stenosis, anal fissure, acute prostatitis, prostatic abscess or an inflammatory pelvic condition (diverticulitis, appendicitis, abscess, Salpingitis) do find the DRE painful and this finding should be noted.
- The perianal skin and the anal sphincter are innervated by S2, 3 and 4. If neurological disease affecting the urinary sphincter is suspected, an assessment is made of perianal sensation and anal tone while performing a DRE. If either or both are reduced, then a lesion affecting these sacral nerves and indeed urinary sphincter function is highly likely.

Investigations

Laboratory Investigations

1. **Biochemical blood tests for renal function**
    - Serum urea
    - Serum creatinine.
    - Serum electrolytes.
    - Arterial blood gas
2. **Urinalysis**
    - For abnormal substances such as blood, protein or signs of infection.

- Dipstick urinalysis, by dipping of a test strip into the urine to detect levels of tell-tale chemicals in the urine.
- Urinalysis can also microscopy, culture and sensitivity

3. **tumor markers: as PSA and acid phosphatase**

Imaging

1. **Ultrasound:**
   Can detect:

   (a) Solid from cystic mass.
   (b) Post voided residual in the bladder
   (c) All types of stones, Radiolucent or Radio-opaque.
   (d) *Trans rectal U/S (TRUS):* For prostatic lesions, especially if PSA is high or abnormal prostatic outline on DRE. can provide access for biopsies.

2. **Radiology**

   (a) KUB

   - It is a plain radiography of the urinary system to detect the stones.
   - Check the presence and position of catheters and stents, and obtain a preliminary view before performing other examinations.
   - Bony abnormalities as spina bifida and sacral agenesis, fractures of the spine or pelvis, osteoplastic metastases (typical of prostate carcinoma), osteolytic metastases (the majority of solid tumors), or manifestations of hematologic disorders (sickle cell anemia, myeloma) or Paget's disease.
   - Abnormal gas collections as gas in the renal parenchyma or collecting system as a result of recent instrumentation or emphysematous pyelonephritis.

   (b) Intravenous pyelogram:

   - Procedure: contrast (Urografin) is given IV.
   - Value: diagnosis of:

   1. Anatomical description of the urinary system.
   2. Stones, tumors (filling defect), diagnose renal artery stenosis.
   3. Differential kidney function.

   - Side effects

   1. Anaphylactic shock.
   2. Acute renal failure (contrast nephropathy).

3. **CT scans and MRI** can also be useful in localizing urinary tract pathology.
4. **Voiding cystourethrogram** is a functional study where contrast "dye" is injected through a catheter into the bladder and urethra. Diagnosis of Vesico-Ureteric Reflux, urethral stricture, posterior urethral valve and Urethral injuries.
5. **Renal arteriography.**
6. **Radionuclide Imaging.**
7. **Surgical procedures**
   - Cystoscopy and biopsy.
8. **Urodynamic tests.**

   Evaluate the storage of urine in the bladder and the flow of urine from the bladder through the urethra. It may be performed in cases of urinary incontinence or neurological problems affecting the urinary system.

Hematuria

Definition: Blood in urine.

Hematuria can be classified in different ways:

Intensity

1. Gross or macroscopic hematuria: Urine is red and hematuria is visible to the naked eye. This is a "**red sign**" for the patient to ask for medical advice.
2. Microscopic hematuria is detected by microscopic urine analysis (the presence of >5 RBCs/hpf).

Origin

1. Systemic disease
2. Urinary tract pathology

Relation to Micturition

1. Total hematuria is present all over the voided urine.
2. Terminal drop hematuria, at the end of micturition
3. Initial hematuria at the beginning of micturition

Associated Symptoms

- Painless hematuria (no other urinary symptoms): Bladder cancer
- Hematuria associated with other symptoms: as in BPH and prostate cancer are associated LUTS (Prostatism).

Etiologic

General or Systemic Causes

- Bleeding disorder: Thrombocytopenia, leukemia, hemophilia
- Liver cirrhosis
- Anticoagulants
- Hypertension

Renal Causes

(a) Nephrologic: Acute glomerulonephritis is the most common cause in children and young adults. It is associated with proteinuria.
(b) Urologic:

  - Congenital: Polycystic kidney
  - Inflammation: Pyelonephritis, TB.
  - Trauma: Accidents, iatrogenic
  - Stones
  - Kidney cancer
  - Vascular: Haemangioma, AV fistulae

Ureteral

- Stones
- Iatrogenic trauma e.g. Uretrescopy.
- Tumors: Urothelial tumors of renal pelvis and ureter

Bladder

- Bladder cancer is the most common cause of gross hematuria in a patient above the age of 50 years.
- Cystitis: Bacterial, Bilaharzial, TB.
- Stones
- Traumas e.g. post tumor resection (TURBT).

Prostate

- BPH
- Prostate cancer
- Prostatitis
- Surgical: After prostatectomy

Posterior Urethra

- Inflammation
- Trauma
- Tumor

Diagnosis

History

- Age: < 40 years: inflammation, stones >40 years: tumors
- Sex: BPH, prostate cancer in elderly men
- Trauma: Violence, accidents → blunt, penetrating
- Bilharziasis and stone disease
- Systemic disease: liver cirrhosis
- Obstructive symptoms: BPH, prostate cancer

Physical Examination

- General: Hypertension, petechial hemorrhages
- Abdominal: Renal mass
- Genital: T.B. thickening and beading of vas
- DRE: Bladder mass, BPH, prostate cancer

Investigations

Laboratory

- Blood: CBC, liver function tests, creatinine, blood glucose
- Attention to platelets, prothrombin, clotting and coagulation times
- Urine analysis and culture

Radiologic

- Ultrasound: Renal masses, stones, polycystic kidneys, bladder mass
- KUB: Radio-opaque stones
- Non-contrast CT: Stone disease
- CT with contrast: kidney, ureteric, bladder and prostate cancer evaluation.

Endoscopic

- Uretrescopy: Stones and tumors of ureter
- Cystoscopy: Diagnostic and therapeutic in bladder cancer

Acute Urinary Retention

- Acute urinary retention (AUR) is a sudden painful inability to urinate inspite of a full bladder due to complete obstruction of lower urinary tract.
- Relief of pain follows drainage by catheterization.

Causes

Mechanical or Obstructive

1. Bladder: - Stone, bladder neck obstruction, cancer
2. Prostate:
   - BPH is the most common cause in men over 50 years.
   - Acute prostatitis and abscess
   - Prostate cancer
3. Urethra: - Stone, stricture, urethritis, injury, Phimosis, posterior urethral valves.
4. Clot retention in severe hematuria e.g. cancer, trauma.
5. Women: pelvic masses, urethral stenosis and diverticulum, pelvic prolapse, hysterical.

Functional and Neurogenic

1. Postoperative AUR is common:
   - Pain, limited mobility, drugs, bladder nerve injury e.g. hysterectomy and abdomin operineal resection.

2. Drugs: Anesthetics, anticholinergic, sympathomimetic
3. Neurogenic: as
   - Spinal cord injury.
   - Intervertebral disc prolapse.
   - Multiple sclerosis.
   - Transverse myelitis.

History

- Cause- related:
  - A complication of BPH
  - Drugs
  - Urethral trauma
  - Stone disease
- Suprapubic bursting pain, no urine, strong desire to urinate.
- Acute urine retention should be differentiated from obstructive anuria.

Abdominal examination: The full bladder is felt as a midline globular tender mass in the Suprapubic region.

Genital examination: Phimosis, severe urethral meatal stenosis.

DRE: BPH, prostate cancer.

Chapter 18
Hernia Sheet

Ahmed Farag, Asif Mehraj, and Patrick Jordan

Abstract This important sheet which is included in the Abdominal Sheet in order to remind the Students and practicing doctors with the abdominal examination as an integral part of the hernia sheet. We proceed to this special form of sheet If the patient has a Swelling at the site of a hernia orifice which gives an Expansile Impulse during cough.

Keywords Hernia · Examination · Sheet · Abdomen · General · Inguinal · Femoral · Umbilical · Obturator · lumbar

General Plan for the Hernia Sheet

This important sheet which is included in the Abdominal Sheet in order to remind the Students and practicing doctors with the abdominal examination as an integral part of the hernia sheet.

We proceed to this special form of sheet If the patient has a **Swelling at the site of a hernia orifice which gives an Expansile Impulse during cough**.

Actually according to the general "Structured" plan of examination mentioned in the General examination sheet in this book all the areas below the diaphragm should be examined namely the Abdomen "Front, Perineum and back" and both LLs are part of the Local examination in addition to the Virchow and Left supraclavicular LNs which may carry metastases from an intra-abdominal malignancy. General

A. Farag (✉)
Kasr Alainy Hospital, Cairo University, Cairo, Egypt

A. Mehraj
Apollo Health City, Hyderabad, India
e-mail: Asifdr80@yahoo.com.in

P. Jordan
SPr SVUH, Dublin, Ireland
e-mail: jordanpr@tcd.ie

A. Farag et al. (eds.), *Clinical Surgical Skills Made Easy*,
https://doi.org/10.1007/978-3-031-69158-4_18

examination of the patient for associated General disease which may affect the result to operate or not to operate on such patient or may affect the healing process and/or infection rate such as Collagen disease hidden thyrotoxicosis "a real life scenario which may cause a thyrotoxic crisis during anesthesia if not detected pre-operatively", Anemia, Hypo-proteinaemia or organ Dysfunction or failure such as Liver Failure or heart failure.

Seven Questions should be answered after examination of a surgical patient:

1. Is it a Hernia or not?
2. Which type of the Hernia? (Inguinal "Direct or indirect" or Femoral? Umbilical or Para-Umbilical? Complete Reaching the bottom of the scrotum or incomplete still in the inguinal Canal?
3. What are the contents of the hernia? "Bowel, Omentum, Tubes and or ovaries, Sliding Bladder "As part of the wall not as content" …etc."
4. Is it Complicated or not? If it is fully reducible it is Uncomplicated. Or not fully reducible "i.e. complicated" and which type of complication? I.e. irreducible, obstructed, incarcerated, Strangulated, inflamed or Hydrocele of hernia Sac. N.B. Ruptured hernia is a special complication after local trauma followed by sudden reduction of the hernia due to rupture of its content from the intestine which retracts into the abdominal cavity and leads to Peritonitis if undiagnosed or suspected.
5. Is there a cause of increased intra-abdominal pressure? Including extra-abdominal causes like chronic cough or an associated intra-abdominal pathology.
6. If the patient fit for surgery or not.
7. Other Hernias "other hernia orifices".

During the Clinical examination in such sheet we leave the General examination to the end.

Present History

- **Age**: Certain Hernias are common at a certain age group e.g. Umbilical hernia in the newborn babies or infants as compared to para-Umbilical hernias and direct Hernia at an older age groups.
- **Sex**: Femoral hernias are more common in females than males.
- **Occupation**: Hard labor is associated with more hernias due to repeated indirect trauma by lifting heavy weights.
- **Special Habits of medical Importance**: Such as chronic smoking associated with chronic cough which repeatedly increase Intra-abdominal pressure.

Complaint: A swelling at the site of a hernia orifice which increase on standing and decreases or disappears on Lying down is a hernia till prove otherwise.

Usually painless if uncomplicated however it may be painful at the start or later on when becomes markedly enlarged "dragging pain", or later on when complicated "Obstruction, inflammation or strangulation.

Present History

- **Onset** "Mode of onset and was it associated with trauma or inflammation":
- Sudden and was associated with indirect trauma such as lifting a heavy weight or during an attack of cough and at this point it may cause sharp pain which draws the patient's attention to the swelling.
- Signs of Inflammation "Local or Systemic" may be due to inflammation of the coverings such as wearing an ill fitted truss "Hernia Belt" or due to inflammation of the contents such as Salpingitis, Diverticulitis, Appendicitis Known as Amyand's Hernia or Meckel's diverticulitis called Littre hernia.
- **Course**: May be stationary but usually progressive "Slow or fast".
- **Duration**: Variable.

Screening for the Symptoms of other Systems such as Cardinal Manifestations of Intestinal obstruction namely Colics, Distension, Vomiting "Projectile due to Mechanical obstruction" and absolute constipation which is manifested as "failure to pass Gases or stools despite the desire to do so" In upper small bowel obstruction the Vomiting is more Pronounced with less distension "upper abdominal" and less obvious and late absolute constipation specially early while vomiting is late in distal small bowel obstruction or in Colonic obstruction in a hernia "Rare" which distension and absolute constipation is more apparent. I.e. In proximal small bowel obstruction vomiting is more pronounced and precedes other obstructive symptoms. In distal bowel obstruction, abdominal distension is more prominent and precedes other obstructive symptoms.

Clinical manifestations of strangulation "Tense and Tender Hernia". Strangulation is usually associated with Intestinal obstruction except when the contents are Omentum, Ovary and/or Fallopian tube, Appendix, Meckel's diverticulum or only part of the bowel wall sparing the bowel Lumen for passage of the intestinal contents called Richter Hernia.

Urinary Symptoms suggestive of a sliding urinary bladder in the hernia namely increase in the size of the hernia before micturition and decrease in its size after micturition and sense of the need for micturition during Local examination of the hernia.

Manifestations of Liver, Kidney, Cardiac, respiratory Problems, Dysfunction or failure and manifestations suggestive of Collagen disease.

Past History

- Medical history:
- Of Systemic diseases such as DM "Type and doses Of insulin and other oral hypoglycemic drugs, which indicates severity of DM", Collagen disease, cigarette smoking "Number of Packets, which indicates the type of habituation e.g. heavy smoking with more than a packet per day. Those affects wound healing especially when skin flaps are needed to raise during surgery as during dermolipectomy, during incisional hernia repair. Anticoagulation treatment past or present for a history suggestive of DVT or recent Angina or cerbro-vascular disease or after recent Coronary stents. History suggestive of advanced vital organ dysfunction or organ failure.
- Surgical History:
- Previous abdominal operation which may lead to incisional hernia even at the port site of laparoscopic or Robotic surgery, though more common after Open surgery or Phantom hernias after extended subcostal, bilateral subcostal incisions or Mercedes Benz upper abdominal incision. They are not true hernias "i.e. no sac or defect" but they result from cutting of the intercostal nerves and subcostal nerve supplying the upper abdominal muscle "Paralytic hernia.
- History of allergies to foods and/or Medications.

Family History

Hernias are more common in some families due to congenitally weal Mesenchyme.

General Examination

Is very important to answer the question number 6 is the patient fit or not?

For Symptoms of anemias, Hypoproteinaemias and collagen disease which may affect infection rate and wound healing. And for the signs of a hidden more dangerous disease like thyrotoxicosis or arrhythmias not reported by the patients during history taking.

And for symptoms suggestive of vital organ dysfunctions, which may affect the decision for surgery or the need to take special precautions before, during or after surgery.

Examination of Inguinal and Femoral Hernia (DD)

N.B. Examination of a hernia is different from examination of any other swelling mentioned in the Chapter of examination of a swelling.

A Swelling at the site of a Known hernia orifice "Or a scar over a cavity" which gives an impulse on cough is a hernia till Prove otherwise.

As mentioned earlier in this chapters the examination sheet has to answer 7 questions:

1. Is it a Hernia or not?
2. Which type of the Hernia?
3. What are the contents of the hernia?
4. Is it Complicated or not?
5. Is there a cause of increased intra-abdominal pressure?
6. Is the patient fit for surgery or not?
7. Is there another Hernias? And marking the side of hernia for medicolegal purpose.
8. DD of this hernia especially in inguinal or femoral hernia?

Inspection

Examine the patient standing and ask him to take-off his clothes from the Lower Chest to the midthigh.

- Site and impulse on cough: This will answer the First question and may answer the fourth question putting in mind that strangulated Hernia may not show an impulse on Cough.
- Size: In Cms or Inches.
- Shape: Direct hernia is rounded in shape and Oblique hernia is oval in shape if purely inguinal but becomes oblong as it descends to the scrotum.
- Surface: Usually.
- Surrounding Structures "including Skin:
  - Skin: Scar of previous operation, inflammation "in Inflamed or strangulated hernia".
  - Pubic Tubercle: Neck of the inguinal hernia is above and medial to the pubic tubercle "PT", while in the Femoral Hernia it is below and lateral the PT.
  - N.B. Alternatively run your index finger over the inguinal Ligament from the ASIS to the pubic tubercle: Hernias above the Line are inguinal hernias while femoral hernias are below this Line "Author's Sign".
  - N.B. There is no need to do the above test If the hernia reaches the Neck of the Scrotum "Funicular hernia", Becomes Inguinoscrotal "Complete acquired hernia" or Complete from the start "Congenital preformed sac".
- Other swellings: Other Hernias

Palpation

In Hernia Sheet we start by putting our hand at the neck of the scrotum "Four fingers behind and the Thumb in Front and ask the patient to Cough. This will determine from the very beginning of palpation if it is a hernia or not and will Classify the swelling into three Categories which are very important in DD:

1. Inguinal "Pubonocele": The swelling is fully above the neck of the scrotum "The Examiner's Hand".
2. Pure Scrotal: The Swelling is fully below the Neck of the scrotum.
3. Inguino-Scrotal: where the Swelling Crosses between the examiners fingers at the neck of the scrotum.

N.B. DD will be discussed for each category.

Palpation proceeds as follows:

- Temperature: Warm in Inflammations which may be due to:
- Inflamed Coverings "due to the wear of an ill-fitting truss.
- An Inflamed Content such as inflamed appendix "Amyand's hernia", inflamed Fallopian tube, an inflamed Meckel's diverticulum "Littre's Hernia" or an inflamed colonic diverticulitis in a hernia.
- Tenderness: in inflamed hernia or strangulation "Tense, Tender and No Impulse on cough"
- Site and Expansile Impulse on cough: Femoral, Inguinal "Pubonocele, Funicular or Complete" according to its position in relation to the pubic tubercle "and the Inguinal Ligament as described above". It gives an expansile impulse on cough "Increase in size in all directions as examined by the two index fingers of the examiner where the distance between the tip of both fingers increases on coughing. "The only exception is strangulated hernia which may lead to confusion in the diagnosis in cases of Femoral hernia DD inflamed L.N.
- Size: in Cms or Inches.
- Shape: As by inspection.
- Surface: Smooth.
- Consistency: Doughy Sensation if it contains Omentum (Table 18.1).
- Special tests:

Table 18.1 DD between omentum and bowel as a content of a hernia

	Omentum	Intestine
Consistency	Doughy 'Like paste" and no gurgle	Soft with a gurgle especially during reduction
Reduction	Easy at the start and difficult at the end	Difficult at start and easy at the end
Percussion	Dull	Resonant
Auscultation	No sounds	Gurgle

Table 18.2 DD. between direct and indirect inguinal hernia

	Direct hernia	Indirect hernia
Site	Inguinal	Inguinal, Funicular or Inguinoscrotal
Shape	Oval	Oblong
Internal ring test	Negative	Positive
Direction of reduction	Direct posterior	Upwards, backwards and laterally
Direction of descend	Direct anterior	Downwards, forwards and medially

N.B. It is important to differentiate Direct and indirect hernia because indirect hernia is Liable to complications mainly "Obstruction and strangulation" and surgery is highly recommended, while Direct hernia is not liable to such serious complications

N.B. The Complete "Inguinoscrotal hernia" may be Congenital into a congenital unobliterated Processus Vaginalis where the Hernia is complete from the start and the testis is felt as a content of the Sac. DD. Acquired Complete hernia which starts as Pubonocele, then Funicular, then Complete with the testis felt separate from the hernia sac and a groove is felt between them

Internal "Deep ring test: if hernia is reducible (Table 18.2):

1. In the Supine position, reduce hernia and notice the direction of reduction, Locate deep ring at midpoint of inguinal ligament "Halfway between ASIS and PT" Occlude deep ring with the Index finger while hernia reduced.
2. Ask the patient to stand while the examiner firmly applying pressure with the thumb to maintain occlusion of the internal ring.
3. Ask patient to cough, if the hernia appears with the thumb closing the internal ring it is a direct hernia "negative internal ring test". "Notice the direction of descent which is directly anterior".
4. Remove your thumb and ask the patient to cough, if the hernia appears it is an indirect hernia "Notice the direction of descend "Downwards, forwards and medially in the direction of the inguinal canal".

- Surrounding structures: Skin, PT and inguinal ligament as mentioned above.
- Other swellings: Other hernia orifices.

Percussion: Resonant if large and containing Bowel.

Auscultation: Gurgle if large and contains bowel.

Complications of a Hernia

Common

1. Irreducibility: The first complication and makes the hernia more Liable to the other more serious complications.
2. Obstruction: when the content of the hernia is whole Circumference of the bowel and presents with acute pain and irreducibility together with cardinal manifestations of Intestinal obstruction namely "Colicky pain, Vomiting which is noisy and explosive "Not silent and regurgitant like that of ileus", Distension and abso-

lute Constipation" in different combinations and sequence according to the level of bowel obstruction.

- In Upper GI obstruction, Pain and Vomiting start early with minimal distension and late absolute constipation where the patient can pass one or two motions before it becomes an absolute constipation "evacuating the stools which passed distal to the obstruction before it happens".
- In Lower GI obstruction Pain and absolute constipation appear early, Distension is marked and Vomiting is late.

3. Obturation: reserved to intestinal obstruction from within. In the case of a hernia it may be with stools or foreign material Such as bezoars, gallstone, worms, or foreign body.
4. Strangulation: It is interference with the blood supply of the hernia which threatens with gangrene of its content:

The Hernia is severely painful and is tense and Tender "In Inflammation it is tender but not tense".

It is accompanied by cardinal manifestations of Intestinal obstruction if it contains the whole Circumference of a bowel loop.

Strangulation without cardinal manifestations of bowel obstruction can happen if the strangulated content is Omentum, appendix, Meckel's diverticulum, Ovary and/or tube or if the hernia contains only a part of the circumference of the bowel "Richter hernia". Most commonly, it is the anti-mesenteric portion of the bowel. These hernias often develop in small Fascial defects.

Less Common

1. Inflammation: Tender, red, hot with or without signs of inflammation which may be due to inflamed coverings or an inflamed content as mentioned above. With or without signs of systemic inflammation "Fever, rigors and tachycardia".
2. Rupture: Which is a rupture of the intestine inside the hernia with its immediate retraction into the general peritoneal cavity due to direct trauma to the hernia especially when irreducible "rare and seen once by the author". It should be suspected by History of direct trauma on irreducible hernia and sudden disappearance "reduction of the hernia. It is an emergency situation because. Emergency abdominal exploration to see, repair the perforated part of the bowel after debridement with or without simultaneous repair of the hernia according to the degree of contamination of the peritoneal cavity especially when a mesh is needed for Hernioplasty.
3. Hydrocele of a hernia Sac: Rare but seen more frequently in patients with massive ascites and narrow neck of the hernia sac which allows only the ascetic flood to go in the hernia sac "No actual content".

Examination of the Scrotum

- Cord "Vas and Vessels "For associated Varicocele due to congenitally weak mesenchyme or Infantile Hydrocele "4 Layered sac hernia which may be confusing for a surgeon in his early training".
- Epidydmis, tunica Vaginalis, Testis and Skin of the Scrotum "Front and back" on both sides.

Examination of the Abdomen

- To Exclude an Intra-abdominal pathology which can cause an increased intra-abdominal pressure.
- Open appendectomy scar which may be the cause of a right direct hernia due to accidental damage of the Ilio-inguinal nerve.

Examination of Umbilical and Para-Umbilical Hernia

Swelling at the Umbilicus which gives an Impulse on cough. It may be True Umbilical which may be Congenital dating since birth or acquired which develop later in Life with marked increase in intra-abdominal pressure e.g. massive ascites "Where the Umbilical scar is seen on the summit of the Hernia sac" or Para-Umbilical "The scar is on one side of the sac and is acquired.

N.B. Congenital true Umbilical hernia usually heals by the age of 2 years using compression band and button.

Inspection of a scar tissue may indicate a recurrence or a scar or previous Laparoscopic surgery "An Incisional Hernia".

Examination of Incisional Hernia

Special points to be addressed during such examination besides answering the above mentioned questions in the Hernia sheet are:

- Is it Complicated or not? If it is reducible it is not complicated.
- The size of the defect as compared to the size of the sac: The larger the defect the less liable are the complications "surgery is done for Cosmetic reasons and on the patient's request"
- If bone forms part of the edge? If bone forms part of the edge this hernia will need a hernioplasty with a mesh "the edges cannot be approximated to each other i.e. not amenable to Herniorrhaphy". The Clearest examples are hernias after Kidney incision, Open Cholecystectomy and after Pfannenstiel Incision.

Rare Types of Hernia

- Abdominal wall Hernias:
  - Spigelian Hernia: It is a type of hernia that occurs along the Spigelian fascia, which is a layer of tissue located along the side of the abdominal wall. This type of hernia typically occurs in the lower abdomen, near the waistline, and can cause pain and discomfort. Spigelian hernias are relatively rare and may require surgical repair to prevent complications.
  - Lumbar hernia: It is a type of hernia that occurs in the lumbar region of the back, which is the area of the lower back on either side of the spine. Lumbar hernias are rare and can be either congenital (present at birth) or acquired (developed later in life). They occur when abdominal contents, such as fat or intestines, protrude through a weakness or defect in the muscles of the lower back.
  - Symptoms of a lumbar hernia may include a visible bulge or lump in the lower back, pain or discomfort in the area, and sometimes difficulty with bowel movements.
- Pelvic Hernias:
  - An obturator hernia is a rare type of hernia that occurs when abdominal contents, such as the small intestine, protrude through the obturator foramen, which is a small opening in the pelvic bone. Obturator hernias are more common in elderly, thin women and are often associated with conditions that cause thinning of the abdominal wall, such as weight loss or chronic illness. Symptoms of an obturator hernia can be nonspecific and may include pain in the inner thigh or groin that worsens with movement, nausea, vomiting, and bowel obstruction. Obturator hernias can be challenging to diagnose because they do not typically cause a visible bulge or lump.
  - Perineal hernia is a type of hernia that occurs in the perineal region, which is the area between the anus and the external genitalia. Perineal hernias involve the protrusion of abdominal contents through a defect in the pelvic floor muscles and connective tissue in the perineal region. These hernias are more common in dogs than in humans, but they can occur in both.
  - Symptoms of a perineal hernia may include a visible or palpable bulge near the anus, difficulty defecating, constipation, straining during bowel movements, pain or discomfort in the perineal area, and in severe cases, urinary or fecal incontinence.
  - Sciatic hernia is a rare type of hernia that occurs through the sciatic foramen, which is a small opening in the pelvis through which the sciatic nerve passes. The sciatic foramen is located in the lower part of the pelvis, near the hip joint. A sciatic hernia involves the protrusion of abdominal contents, such as fat or intestines, through this opening, causing a bulge in the buttock or thigh area. Symptoms of a sciatic hernia may include a visible or palpable mass in the buttock or thigh, pain or discomfort in the affected area, and in some cases, symptoms of bowel obstruction if the hernia compresses the intestines.

Chapter 19
D.D. of Inguinoscrotal Swelling

Ahmed Farag, Asif Mehraj, and Patrick Jordan

Abstract Oblique inguinal Hernia: Commonest, Varicocele: It is a condition characterized by the enlargement of the veins within the scrotum, which is the pouch of skin that holds the testicles. Varicocele are similar to varicose veins that occur in the legs, and they are most commonly found on the left side of the scrotum. Varicocele can cause pain, discomfort, and swelling in the scrotum, and they may also affect fertility in some cases.

Keywords Inguinal · Scrotal · Inguinoscrotal · Swelling · Examination · Sheet · Hernia · Varicocele · Hydrocele

1. Oblique inguinal Hernia "Commonest": AS above.
2. Varicocele:

   It is a condition characterized by the enlargement of the veins within the scrotum, which is the pouch of skin that holds the testicles. Varicocele are similar to varicose veins that occur in the legs, and they are most commonly found on the left side of the scrotum. Varicocele can cause pain, discomfort, and swelling in the scrotum, and they may also affect fertility in some cases.

   Symptoms of Varicocele may include a dull ache or pain in the scrotum, swelling or enlargement of the scrotum, and a feeling of heaviness or dragging sensation in the scrotum. Some men with Varicocele may also experience fertility issues, as the increased blood flow and higher temperature in the scrotum can affect sperm production and quality.

A. Farag (✉)
Kasr Alainy Hospital, Cairo University, Cairo, Egypt

A. Mehraj
Apollo Health City, Hyderabad, India
e-mail: Asifdr80@yahoo.com.in

P. Jordan
SPr SVUH, Dublin, Ireland
e-mail: jordanpr@tcd.ie

A. Farag et al. (eds.), *Clinical Surgical Skills Made Easy*,
https://doi.org/10.1007/978-3-031-69158-4_19

On Examination as in case of a Hernia where the hand of the examiner examines the Neck of the Scrotum with the thumb anterior to the neck of the scrotum and the rest 4 Fingers behind it. Try to roll the Cord between your fingers and the thumb gently without hurting the patient. Normally you can feel the Vas difference as a tough robe and the veins few and soft vertical structures. In Varicocele they are many tortuous and engorged which give the classic sensation of a "bag of Worms" used for fishing. They are normally compressible, gives a thrill on cough and decrease in size or disappear on Lying down "Primary varicose veins".

DD. is Secondary Varicocele which is due to obstruction of those veins at the Level of their drainage into the left renal vein or into the IVC on the right side due to Tumor thrombus from a Hypernephroma. Characteristically they are always engorged and does not disappear or decrease on Lying down and no thrill on Cough.

3. Funiculitis: It is a medical term that refers to inflammation of the spermatic cord, which is the cord-like structure that contains blood vessels, nerves, and the vas deferens that connects the testicles to the rest of the reproductive system. Funiculitis can be caused by various factors, including infections and trauma.

   Symptoms of funiculitis may include pain or discomfort in the scrotum or groin area, swelling or redness in the scrotum, and sometimes fever or other signs of infection. In some cases, funiculitis may be associated with conditions such as epididymitis. Infection may be non-specific with reflux of the infected Urine into the Vas Deference or specific "Now rare" Characterized by matting of the Cord in Filariasis or Beaded Cord in T.B.
4. Encysted hydrocele: It is a specific type of hydrocele that involves the presence of a cyst or sac-like structure within the spermatic cord. This condition is characterized by the accumulation of fluid within a localized area of the spermatic cord, leading to a cystic swelling.

   Encysted hydrocele of the cord typically presents as a painless, firm, and sometimes palpable mass along the spermatic cord. The cystic structure may contain clear fluid and can vary in size. It is important to differentiate encysted hydrocele of the cord from other scrotal masses, such as hernias or tumors, through physical examination. A Characteristic sign is that the Cyst moves up and down freely except with pulling down of the testis "Which makes the Cord tense "the cyst can be moved side—side with the cord but not vertically across the cord".
5. Diffuse Hydrocele of the Cord: It is like the encysted hydrocele of the Cord but longer and oblong in shape.
6. Congenital Hydrocele: It is a common condition in newborns and infants characterized by the accumulation of fluid around the testicle within the scrotum. It is often referred to as a "communicating hydrocele" because it is typically associated with a persistent connection between the abdominal cavity and the scrotum, known as the Processus Vaginalis.

   In infants, the processus vaginalis is a normal structure that allows the testicles to descend into the scrotum during fetal development. In some cases, this connection remains open after birth, leading to the accumulation of fluid and the formation of a hydrocele.

Infantile hydroceles are usually painless and may present as a soft, fluid-filled swelling in the scrotum. They are typically non-tender and may change in size throughout the day. In most cases, infantile hydroceles are harmless and tend to resolve on their own within the first year of life as the processus vaginalis closes off.

7. Infantile Hydrocele: is like congenital hydrocele but its connection to the abdominal cavity is closed "DD. It does not change in size over the day. When encountered during hernia repair it is called 4 layered sac hernia "The 2 walls of the Hydrocele overlapping the 2 walls of the hernia sac. And hernia is called infantile hernia "see above'.
8. Tumors of the Cord are usually benign "Lipoma or diffuse lipomatosis of the Cord but rarely malignant.

D.D. of Pure Inguinal Swelling

1. Swellings n the femoral triangle. See in the relevant Chapter.
2. Swellings in the right Iliac fossa. "See in the Abdominal Sheet"

D.D. of Scrotal Swelling

1. Vaginal hydrocele "Commonest": including the variants e.g. Haematocele, Pyocele or Chylocele. Vaginal hydrocele can be primary or secondary. Primary Vaginal hydrocele usually presents with heaviness, and enlargement in size. On inspection and palpation it is a purely scrotal swelling "Below the examining hand at the neck of the scrotum. It shows a bipolar fluctuation test positive. Alternating squeeze of the hydrocele between the examiner's hands on at the neck of the scrotum and the other at the lower pole of the testis the other hands and fingers will receive and expansile pulsation on the negative "Receiving hand". Characteristically we cannot feel the other contents of the scrotum "Testis and epidydmis" due to tense fluid inside the Tunica. It shows a positive trans-illumination test.

   On the other hand the Secondary hydrocele can develop after trauma including hernia surgery, inflammation or tumors. Secondary hydrocele is usually Lax, we can palpate the Testis and Epidydmis well and the tunica vaginalis can be felt by gentle rolling of the skin of the scrotum below the lower pole of the testis where it is felt like a shirt under the jacket 'i.e. 2 layers under the skin of the scrotum.

Pyocele and Haematocele may be felt as severe pain, tense tunica V. which is tender with or without Systemic manifestations of inflammation. Negative trans-illumination test.

N.B. Trans-Illumination test: By holding an electric Torch light externally to the scrotum "e.g. from behind, one can easily determine whether the mass is cystic (light shines through and can locate the position of the testis and epidydmis in order to avoid injuries to the testis if anteriorly located during an operation for primary hydrocele) or solid (light blocked by the mass, Pyocele or Haematocele).

Chylocele is another variant which can only be diagnosed with aspiration. The Milky fluid drained has a very low Specific gravity and becomes clear by adding ether "As a fat solvent".

2. Epidydmo-orchitis "Second most common": DD. Torsion testis". It presents as in Funiculitis above but infection extends into the epidydmis and testis. Torsion testis is an emergency operation which should be done before gangrene of the testis by fixation of the testis to the bottom of the scrotum and exploration of the other side is important to avoid torsion of the other side"

   In Torsion testis the testis Lie high at the neck of the scrotum "due to shortening of the cord by torsion" and pain increases with elevation. In Epidydmo-orchitis, the testis Lie down and hanging lower than the normal side and elevation relives pain. If in doubt US and duplex are very helpful, if not available explore as torsion testis.
3. Spermatocele: typically arise from the head of the epididymis, which is located on the superior aspect of the testicle. During trans-illumination it is Cystic with septae inside "Chinese Lantern appearance".
4. Tumors of the Testis: of different types and stages usually the testis is heavier than the normal side and characteristically there is loss of testicular sensation when touched by the Examiners hand "This should be done very carefully because when done with reluctance or frequently, it can lead to spread of the tumor.
5. Chronic Epidydmo-orchitis: Nonspecific, Syphilis, TB or Bilaharzial: As mentioned in Funiculitis but the Symptoms of inflammation are milder than acute inflammation in Non-specific infections. In T.B. the cord and head are beaded and the epidydmis "Which is normally behind the scrotum can invade the skin of the scrotum and cause a T.B. sinus at the back of the Scrotum In Syphilis a Gumma of the testes may be mistaken for malignancy but it can cause interstitial orchitis without Gumma. Bilaharzial infection being a venous disease it may affect the head of the epidydmis causing a Mass "Bilaharzial granuloma"
6. Tumors of the epidydmis and Cord specially Lipomas and Fibromas.

D.D. of Swelling in the Skin of the Scrotum

- **Localized swelling**:

1. Sebaceous cyst. "Cystic, Rounded with a punctum over it.
2. Lipoma.
3. Wart.
4. Carcinoma. In the Squamous Cell carcinoma SCC was common as occupational disease in Chimney Sweepers and in Mule spinners due to repeated and prolonged exposure of the skin of their scrotum to the carcinogenic material in Soot and in the mineral oils used by those workers and heavily soak their undergarments.

- **Diffuse swelling:**

1. Erysipelas: pain, Redness, hotness, swelling, tenderness and marked systemic toxic manifestations "DD. Fournier gangrene".
2. Hematoma and/or Urinary extravasation after trauma:
3. Filarial Elephantiasis.
4. Bilaharzial Pseudo-elephantiasis.

Chapter 20
Vascular Examination Sheet

Mohammed Elkassaby

Abstract The clinical examination of the vascular system is a crucial aspect of assessing and managing a wide range of medical conditions. From identifying arterial and venous disorders to evaluating perfusion and circulation, a thorough vascular clinical examination provides valuable insights into a patient's cardiovascular health. This chapter will guide healthcare professionals through the essential components of a vascular clinical examination, emphasizing the importance of a systematic approach to ensure accurate diagnosis and appropriate treatment.

Keywords Vascular · System · Examination · Sheet · Arterial · Venous · Lymphatic · Clinical

Introduction

The clinical examination of the vascular system is a crucial aspect of assessing and managing a wide range of medical conditions. From identifying arterial and venous disorders to evaluating perfusion and circulation, a thorough vascular clinical examination provides valuable insights into a patient's cardiovascular health. This chapter will guide healthcare professionals through the essential components of a vascular clinical examination, emphasizing the importance of a systematic approach to ensure accurate diagnosis and appropriate treatment.

The arterial System: Deciphering the pulses.

M. Elkassaby (✉)
Vascular Surgery Department, University Hospital Waterford, Waterford, Ireland

Vascular Surgery Department, Mansoura Faculty of Medicine, Mansoura, Egypt

A. Farag et al. (eds.), *Clinical Surgical Skills Made Easy*,
https://doi.org/10.1007/978-3-031-69158-4_20

Patient History

- Age and Gender:
- Atherosclerosis is a disease primarily associated with advanced age, affecting individuals in their later years. It is more prevalent in men than in women. Buerger's disease, also known as Thromboangiitis obliterans, is commonly observed in heavy smokers between the ages of 20 and 40. On the other hand, Raynaud's disease predominantly affects young women. Diabetic arteriopathy is more frequently seen in middle-aged individuals.
- Affected Limbs:
- Buerger's disease and atherosclerotic gangrene typically impact the lower limbs, while Raynaud's disease primarily affects the upper limbs. When a patient presents with superficial gangrene in the finger, several potential causes should be considered, including Raynaud's disease, the presence of a cervical rib, Thoracic outlet syndrome, and auto-immune vasculitis.
- Laterality of the affected limbs:
- Atherosclerotic gangrene may initially manifest as unilateral, but it often progresses to become a bilateral condition. Gangrene caused by embolism, however, is predominantly unilateral. In Buerger's disease and Raynaud's disease, the involvement of limbs is usually bilateral. Diabetic gangrene can occur either unilaterally or bilaterally.
- Onset Pattern
- Gangrene secondary to atherosclerosis, Buerger's disease, and Raynaud's disease typically develop gradually and spontaneously, usually preceded by rest pain or claudications. In contrast, embolic gangrene has a sudden onse. Diabetic gangrene may initiate from minor trauma, such as careless trimming of the toenail or a mild infection.
- Pain
- It is important to note the location, nature, radiation, response to walking or exercise, cessation upon discontinuation of exercise, and exacerbation upon application of heat. When there is impaired circulation in the limb, two types of pain are commonly observed: intermittent claudication, which is characterized by pain during physical activity or exercise, and rest pain, which occurs even in the absence of any significant physical activity.

Intermittent Claudication

Although the term 'Claudio' in literature signifies 'I limp', in this context, claudication refers to the muscle pain caused by the accumulation of excessive metabolic waste products due to insufficient blood flow. Typically, this pain manifests in the bulky muscles, particularly in the calf, and is described by patients as a cramp. The specific location of the pain varies depending on the level of arterial occlusion. For instance, in Buerger's disease, where arterial occlusion primarily affects the lower tibial or plantar arteries, the pain is felt in the feet. In cases of arterial occlusion at the femoro-popliteal junction, which is quite common, the pain is experienced in the calf. Similarly, occlusion at the ilio-femoral level leads to pain in the thigh, while occlusion at the aorto-iliac segment results in buttock claudications. Characteristically, the pain develops and intensifies with muscle activity and subsides gradually upon resting, even in standing position.

Patients often report that the pain begins after walking a certain distance, referred to as the 'claudication distance'. In some instances, if the patient continues walking, the metabolites increase blood flow to the muscles, effectively eliminating the metabolic waste products produced during exercise and causing the pain to dissipate (Grade I). Grade II pain often persists and the patient may still be able to walk with effort. However, Grade III pain, according to Boyd's classification, typically forces the patient to rest. Rest pain is characterized by continuous and aching sensations. It is believed to be caused by ischemic changes in the somatic nerves, representing the distress of dying nerves. It is usually more severe at night and is exacerbated when the leg is elevated above the level of the heart. Conversely, hanging the leg below the level of the heart can provide relief. Initially, the pain primarily affects the most distal part of the body, such as the tip of the toes. The affected area becomes highly sensitive, and any movement or pressure can trigger an acute worsening of the pain.

- Associated symptoms:

- Diabetic patients with chronic ischemia frequently experience sensations of numbness, pins and needles, and other forms of paraesthesia in the skin of their foot. This is typically attributed to diabetic peripheral neuropathy, and should be differentiated from paraethesia secondary to severe limb threatening ischaemia.

- Buerger's disease is commonly associated with superficial phlebitis, characterized by swelling, redness, and mild pain in the affected area.
- Systemic affection:
- It is important to inquire about symptoms such as fainting, transient blackouts, chest pain, weakness or paraesthesia in the upper limbs, blurred vision, and abdominal pain. Impotence resulting from the inability to achieve an erection is a common symptom in cases of bilateral internal iliac artery occlusion. Patients with arterial occlusion may have a history of previous cardiac attacks or embolic syndromes.
- Smoking history:

- Excessive smoking has been implicated as a causative factor in thromboangiitis obliterans and the progression of atherosclerotic disease. It is imperative to document patients smoking history and provide support for smoking cessation.

Family History

It is noteworthy that arterial disease, particularly atherosclerosis, often has a familial predisposition. Therefore, it is prudent to inquire about the presence of the same disease in other family members, as some may have been or currently are affected by this condition, as evidenced by the occurrence of gangrene in the great and middle toes of the left leg. Aortic aneurysms also have familial.

Tendency, and screening should be applied at earlier age to those who are first degree relatives of patients with aortic aneurysms.

Local Examination

Inspection

The most noticeable feature of an ischemic limb is a change in color. To detect even minor changes in color, the clinician should compare the affected limb to its unaffected counterpart. A significant pallor is a remarkable feature of sudden arterial obstruction, as seen in cases of embolism or arteriole spasm in Raynaud's disease. Congestion and a cyanosed appearance are characteristic features of severe ischaemia and the pre-gangrenous stage. When the limb is elevated, it quickly becomes pale or purple-blue.

When examining a case of arterial insufficiency, it is important to be aware of the signs of ischaemia. These signs include thinning of the skin, diminished hair growth, trophic changes in the nails and minor ulceration in pressure areas and tips of the toes.

In a healthy individual, the color of the legs remains pink even when raised to a 90° angle. However, in the case of an ischemic limb, raising it to a certain degree will result in significant paleness, with empty and constricted veins. This point at which paleness occurs is referred to as 'Buerger's angle'. An angle measuring less than 30° indicates severe ischemia.

Regarding venous refilling, when a limb is elevated for a period of time and then placed flat on the bed, the veins normally refill within 5 seconds. However, in an ischemic limb, this refilling process is delayed. When a healthy limb is raised to approximately 90°, there is a gradual collapse or guttering of the veins. Conversely, in an ischemic limb, the veins appear collapsed either in the horizontal position or as soon as it is lifted even 10° above the horizontal level.

In cases of established gangrene, several observations are made. Firstly, the extent and color of the gangrenous area are important in determining the level of arterial occlusion. In gas gangrene, in addition to the characteristic odor of sulphurated hydrogen, the muscles also undergo color changes, ranging from brick-red to green or even black, depending on the stage of the disease. Secondly, the type of gangrene should be noted, whether it is dry, resulting in mummification of the affected part, or wet and putrefying, as seen in diabetic gangrene. Lastly, the presence of a line of demarcation is often observed between the dead gangrenous tissue and the normal living limb.

Palpation

When palpating the affected limb, it is important to assess the skin temperature using the back of the fingers. Comparing the temperature of both limbs is crucial.

Capillary refilling can be assessed by applying pressure to the tip of the nail or the pulp of a toe or finger for a few seconds and then releasing the pressure. The time it takes for the blanched area to regain its pink colour after pressure release provides a rough indication of capillary blood flow. In the case of an ischemic limb, this time will be noticeably longer.

Several arteries are commonly examined for evaluation. The Dorsalis Pedis artery can be felt just lateral to the tendon of the extensor halluces Longus. It can be normally absent in 10% of the population. The posterior tibial artery is palpated midway between medial malleolus and the tendo Achilles. The anterior tibial artery is felt anteriorly, midway between the two malleoli, just lateral to the tendon of the extensor hallucis longus. The popliteal artery is challenging to detect due to its deep location behind the knee. To facilitate the examination, the knee is flexed to approximately 40 degrees, and palpating the popliteal artery against the posterior aspect of the tibial condyles. The femoral artery can be palpated below the inguinal ligament, midway between the anterior superior iliac spine and the symphysis pubis. To locate the radial and ulnar arteries, one must feel the wrist. The radial artery is found on the lateral side of the volar aspect of the wrist, while the ulnar artery is located on the medial side. The brachial artery is felt in front of the elbow, just medial to the tendon of the biceps.

During the examination of the artery, several points are noted. These include assessing the pulse's volume and tension, examining the condition of the arterial wall for any signs of athermanous changes, and checking for thrombosis of the vessels.

Elevated arms test is conducted when there is suspicion of thoracic outlet syndrome. The patient is instructed to raise their shoulders to a 90-degree angle while fully externally rotating their upper limbs. Subsequently, the patient is asked to repeatedly open and close their hands for a duration of 5 min. Individuals with thoracic outlet syndrome will experience fatigue and pain in the forearm muscles, as well as paraesthesia and numbness in the fingers.

Adson's test is a diagnostic procedure used to identify the presence of a cervical rib or scalenus anterior syndrome, which can compress the subclavian artery. During the test, the patient sits on a stool and is instructed to take a deep breath and turn their face towards the affected side. The examiner then checks the radial pulse, which is often diminished due to the compression of the subclavian artery.

Allen's test for assessing the patency of the radial and ulnar arteries involves a series of manoeuvres. Initially, the patient is instructed to tightly clench their fist.

The surgeon then applies pressure on both the radial and ulnar arteries at the wrist. After one minute, the patient is asked to open their fist, resulting in a white appearance of the palm. Subsequently, the pressure on one of the radial and ulnar arteries is released to observe hand reperfusion, or Doppler signals are examined on the palmer arch "Modified Allen's test" to establish patency of the released artery.

Palpating the blood vessels is a crucial aspect of examining an ischemic limb. The absence of arterial pulsation below the site of occlusion is typically observed. However, in cases where there is adequate collateral circulation, the pulse may be diminished but not completely absent. In some instances, a seemingly normal peripheral pulse may disappear after the patient exercises to the point of claudication. This phenomenon, known as the "disappearing pulse," signifies the initial stage of arterial occlusion being unmasked. This is typically observed with significant fall in exercise ABI test.

An aneurysm can be identified by the presence of an arterial pulsation that is Expansile. This should be differentiated from transmitted pulsations through a swelling overlying an artery, where the pulsations are not Expansile.

Auscultation

Auscultation, or listening with a stethoscope, is a crucial part of the examination. It is recommended to listen along the course of major arteries. The Presence of a systolic bruit, or turbulent blood flow, beyond a stenosis can be detected through auscultation. A systolic murmur may also be heard over an aneurysm.

General Examination

Atherosclerosis is a systemic condition, and it is crucial to conduct a comprehensive examination of the patient to rule out other associated conditions such as ischemic heart disease, cerebrovascular disease, hypertension, and renal artery stenosis. When assessing for embolic manifestations, it is important to examine the heart for the presence of cardiac murmurs. Diabetes often coexists with atherosclerosis, highlighting the need for thorough evaluation in patients with both conditions.

Measurement

Circumference Measurements:

Limb circumference should be assessed to detect oedema or atrophy.

Ankle-Brachial Index (ABI)

A non-invasive test comparing blood pressure in the arms and ankles to assess peripheral arterial disease. An ABI of 0.9 to 1.2 is normal. Higher values indicate calcified arteries, commonly in diabetic patients with non-reliable results, while lower values indicate arterial insufficiency. Values of 0.3 and lower indicate impending gangrene.

Special Investigations

Blood tests play a crucial role in the diagnostic process. Routine examination of blood, along with sugar levels (for diabetes), urea, and electrolytes, can provide valuable insights into the diagnosis. Additionally, estimation of serum P-lipoprotein, triglyceride, and cholesterol levels should be conducted when atherosclerosis is suspected.

X-ray imaging can be instrumental in diagnosing various conditions. These include arteriosclerosis. X-rays can help identify aneurysms by highlighting flecks of calcium that outline the affected area. Gas gangrene, characterized by the presence of gas as dark spots in soft tissue, can also be identified through this imaging technique. Osteomyelitis associated with ulcers and diabetic foot infections can also be diagnosed with X rays. Lastly, X-rays can aid in the detection of cervical rib.

Arteriography stands as the most reliable method for assessing the condition of the main arterial tree. It is a minimally invasive test involving live imaging of contrast flow when injected into the arterial tree of interest. The common femoral artery is typically used for aortoiliac, renal, mesenteric, and femoropopliteal arteriography, while the brachial artery is utilized for subclavian, vertebral, carotid, and thoracic angiography.

Duplex Ultrasound combines traditional ultrasound with Doppler to visualize blood flow and detect vascular abnormalities. Magnetic Resonance Angiography (MRA) or Computed Tomography Angiography (CTA) imaging techniques provide detailed views of blood vessels. Both are more reliable than duplex scans but carry the side effects of contrast injection which may affect the renal function and in some rare cases with severe renal impairment may induce fatal systemic fibrosis after injection of Gadolinium based contrast for MRA imaging.

The Venous System

Navigating the Tributaries

Chronic Venous Insufficiency (CVI) stands as a multifaceted vascular disorder with a complex interplay of physiological, anatomical, and hemodynamic factors. This condition, characterized by the compromised ability of venous circulation to adequately return blood from the lower extremities to the heart, manifests as a spectrum of clinical presentations that span from subtle discomfort to debilitating complications. As we delve into the intricate landscape of CVI, it becomes evident that a comprehensive understanding of the underlying mechanisms is indispensable for unravelling the complexities associated with this chronic vascular pathology. This chapter will concentrate on the examination of the most common conditions compromising CVI, which are varicose veins and venous thrombosis.

Varicose Veins

Varicose veins are characterized by the dilation and tortuosity of a vein. This condition can occur in various parts of the body, such as the veins of the lower limb, spermatic veins, oesophageal veins, and haemorrhoidal veins. However, this chapter will specifically focus on varicose veins of the lower limbs.

The primary cause of varicose veins is the incompetence of the valves within the veins. Interestingly, this condition is unique to humans and is believed to be a consequence of our upright posture. Individuals who engage in occupations that require prolonged standing are more prone to developing varicose veins. Nevertheless, it is not uncommon for women to also experience this condition, suggesting the involvement of other contributing factors. Varicosity can also be secondary, predisposed by any obstruction that impedes venous return, such as abdominal tumors, fibroids, ovarian cysts, abdominal lymphadenopathy, pregnancy, loaded colon, retroperitoneal fibrosis, and ascites. Furthermore, there is an indication that a hormonal factor, possibly progesterone, plays a role in the occurrence of this disease in females. In some cases, varicose veins in younger individuals may be caused by congenital arteriovenous fistula.

Patient History

- Age and gender
- Although varicose veins can affect individuals of all age groups, it is more commonly observed in middle-aged individuals. Women are significantly more affected by varicose veins compared to men, with a ratio of 10:1.

- Occupation:
- Certain occupations that require prolonged standing, such as tram drivers and policemen, often contribute to the development of varicose veins. However, it remains uncertain whether these occupations directly cause varicose veins or simply worsen pre-existing symptoms.

Presenting Complaints

The most common symptom associated with varicose veins is pain, which manifests as an aching sensation throughout the leg or in the lower part of the leg, depending on the location of the varicose vein. This pain tends to worsen towards the end of the day, particularly when the patient has been standing for an extended period, and is relieved when the patient lies down. Patients may also report a sensation of bursting pain while walking, which could indicate the presence of deep vein thrombosis.

Past History

It is crucial to inquire whether the patient has undergone any injection treatments or operations for varicose veins. Additionally, it is important to ask about any serious illnesses or previous complicated operations, as these factors may contribute to the development of deep vein thrombosis, which is now causing the varicose vein.

Personal History

It is necessary to ask women about their obstetric history, including details of previous pregnancies. Furthermore, if the patient has been taking contraceptive pills for an extended period, it is essential to consider the potential risk of deep vein thrombosis.

Family History

Varicose veins often have a familial tendency. Therefore, it is not uncommon for the patient's mother and sisters to have also experienced this condition.

Local Examination

Inspection

Take note of which vein is affected by varicosity, either the long saphenous vein, the short saphenous vein, or both. In the case of the former, a prominent venous trunk can be observed on the inner side of the leg, extending from the front of the medial malleolus to the inner side of the knee and continuing along the inner side of the thigh up to the saphenous opening. This venous trunk receives tributaries along its course. In the case of short saphenous vein varicosity, the dilated venous trunk is visible on the back of the leg, starting from behind the lateral malleolus and extending upwards in the posterior aspect of the leg, terminating in the popliteal fossa.

Swelling can manifest in two ways: localized swelling, as seen in varicose veins affecting a segment of a superficial vein in cases of superficial thrombophlebitis, or generalized limb swelling, mostly attributed to deep vein thrombosis.

Local redness is typically indicative of superficial thrombophlebitis or venous eczema. Generalized change in color may appear as brown discoloration of the skin resulting from chronic venous insufficiency, a condition named "Lipodermatosclerosis" with characteristic thickened leathery brown skin with muscle atrophy, rendering the leg into the shape of "inverted Champaign bottle" appearance.

The presence of ulceration, commonly observed on the inner side of the lower leg, is referred to as venous ulceration. Ulcers are commonly irregular in shape, superficial, moist with necrotic floor and commonly secondary infected.

Scarring may be visible on the lower leg, which could be a result of a healed venous ulcer or a previous surgical procedure for varicose veins.

Palpation

The examination of varices holds significant importance. The primary objective is to identify the incompetent valves that connect the superficial and deep veins. The Brodie-Trendelenburg test is conducted to assess the incompetence of the sapheno-femoral valve and other communicating systems. There are two methods to perform this test. In both methods, the patient is initially positioned in a lying down position, and their legs are elevated to facilitate the emptying of the veins. This process can be expedited by gently squeezing the veins closer to the body. The clinician then applies pressure on the sapheno-femoral junction using their thumb or by applying a tourniquet just below the junction. Subsequently, the patient is instructed to stand up quickly.

In the first method, the pressure is released. If the varicose veins rapidly fill with blood from above, it indicates the incompetence of the sapheno-femoral valve. This outcome is referred to as a positive Trendelenburg test.

To evaluate the communicating system, the pressure is not released but maintained for approximately one minute. If the veins gradually fill during this period, it suggests the incompetence of the communicating veins, which are typically located on the medial side of the lower half of the leg and are associated with long saphenous varicosity. This outcome is also considered a positive Trendelenburg test. Positive test results serve as indications for surgical intervention.

The Tourniquet test, which can be considered as a variation of the Trendelenburg test, involves the application of a tourniquet around the thigh or leg at various levels. Prior to performing the test, the superficial veins are emptied by elevating the leg while the patient is in a lying position. Subsequently, the patient is instructed to stand up. If the veins located above the tourniquet become filled while those below it remain collapsed, this indicates the presence of an incompetent communicating vein above the tourniquet. Conversely, if the veins below the tourniquet rapidly fill while the veins above it remain empty, the incompetent communicating vein is likely situated below the tourniquet. By adjusting the position of the tourniquet downwards, the healthcare professional can further assess the location of the incompetent communicating vein.

To definitively confirm short saphenous incompetence, a specific examination is conducted. First, the saphenopopliteal junction is marked with a pen while the patient is standing. Then, the short saphenous vein is emptied by elevating the leg, and firm thumb pressure is applied to the ink mark. The patient is then made to stand, and the pressure is released. If the vein immediately fills, it provides final and conclusive proof of short saphenous incompetence.

Modified Perthes' test is primarily used to assess the normalcy of deep veins. To conduct this test, a tourniquet is tightly secured around the upper thigh to prevent any backward flow in the vein. The patient is then instructed to walk briskly while the tourniquet remains in place. If both the communicating and deep veins are functioning properly, the varicose veins will decrease in size. However, if there is a blockage, the varicose veins will become more distended.

The Schwartz test is applicable in cases of long-standing varicose veins. By tapping on the long saphenous varicose vein in the lower leg, an impulse can be felt at the saphenous opening with the other hand.

Pratt's test is performed to determine the locations of leg perforators. Initially, an Esmarch elastic bandage is wrapped from the toes up to the groin. A tourniquet is then applied at the groin, causing the varicose veins to empty. The tourniquet is maintained in position while the elastic bandage is removed. Subsequently, the same elastic bandage is reapplied from the groin downwards. At the sites where the perforators "blow out" or visible varices are present, they can be observed.

The Morrissey's Cough Impulse Test involves raising the limb to drain the varicose veins, followed by placing the limb in a resting position and instructing the patient to cough forcefully. This manoeuvre elicits an expanding impulse in the long saphenous vein, particularly at the saphenous opening, indicating incompetence of the sapheno-femoral valve. Additionally, a bruit may be audible upon auscultation.

Fegan's test is employed to identify the locations of perforators in patients with varicose veins. Initially, the patient stands upright, and areas of excessive bulging within the varicosities are marked. Subsequently, the patient lies down, and the affected limb is elevated to empty the varicosed veins. The examiner then carefully palpates along the line of the marked varicosities, searching for gaps or pits in the deep fascia that transmit the incompetent perforators.

Percussion

Percussion can be utilized to evaluate varicose veins by tapping on the most prominent areas. This technique, known as the Schwartz test, elicits an impulse that can be felt at the saphenous opening. In certain instances, the percussion wave may be transmitted from above downwards, indicating the absence or incompetence of valves between the tapping finger and the palpating finger.

Auscultation

Auscultation is primarily relevant in cases of arteriovenous fistula, where a continuous machinery murmur may be audible.

General Examination

The examination of the other limb is essential to assess for the presence of varicose veins and to perform different tests aimed at excluding deep vein thrombosis, incompetent perforators, and venous ulcers. This comprehensive evaluation aids in planning the appropriate treatment approach.

Examination of the abdominal region is of utmost importance when considering a case of varicose veins. Among the various general examinations, this particular examination holds significant value. It is crucial to assess the abdomen as conditions such as a pregnant uterus, Intrapelvic tumors (such as fibroids, ovarian cysts, or cancer of the cervix or rectum), or abdominal lymphadenopathy can exert pressure on the external iliac vein. This pressure can subsequently lead to the development of secondary varicosity.

Venous Thrombosis

Venous thrombosis can manifest in different forms. One common type is deep vein thrombosis (phlebothrombosis), which often occurs after surgical procedures performed under general anesthesia. In such cases, the calf muscles remain inactive, leading to a disruption in the normal blood flow within the deep veins and resulting in the formation of blood clots. Additionally, deep vein thrombosis can also occur following childbirth, prolonged immobility, or certain debilitating diseases. It is important to note that deep vein thrombosis (DVT) is predominantly an asymptomatic condition. Only a quarter of DVT cases manifest with minor symptoms. To detect asymptomatic DVT, various diagnostic techniques have been introduced due to the potential danger it poses in causing pulmonary embolism.

Superficial vein thrombosis, also known as thrombophlebitis, is an inflammatory condition that typically occurs after intravenous transfusion or in individuals with varicose veins. The main symptom experienced by patients is pain, often accompanied by an increase in body temperature. The affected skin may appear inflamed, and the vein itself feels hard and tender to the touch. Unlike phlebothrombosis, the resulting blood clot is firmly attached to the vein, reducing the likelihood of pulmonary embolism. In some cases, thrombophlebitis may exhibit migratory characteristics, known as thrombophlebitis migrans, which can be associated with conditions such as Buerger's disease, polycythemia, polyarteritis, and certain types of visceral carcinoma (such as bronchus, pancreas, stomach, or lymphoma). Occasionally, thrombophlebitis may have no identifiable cause (idiopathic), or it may be iatrogenic, resulting from intravenous injections or injuries. Even if a patient has varicose veins, a thorough examination should be conducted to rule out any underlying occult cancer.

Patient History

Patients with DVT may experience pain and swelling in the leg. There might also be a slight elevation in body temperature. In cases where the patient has previously suffered from pulmonary embolism, they may complain of chest pain, shortness of breath, and coughing up blood (hemoptysis).

Local Examination

Inspection

The most prominent aspect of the physical examination is the presence of swelling in the leg. This swelling is typically localized around the ankle or slightly higher. In some cases, the swollen leg can be extremely painful, a condition known as "Phlegmasia Alba Dolens". When all the deep veins are obstructed, the skin may appear congested and blue, a condition referred to as "Phlegmasia Cerulea Dolens".

Palpation

Historically, Homan's sign was elicited during palpation to check for DVT by forcefully dorsiflexing the foot while the knee is extended, tenderness can be elicited in the calf. Additionally, applying gentle pressure directly on the calf muscles in a relaxed position can also cause pain. It is currently advised to abstain from performing this test to avoid dislodging a clot, which could potentially lead to pulmonary embolism. Measurements of leg circumference at different levels and comparing to the other limb frequently indicate the presence of swollen calf muscles.

Special Investigations

If one solely relies on clinical findings, there is a 50% chance of failing to diagnose this condition. In some cases, a fatal pulmonary embolus may be the first indication of thrombosis. On the other hand, there may be extensive involvement of veins by the thrombotic process without any clinical signs. In such instances, the destruction of venous valves can lead to the development of varicose veins, varicose eczema, ulceration, and other trophic changes.

Phlebography is a diagnostic procedure that involves injecting a contrast medium into a vein to visualize the deep veins in the leg. During the procedure, the patient lies on a movable table in a horizontal position. The contrast medium, is slowly injected into a vein on the dorsum of the great toe. To direct the contrast medium into the deep veins, a pneumatic cuff is placed just above the ankle. Another cuff at the mid-thigh position initially confines the contrast medium to the lower leg. Once the veins are adequately filled, films are taken of the leg.

Duplex Imaging is a technique that combines B mode ultrasound with a Doppler probe. It allows for direct visualization of the deep veins and provides information about both anatomical and physiological variations. Although it is a more expensive method, it is gradually replacing venography.

Ultrasound and CT scan are recommended when there is suspicion of secondary varicose veins caused by abdominal tumors. These imaging techniques can help identify any underlying pathology that may be contributing to the development of varicose veins.

The Lymphatics: Exploring the Drainage System

The lymphatic system consists of lymph nodes and lymphatics. For the purpose of vascular diseases examination discussed in this chapter we will concentrate on diseases of the lymphatics.

Lymphedema is a condition characterized by the accumulation of lymph within the tissues, primarily affecting the subcutaneous tissues of the limbs. This occurs as a result of lymph stagnation within the lymphatics. The causes of lymphoedema can be classified into two categories: congenital malformation, also known as primary lymphoedema, and acquired obstruction, referred to as secondary lymphoedema.

Patient History

- Age and gender
- In terms of the history of lymphoedema, there are several factors to consider. Firstly, primary lymphoedema may manifest at a young age, while secondary lymphoedema is more commonly observed in middle-aged and older individuals. Secondly, there is a notable gender difference in the prevalence of primary lymphoedema, with females being more affected than males. Additionally, secondary lymphoedema is more frequently seen in women who have undergone radical mastectomy or have been affected by malignant tumours of the uterus or ovary that involve the iliac and inguinal nodes.
- Ethnicity and geographical factors:
- The distribution of lymphoedema can vary depending on the underlying cause. For instance, lymphoedema resulting from filariasis is more prevalent in tropical countries
- Onset and duration:
- The progression of this condition is gradual enlargement of the limb and the reproductive organs, which may take several years to manifest, is characterized by the presence of secondary oedema. This condition is often accompanied by various symptoms, such as those seen in malignant filariasis or following the removal of lymph nodes, such as in radical mastectomy. Additionally, this condition is often associated with the opposite effect of lymphatic growth, resembling lymphatic fluid.

Local Examination

During a local examination, it is important to observe the presence of prominent lymphatic vessels, which can be identified as red streaks progressing towards the regional lymph nodes. Additionally, one may notice the presence of brawny oedema in the surrounding area. This particular manifestation is indicative of acute lymphangitis. Furthermore, subcutaneous nodules may be observed along the lymphatics, resembling those found in cases of malignant melanoma and carcinoma. In instances of malignant melanoma, these nodules often exhibit a deep brown to black coloration.

Initially, the oedema in the affected area may exhibit pitting upon pressure. However, over time, the subcutaneous tissue undergoes fibrosis, resulting in the skin becoming keratotic, a condition known as Elephantiasis. In cases of secondary lymphedema, the examination should encompass an evaluation of the regional lymph nodes, as well as a general examination to aid in the diagnosis.

General Examination

It is imperative to perform a thorough general examination, comparing contra lateral limbs to detect generalised causes of lymphedema versus localized ones. It is also very crucial to examine different lymph node groups, looking for possible signs of malignancy, generalised or local infective causes of lymphedema or signs of iatrogenic obstructions secondary to lymph nodes removal or scarring after irradiation.

Special Investigations

Blood analysis is a crucial component of routine examinations in medical investigations. It serves various purposes, such as identifying leucocytosis, particularly polymorphs, which can indicate acute lymphadenitis. Additionally, lymphocytosis may be observed in cases of tuberculosis, leukaemia, and other related conditions. Eosinophilia, on the other hand, is commonly associated with filariasis. Raised erythrocyte sedimentation rate (E.S.R.) levels may indicate tuberculosis, secondary carcinoma, or primary malignant lymphadenopathy. Furthermore, the W.R. and Kahn test is employed for diagnosing syphilis, while the presence of microfilaria in peripheral blood vessels during sleep suggests filariasis. Complement fixation tests are recommended for detecting lymphogranuloma inguinale and syphilis.

Aspiration of abscesses plays a vital role in diagnosing conditions such as cold abscesses or lymphogranuloma inguinale. In the case of cold abscesses, acid-fast bacilli are sought after. For lymphogranuloma inguinale, pus from an unruptured bubo is diluted with normal saline and sterilized before being injected intradermally.

The Mantoux test and guinea pig inoculation test are both specific to tuberculosis and are employed for diagnostic purposes.

Biopsy is considered one of the most crucial special investigations in this field. In many cases, clinical diagnosis alone may not be sufficient, necessitating the use of additional special investigations. Biopsy is recommended in such cases.

In the case of secondary carcinoma, the tumor cells reach the lymph nodes through the lymphatics using two methods: permeation or embolism. Initially, the carcinomatous cells enter the peripheral lymph sinuses and gradually permeate the sinuses between the follicles and cords, ultimately disrupting the normal architecture of the nodes. Microscopically, the structure of secondary carcinoma closely resembles that of the primary carcinoma, whether it is epidermoid, adenocarcinoma, anaplastic, or other types. In fact, the secondary growth often exhibits a more typical and characteristic appearance than the primary tumour.

Lymphangiography is an invaluable test for determining the causes of lymphedema and lymph node enlargement.

Chapter 21
Breast Examination Sheet

Tim Harding

Abstract The ability to perform a comprehensive and reproducible breast examination is an essential skill for physicians and healthcare professionals. Physicians should have a detailed process by which a thorough history and examination can be performed predominantly in the outpatient setting. Although, regularly used as an adjunct to a multimodal investigation process, a well-performed breast examination can provide key information with regard to both benign and malignant disease.

Keywords Breast · Examination · Sheet · Axilla · Benign · Malignant · Discharge · Nipple · Discharge

Introduction

The ability to perform a comprehensive and reproducible breast examination is an essential skill for physicians and healthcare professionals. Physicians should have a detailed process by which a thorough history and examination can be performed predominantly in the outpatient setting. Although, regularly used as an adjunct to a multimodal investigation process, a well-performed breast examination can provide key information with regard to both benign and malignant disease.

Prior to performing a breast examination an in-depth history should be obtained from the patient. Patient's will provide important information regarding timing and symptomology. This information can aid in a focused examination and more timely diagnosis.

Although the step wise process to the breast exam may vary amongst clinicians, the components of the examination and patient history remain constant.

Timing and use of concurrent breast imaging varies across centers; however, a methodical breast examination will aid in identifying patients who require subsequent imaging or can be safely discharged from the service. It is vital for clinicians

T. Harding (✉)
Breast and Endocrine Surgery SpR, St. Vincent's University Hospital, Dublin, Ireland

A. Farag et al. (eds.), *Clinical Surgical Skills Made Easy*,
https://doi.org/10.1007/978-3-031-69158-4_21

to remember this is an intimate examination and all efforts to ensure patient comfort throughout should be sought.

Anatomy and Physiology

Although a great variation in breast size and shape amongst patients, breast anatomy and landmarks remain constant. This variation is due to the differing volumes of fatty tissue and stroma.

Anatomy:

- Overlie the 2nd to 6th ribs
- Comma or teardrop shaped with the tail extending toward the axilla
- Overlying fascia (Scarpa's fascia)
- Base of the breast primarily overlies the pectoralis major. Laterally, part of the breast extends over the latissimus dorsi and inferiorly the rectus sheath.
- Multiple suspensory ligaments run through the breast connecting the skin to the deep layer of the superficial fascia, known as Cooper's ligaments.
- The female breast contains roughly 15–20 lobes, each of which contains multiple lobules. Contained within these lobules are the terminal duct lobular units (TDLU) which are responsible for milk production.

Given roughly 80% of the lymphatic drainage of the breast is preferential to the axilla, an in-depth knowledge of the axilla is fundamental.

- Pyramidal in shape
- From a surgical perspective the axilla can be separated into 3 distinct levels.
  - Level 1: lateral to the pectoralis minor,
  - Level 2: deep to the pectoralis minor
  - Level 3: above and medial to the pectoralis minor.

The number of nodes lying within each level is highly variable within level 1 containing round 10–20 lymph nodes, whereas level 3 may only contain 4–5 lymph nodes.

The Breast Clinic

The breast clinic is a busy element of working in any symptomatic breast unit. In many units overcrowding and staffing issues are a regular occurrence. Depending on the type of clinic, patients may be offered triple assessment during the index visit or simply a history and examination with radiological examination completed at a later date. In recent years, some units have began to offer imaging first outpatient clinics where a patient will receive a mammogram prior to an initial clinic appointment. Irrespective of imaging results, clinicians must allow the patient to provide their history and complete a thorough examination. Although mammography may reassure the patient and clinician alike, like all forms of radiological examination it is not an exact science and subtle irregularities may become apparent on examination that are not evident on imaging.

Patients of varying ages will present with a multitude of conditions, so an in-depth knowledge of both benign and malignant appearing conditions is vital. For the clinician, having a personalized systematic and reproducible history and examination will aid in an accurate and timely diagnosis. Clinicians should allow ample opportunity for the patient to express their concerns, while guiding the patient to provide all pertinent information that will aid in a diagnosis and discharge if appropriate.

It is essential to remember in the symptomatic breast setting, only 1 in 12–13 patients will be diagnosed with a new breast cancer. Being empathetic and having good communication skills are qualities that are paramount for a breast physician with emphasis on reassuring the worried well.

Clinical History Taking

Communication

First and foremost, do not forget communication skills. The consultation should be at all times patient focused, and demonstrating good general communication skills will help the patient relax and aid in a seamless consultation. Maintain relaxed body language while remaining professional. Allow the patient to speak and try to not interrupt the patient while speaking.

Discovering Symptoms

While there are many methods of exploring the symptomology the patient may be experiencing, following a structured approach, such as the SOCRATES acronym, will assist in providing the important information. The components of the SOCRATES acronym are listed below:

- Site: Location of the symptom (Lump, pain etc)
- Onset: How long has the symptom/ lump been present
- Character: The subjective view of the patient regarding the symptom/ lump
- Radiation: Do any of the associated symptoms move elsewhere
- Associated symptoms: Is there other symptoms/signs associated. Further discussed below
- Time: Has this symptom/sign evolved over time

- Exacerbating factors: Especially important when discussing mastalgia
- Severity: A subjective rating can be attained from the patient

Breast Specific History

Special emphasis must be paid to a well-defined, but not limited to, list of breast specific signs and symptoms. Not only will this aid the clinician in forming a preliminary diagnosis, but will assist the radiologist in focusing on the area of concern. Key symptoms regarding a breast lump include:

- Pain/mastalgia
- Lump (Location, consistency, size, shape, mobility, discovery)
- Skin changes (Color changes/ ulceration/ dimpling)
- Nipple changes (Retraction, inversion, color changes)
- Nipple discharge (Color, unilateral/ bilateral/ concurrent mass)
- Associated Lymphadenopathy (Axillary or distant)
- Systemic symptoms

Medical History

A key element of any systems history is exploring the patient's past medical and surgical history. Vital components of a past medical history include:

- Past medical conditions:
    - When was this diagnosed?
    - How well is the controlled?
    - Is the patient taking any medication?
- Past surgical procedures:
    - When was this performed?
    - What procedure (including biopsies) was performed?
    - Any associated complications?
- For the purpose of a breast specific history, it is imperative to take a focused gynecological and obstetric history. Elements of this history may identify risk factors for breast cancer such as:
    - Nulliparity
    - Early menarche
    - Late menopause
    - Previous/ current use of hormone replacement therapy (HRT)

- Given the increased utilization of genetic testing and identification of breast cancer associated genetic mutations, a thorough family history of any benign or malignant breast disease as well as ovarian cancer should be explored with the patient. Having a first degree relative or a number of second-degree relatives with a previous diagnosis of breast cancer is a significant risk factor for breast cancer.
- Finally, although not to be specifically undertaken as a formulaic element of the patient's history, it is important to address any ideas, concerns and expectations (ICE) from the patient. Allowing the patient ample time to discuss any ideas, concerns, expectations will gain insight into what the patient hopes or expects to gain from the consultation as well as what they currently perceive to be the primary issue.

Closing the Consultation

In closing the consultation, it is vital to summarize the breast specific history provided by the patient as well as any pertinent findings. Allow the patient time to ask any further questions that have not been addressed. To allow for realistic expectations, outline any further investigative plans with a realistic timeframe. Be honest with the patient, if you are unsure or concerned, discuss this with the patient. Finally thank the patient for their time.

Examination

Breast Examination

General Plan (Fig. 21.1):

Includes Inspection and Palpation with no place for Percussion or Auscultation.

In three positions after exposure of the whole upper part of the body including the abdomen:

- During Sitting.
- During elevation of the hand above the head.
- During leaning forwards.

Inspection is done in Circles:

- Inner Circles:
  - Nipple in the center:
  - Areola:
  - Breast proper including back of the breast.

- Outer Circle including:
  - Axilla and Ipsilateral upper Limb.
  - Supraclavicular area.
  - Contralateral breast and Axilla.
  - Upper Abdomen.

Palpation in Circles:

By the Flat of the Fingers “Not by the flat of the Hands” and By Tips of the Fingers starting with the Normal Breast:

- Nipple.
- Centre of the breast.
- Quadrants of the breast.
- Axilla.
- Supraclavicular Lymph nodes.
- Parasternal, Contralateral breast and contralateral axilla.
- Upper abdomen including Liver and Umbilicus.

N.B. The axilla is a Pyramid like structure when the arm is in its natural adducted position with:

Anterior wall made of Pectoralis muscles “Minor and major”.

- Posterior wall made of the Latissimus dorsi muscle.
- Medial wall is made by the first three intercostal spaces and ribs.
- Lateral wall made of the humerus.
- Base made by the skin of the floor of the axilla.

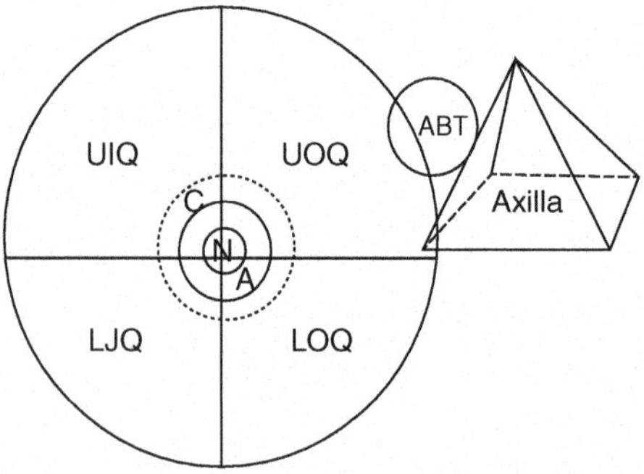

UOQ “Upper Outer Quadrant” . UIQ “Upper Inner Quadrant, LOQ ”Lower Outer quadrant” . LIQ “Lower Inner Quadrant. C ” Central Part of the breast is the breast tissue deep to the Nipple and Areola“ A ‘Areola” . N “Nipple” ABT ‘Axillary Breast Tail”

Fig. 21.1 General plan for examination of the breast and Axilla

- Apex which is the interval between the superior border of the scapula, the posterior border of the clavicle, and the external border of the first rib.

The Axillary space "The pyramid of the axilla" disappears when the arm on elevation of the hand over the head when the floor of the axilla touches the apex and the Pectoralis and Latissimus dorsi muscles slip over the head of the humerus anteriorly and posteriorly respectively.

A thorough and reproducible breast examination is essential while working in any breast unit. Although the timing of the various elements of the exam may vary amongst clinicians, the components are constant.

Introduction

- Introduce yourself and explain your role with the team/ unit.
- Explain to the patient what the examination will involve and why you are performing it.
- Irrespective of gender, always have a chaperone present.
- Provide the patient with a disposable gown or blanket during the examination. This will allow the patient to be covered and most importantly comfortable.
- Before beginning the examination, check with the patient that they fully understand the purpose and process of the examination.
- Ask the patient if they currently have any pain.
- Ask the patient to point with one finger to any area of concern. Remember, it is not uncommon for patients to present with vague symptoms or to no longer be able to feel a previously discovered lump.
- Finally, sit the patient on the edge of the bed with their arms resting comfortably by their side.

Inspection

- With the patient sitting comfortably on the side of the bed inspect the breasts. Inspect for:
  - Asymmetry of the breasts—Although asymmetry of the breasts is normal, gross distortion by comparison may help in identification of pathology.
  - Visible masses—Any visible lumps should be documented.

- Skin changes—Dimpling of the skin, erythema and discoloration of the breast should be noted.
- Nipple abnormalities—Retraction, inversion and discharge from the nipple.
- Scars from previous procedures—Special attention should be paid to any previous biopsy sites, lumpectomy or mastectomy scars.

- While seated, the patient should be asked to place their hands on their hips and squeeze. This maneuverer will contract the underlying pectoral muscles. The clinician should observe if any masses become apparent or if any masses have been previously noted, observe for tethering to underlying muscle. Puckering of the overlying skin may be accentuated during this maneuverer.
- Ask the patient to now place their hands behind their head. This will expose all of the breast and also help to exaggerate any dimpling or puckering.

Palpation

- The patient should now be asked to lie supine at a 30-degree angle with a pillow behind their head.
- Ask the patient to firstly place both arms by their side.
- Prior to commencing the examination, confirm the side of concern to the patient.
    - Beginning with the asymptomatic side, ask the patient to place their hand behind their head.
    - Palpation should be undertaken using the pads of digits 2, 3 and 4 (index, middle, ring fingers).

It is important to have a systematic approach to palpation of the breast.

(a) Spiral method
(b) Up and down method
(c) Quadrant method

- Gently compress the underlying breast tissue onto the chest wall paying particular attention to any masses apparent.
- Ensure to examine the entire breast including the sternum and inframammary fold.
- Prior to repositioning the patient to examine the axilla, ensure to examine the axillary tail. The breast is teardrop shaped and there is a projection of breast tissue from the upper outer quadrant of the breast into the axilla. As the majority of breast cancers develop in the glandular upper outer quadrant of the breast, it is vital to ensure the whole breast is examined.
- Nipple areolar complex (NAC): Ask the patient to gently press on the areola. This may exacerbate any discharge.

- Following examination of the entirety of the breast tissue, regional lymph nodes should be examined, for the purpose of the breast examination special consideration should be paid to the axillary lymph nodes.
  - Begin the examination on the contralateral side of concern
  - Assess for any pain prior to lifting the arm
  - Similar to the breast examination, inspect for scars, visible masses or skin changes
  - Hold the patients right arm with your right hand. Ask them to completely relax the arm which will allow the pectoral and axillary muscles to relax. The reverse is applied when examining the left-hand side.
  - To entirely assess the axillary lymph nodes, the anterior, central, medial and posterior lymph node groups of the axilla should be palpated.
    (a) Anterior: Posterior to lateral edge of pectoralis major
    (b) Posterior: Lateral edge of the latissimus dorsi
    (c) Medial: Wall of the thorax
    (d) Lateral: Inner aspect of the humerus in the axilla
- Repeat the examination on the contralateral side
- For completion, the cervical, supra and infraclavicular lymph nodes should be examined.

Completion

- Advise the patient that the examination is now complete.
- Allow the patient ample time and privacy to re-dress.
- Begin documentation of the examination.

Documentation

Precise documentation of the breast examination is vital for several reasons. Firstly, many patients will require multiple consultations from the time of index visit to final diagnosis. It is not uncommon for multiple clinicians to be involved with any one case. Accurate and detailed note taking will allow seamless and fluid further consultations. Secondly, it is imperative to provide the radiologist with a detailed description of the location of concern. Size, mobility, consistency and most importantly accurate location of the lesion should be clearly documented. Finally, from a medico-legal standpoint it is essential to legibly and clearly describe your findings during examination. It is important on retrospective review of notes to be confident and clear in your findings.

Although documentation or proforma use will vary amongst breast units, documentation will be similar or the same in many instances. It is important to illustrate findings with a drawing of both breasts.

Common terminology and elements of the breast examination that should be documented includes:

- Side of concern: unilateral or bilateral
- Symmetrical or asymmetrical breast shape
- Shape of the breast—Grade of ptosis, previous scars
- Location of area of concern—This may include location on a clock face and distance from nipple
- Description of the mass—Shape, size, consistency, fluctuance, mobility, overlying skin changes
- Description of the nipple areolar complex (NAC)
- Documentation of axillary exam as described above—Palpable lymphadenopathy, gross deformities.

Common Breast OPD Conditions

Benign breast disease will account for most referrals to the breast outpatient clinic. Although these may cause significant distress and concern for patients, few, if any of benign breast conditions are associated with an increased risk of malignant transformation. Breast pain and lumps are synonymous with cancer for many patients, so for the clinician the ability to reassure and adequately explain the benign nature of the conditions is vital.

Some of the most common breast conditions encountered, but not limited to, include:

Fibroadenoma:

- Characterized by cellular proliferation of both connective and stromal tissues.
- Typical in younger female (18–30).
- Do not invade the surrounding tissue.
- Management of these lesions includes simple reassurance, however in certain instances surgical management may be preferable. Surgical excision may be recommended if the Fibroadenoma is larger than 3.5/4 cm or if any suspicious features are present.

<u>Breast Cysts:</u>

- Typically, present as soft well circumscribed mobile lump.
- Affect females aged 40–60 years and may present with bilateral palpable lumps.
- Overall, will affect roughly 7–10% of the female population.

- Management includes reassurance as many of these lesions will involute over time, however if the cyst is increasing in size or causing discomfort the patient may be offered cyst aspiration.

Fat necrosis:

- Characterized by necrosis of the underlying adipose tissue and associated surrounding inflammatory response.
- Typically a direct result of trauma to the breast
- Given the similarity to carcinoma on presentation it is essential formally out rule a malignant process.
- Treatment involves simple reassurance of the benign nature of this condition. Patients can be advised that areas of fat necrosis will resolve over time.

Mastalgia:

- The most common presenting complaint to breast OPD is that of mastalgia (breast pain) accounting for roughly 40–50% of all referrals.
- The relationship to the patient's menstrual cycle will differentiate this into cyclical and non-cyclical breast pain.
- Patients should receive formal imaging of their breasts.
- Treatment involves information regarding breast pain triggers as well as breast pain journaling. Medications such as Evening Primrose Oil may be prescribed.

Duct Ectasia/Peri-Ductal Mastitis

- Characterized by dilation of the terminal ducts toward the NAC. Inflammation will cause shortening and fibrosis of these ducts which may in turn be associated with abscess formation
- Smoking is a significant risk factor for the development of periductal mastitis (8 times more likely to develop in smokers than in general population).
- Smoking cessation and broad-spectrum antibiotics are traditionally the mainstay of treatment.
- Fistulectomy may be required in patients with multiple episodes of periductal mastitis and fistula formation.

Mastitis

- Mastitis refers to infection of the underlying breast parenchyma.
- Examination will reveal an erythematous tender breast which may be hotter to touch than the non-affected side.
- Progression from severe or untreated mastitis may result in abscess formation.
- Common organisms isolated may include Staphylococcus Aureus and Staphylococcus epidermis.
- The mainstay of treatment for both mastitis and abscess formation includes broad spectrum antibiotic therapy. Depending on abscess formation, ultrasound guided aspiration +/− incision and drainage may be required.

Chapter 22
Examination of the Axilla

Alexandra M. Zaborowski and Arnold D. K. Hill

Abstract The ability to perform a comprehensive and reproducible breast examination is an essential skill for physicians and healthcare professionals. Physicians should have a detailed process by which a thorough history and examination can be performed predominantly in the outpatient setting. Although, regularly used as an adjunct to a multimodal investigation process, a well-performed breast examination can provide key information with regard to both benign and malignant disease.

Keywords Breast · Examination · Sheet · Axilla · Benign · Malignant · Discharge · Nipple · Discharge

Basic Anatomy of the Axilla

The axilla is an anatomical region under the glenohumeral joint, at the junction between the thorax and upper limb. The anatomic borders are the clavicle, scapula and first rib superiorly, serratus anterior and the first four ribs medially, coracobrachialis and short head of the biceps muscle laterally, pectoralis major and minor muscles anteriorly, and subscapularis, teres major and latissimus dorsi muscles posteriorly. The axilla contains the axillary artery and vein, the brachial plexus, lymph nodes, fat, accessory breast tissue, subcutaneous glands and skin.

The primary blood supply of the upper limb is provided by the subclavian artery, which lies beneath the clavicles bilaterally. Beyond the border of the first rib, the subclavian artery becomes the axillary artery which becomes the brachial artery

---

A. M. Zaborowski (✉)
Department of General, Breast and Endocrine Surgery, Beaumont Hospital, Dublin, Ireland
e-mail: zaborowa@tcd.ie

A. D. K. Hill
Department of Surgery, The Royal College of Surgeons in Ireland, Dublin, Ireland
e-mail: adkhill@rcsi.com

A. Farag et al. (eds.), *Clinical Surgical Skills Made Easy*,
https://doi.org/10.1007/978-3-031-69158-4_22

beyond the inferior margin of teres major. The largest branch of the axillary artery is the subscapular artery which supplies the intercostal muscles, latissimus dorsi, and the serratus anterior. The suprascapular artery, a branch of the thyrocervical trunk, supplies the rotator cuff muscles. The axillary artery also gives rise to the anterior and posterior humeral circumflex arteries which supply the head of the humerus, and teres major, teres minor, deltoid, and triceps muscles respectively.

The brachial plexus, formed by the anterior primary rami of C5 to T1, provides sensory and motor innervation of the upper limb. It consists of 5 roots, 3 trunks, 6 divisions, 3 cords, and 5 branches. The 3 cords are described in relation to their position relative to the axillary artery (medial, lateral, and posterior). The five branches include the musculocutaneous, axillary, radial, median, and ulnar nerves.

Lymph nodes in the axilla are arranged into 5 groups as follows: anterior (pectoral), lateral, central, apical and posterior (subscapular). Collectively, they drain the breast, thoracic wall, arm, and upper abdominal wall above the level of the umbilicus. Axillary lymph nodes are of particular clinical importance as they may harbor metastases from breast cancer. Patients diagnosed with breast cancer who have clinically or radiologically normal axillary lymph nodes should undergo a sentinel lymph node biopsy to stage the axilla. The sentinel lymph node is the first node into which the breast tumour drains. The status of the sentinel node provides important prognostic information and is used to guide further management e.g. surgery in the form of an axillary lymph node dissection or radiotherapy. Patients with biopsy confirmed axillary metastases may require an axillary lymph node dissection. The anatomical levels of axillary lymph nodes are defined by their relationship to pectoralis minor and are used to describe the extent of surgery in an axillary lymph node dissection (level I: inferolateral to pectoralis minor, level II: posterior to pectoralis minor, level III: superomedial to pectoralis minor). The long thoracic nerve and thoracodorsal neurovascular pedicle should be identified and protected. Injury to the long thoracic nerve may cause winging of the scapula. Axillary lymph nodes may also be enlarged in the setting of haematological malignancy, infection, autoimmune conditions, and post-vaccination.

Examination of the Axilla

Introduction

- Introduce yourself to the patient, explain what the examination involves and obtain consent. Ensure a chaperone is present.
- Ask the patient to remove their clothing from above the waist to expose the chest. Provide a surgical gown for the patient to cover themselves when not required to expose the breasts.
- Ask the patient to sit upright on the examination table.

Inspection

- Inspect the patient from the end of the bed and assess for any obvious asymmetry, masses, scars or skin changes.
- Ask the patient to place both hands behind their head and repeat the inspection of both axillae.
- Ask the patient to place both hands on their hips and repeat the inspection.

Palpation

- Examine both axilla in turn.
- Support the arm on the side being examined and abduct the arm to an angle of approximately 45°. Ask the patient to fully relax the arm to aid identification of any enlarged lymph nodes.
- Palpate the axilla with the tips of your 2nd, 3rd and 4th fingers for any lymphadenopathy. There are 5 stations of axillary lymph nodes: apical, anterior, central, posterior, and medial.
- Palpate the supraclavicular and infraclavicular lymph nodes. The right supraclavicular nodes may be involved in thoracic or oesophageal carcinoma. Metastases to left supraclavicular nodes may occur in gastric carcinoma (Virchow's node, Troisier's sign).
- Complete the examination by examining the breasts and all lymph node groups, the abdomen for hepatomegaly and splenomegaly, the testes for testicular masses, and the skin and nails for melanoma.

Lymph Node Characterization

Assess for the following characteristics during examination.

- Site: localized vs. generalized.
- Size: >1 cm is abnormal.
- Consistency: hard lymph nodes suggest malignancy whilst rubbery lymph nodes suggest lymphoma.
- Mobile or fixed: lymph nodes fixed to underlying or surrounding structures suggest malignancy.
- Tenderness: tender lymph nodes are typically found in the setting of infection or acute inflammation. Abnormal lymph nodes due to malignancy are usually non-tender.
- Overlying skin changes: erythema of the skin suggests infection or inflammation, whilst tethering suggests malignancy.

Differential Diagnosis of an Axillary Mass

1. Lymphadenopathy
   - Haematological malignancy such as lymphoma or leukaemia.
   - Metastases from invasive carcinoma e.g. breast.
   - Infection (acute or chronic).
     - Bacterial e.g. tuberculosis, staphylococcus or streptococcal cellulitis, bartonella henselae (cat scratch disease).
     - Viral e.g. human immunodeficiency virus, cytomegalovirus, infectious mononucleosis.
     - Protozoal e.g. toxoplasmosis.
   - Autoimmune disorders such as systemic lupus erythematosus, rheumatoid arthritis.
   - Sarcoidosis.
   - Post-vaccination.
2. Subcutaneous lesions such as lipomas or accessory breast tissue.
3. Cutaneous lesions such as sebaceous cysts or hidradenitis suppurativa.

Radiological Assessment of the Axilla

Ultrasonography (US) is the most commonly used imaging modality to assess the axilla. It is widely available, well tolerated, and does not involve ionizing radiation. The patient is positioned supine with the arm above the head, abducted and externally rotated. If imaging reveals a suspicious finding e.g. abnormal lymph node, percutaneous sampling techniques such as fine needle aspiration (FNA) or core biopsy can be performed under US guidance with local anaesthetic. FNA specimens provide a sample for cytological assessment whilst core biopsy specimens provide tissue for histological assessment. Limitations of FNA include that it is operator dependent and has a relatively high false negative rate of up to 25%. A repeat FNA or core biopsy should be performed if there is high clinical or radiological suspicion despite normal cytology. Core biopsy is highly accurate and can provide information on the type and grade of carcinoma as well as molecular subtype. Further imaging should be guided by clinical findings and the differential diagnosis e.g. mammography for suspected breast cancer or computed tomography of thorax, abdomen and pelvis for a potential lymphoproliferative disorder.

Chapter 23
Examination of the Head and Neck

Husam Hosny and Ahmed Farag

Abstract The Face is attached to the undersurface of the Cranium hanging in front of the cervical spine where the hard palate is opposite the C1 Vertebra and the Lower border of the Mandible is opposite C2. The Pharynx is attached to the back of the nose——Naso-Pharynx|| and back of the mouth——Oro-pharynx|| like a mask placed on the nose and mouth but opposite the Cervical Vertebrae. Lower down It is opposite the Larynx "Laryngo-pharynx".

Keywords Face · Neck · Examination · Sheet · Mass · Ulcer · Pharynx · Larynx · Lymph · Node

Anatomical Background (Figs. 23.1 and 23.2)

The Face is attached to the undersurface of the Cranium hanging in front of the cervical spine where the hard palate is opposite the C1 Vertebra and the Lower border of the Mandible is opposite C2. The Pharynx is attached to the back of the nose "Naso-Pharynx" and back of the mouth "Oro-pharynx" like a mask placed on the nose and mouth but opposite the Cervical Vertebrae. Lower down It is opposite the Larynx "Laryngo-pharynx".

Just above the Larynx is the Hyoid bone opposite C3 Vertebra.

Larynx is opposite C\4 and C5 Vertebrae, and Cricoid Cartilage is opposite the C 6 Level, which is a Very important landmark in the Neck both anatomically and clinically.

Knowledge of the Lymphatic drainage of the Neck is of paramount importance in Clinical Examination both the drainage area s and Lymphatic groups:

H. Hosny
Cairo University, Cairo, Egypt
e-mail: husamhosny@kasralainy.edu.eg

A. Farag (✉)
Kasr Alainy Hospital, Cairo University, Cairo, Egypt

A. Farag et al. (eds.), *Clinical Surgical Skills Made Easy*,
https://doi.org/10.1007/978-3-031-69158-4_23

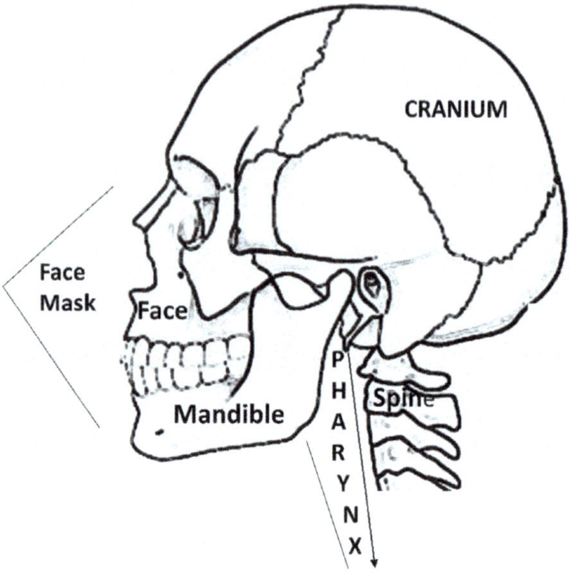

Fig. 23.1 The Cranium is above the spine and the face is hanging from the base of the skull in front of the cervical vertebrae

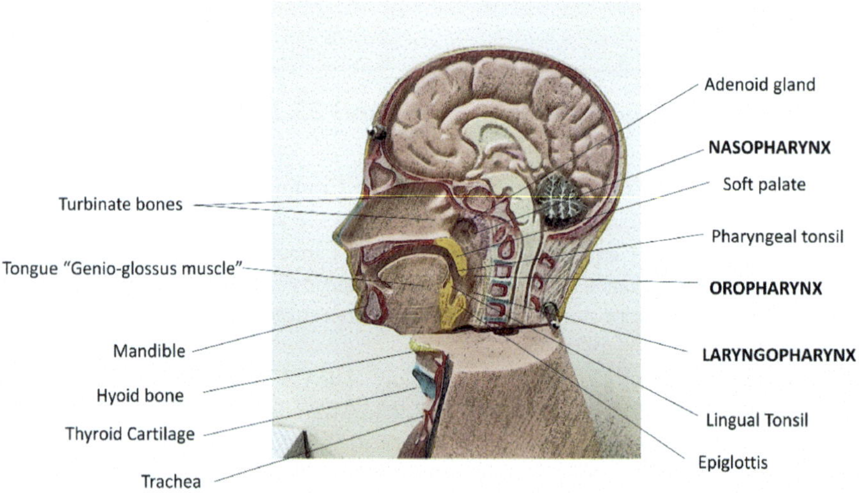

Fig. 23.2 The Pharynx occupies the space between the back of the face in front of the cervical vertebrae

Neck Examination

Introduction

Neck masses are frequent presentation to the clinician and include plethora of possible causes as many anatomical structures in the neck or adjacent areas e.g. scalp, face and thorax that may present their pathological abnormalities in the neck. It is always the clinician duty to limit those possibilities into a one or two most likely possible causes (provisional diagnosis) to help formulating a targeted plan of management without exhausting the patient or the financial system resources with undue investigations.

Key Points

- **Age** is a risk factor by itself. While most masses in children are benign, those presenting in adults have higher incidence of malignancy and should be considered malignant until proved otherwise.
- Thorough knowledge of neck anatomy including **neck triangles** is essential to predict possible causes of neck abnormalities. However for purposes of simplicity, dividing the neck into **central and lateral parts** is practical in restricting differential diagnosis possibilities.
- ***"Common things occur commonly, but uncommon diagnoses do occur".*** So it is always judicious to assess common pathologies before embarking in searching for an uncommon or rare disease.
- Neck masses are common in children and adults. The etiology can be generally classified into congenital, inflammatory/infectious or neoplastic. However those occurring in children vary much from those in adults.
- Lymph node enlargement is the commonest swelling in the neck in all ages. Failure to respond to treatment for 2–3 weeks mandates further procedures to detect a specific infection or reveal a hidden malignancy.
- **Hidden areas** e.g. base of the tongue, hard palate, tonsils, nasopharynx, oropharynx and the submucosa should always be in mind especially when a primary cause cannot be identified.
- Fine needle aspiration cytology (FNAC), is useful in identifying the nature of neck masses and avoid complications of open wound biopsy. In cases of metastatic disease of unknown primary, PET-CT should be done first to identify areas of high metabolic activity (suspicious areas) then endoscopic or open biopsies can be done accordingly, otherwise false positive results may be obtained from sites of previous biopsies if done first.

Triangles of the Neck

The neck is bordered by the inferior border of the mandible (above), the midline of the neck (in front), the superior border of the clavicle (below), and the anterior margin of the trapezius muscle (behind).They are of paramount importance for anatomical DD in neck swellings. The neck is divided by the sternocleidomastoid muscle into.

Anterior Triangle

The anterior triangle of the neck is bordered by the inferior border of the mandible (superiorly), the midline of the neck (medially), and the anterior border of the sternocleidomastoid muscle (laterally). It is further subdivided into three paired triangles (submandibular, carotid, and muscular) and one unpaired submental triangle.

- ***Submental Triangle:***
- Bordered inferiorly; by hyoid bone, laterally; by the anterior belly of the digastric muscle, medially; by midline of the neck. Its floor is made by the mylohyoid muscle.
- *Contents*: the most important is the submental group of lymph nodes. These lymph nodes are responsible for the central wedge of the face i.e. central lips, tongue, floor of the mouth and mandibular symphysis menti.
- ***Digastric/Submandibular Triangle:*** The submandibular triangle is a triangular region of the neck bordered by the inferior border of the mandible (above), the anterior belly of the digastric muscle (in front), the posterior belly of the digastric muscle (behind), and the hyoid bone (below). The floor of the triangle is formed by the mylohyoid muscle.
- *Contents:* the most important structures include the submandibular salivary gland, submandibular lymph nodes, the facial artery and vein, the marginal mandibular nerve underneath the Platysma muscle, the hypoglossal and the lingual nerves deep in the triangle.
- The submandibular triangle is clinically significant because it is a common site for neoplasms, infections, and immunologic pathologies. The submandibular salivary gland can be affected by sialadenitis or neoplasms (50% malignant), lymph node enlargement can occur with facial middle wedge infections or tumors, marginal mandibular nerve can be affected by trauma or iatrogenic injury during previous surgery in this area.
- ***Carotid Triangle:*** is bounded by the posterior belly of digastric muscle, the superior belly of omohyoid muscle and the anterior border of sternomastoid muscle.
- *Contents*:

- Arteries: common carotid artery and its bifurcation into internal and external carotid arteries, and the latter branches namely; superior thyroid, lingual, facial, occipital, and ascending pharyngeal arteries.
- Veins: internal jugular vein, superior thyroid, lingual, facial, ascending pharyngeal, and occipital veins.
- Nerves: external and internal branches of the superior laryngeal nerve arising from the Vagus nerve (CN X), hypoglossal nerve (CN XII).It worth mentioning that the carotid triangle is a very important region of the neck, as it contains many vital structures. The internal jugular vein, for example, is a major vein that drains blood from the brain and neck. The common carotid artery is also a major artery that supplies blood to the brain and face. The hypoglossal nerve is responsible for controlling the tongue muscles.
- ***Muscular Triangle:*** bounded anteriorly by midline of the neck from the hyoid bone above to the sternum below, the anterior margin of sternomastoid infero-posterior, and the superior belly of omohyoid posterosuperior.
- Contents:
- Organs: esophagus, trachea, thyroid gland, and the lower part of the larynx.
- Blood vessels: superior thyroid artery, anterior jugular and inferior thyroid veins.
- Lymphatics: anterior cervical, infrahyoid, prelaryngeal, thyroid, pretracheal, paratracheal lymph nodes.
- Muscles: thyrohyoid, sternothyroid, sternohyoid, omohyoid muscles.
- Nerves: ansa cervicalis (C1-3).

Posterior Triangle

Bounded by posterior border of sternomastoid muscle anteriorly, anterior border of trapezius muscle posteriorly and middle third of the clavicle inferiorly. It is further subdivided into occipital and supraclavicular triangles.

- ***Occipital Triangle:***
- Anterior border: posterior margin of sternocleidomastoid muscle.
- Posterior border: anterior margin of trapezius muscle.
- Inferior border: the inferior belly of the omohyoid muscle.
- Floor: levator scapulae, splenius capitis, and middle and posterior scalene muscles.
- *Contents:*

- Artery: transverse cervical artery.
- Lymphatics: accessory lymph nodes and inferior deep lateral cervical lymph nodes.
- Nerves: accessory nerve (CN XI), cutaneous and muscular branches of the cervical plexus, the uppermost part of brachial plexus, supraclavicular nerves.
- *Clinical Significance:* It houses major nerves that innervate muscles vital for head and neck functions
- ***Subclavian (supraclavicular) Triangle***:
- Superior border: the inferior belly of the omohyoid muscle.
- Anterior border: posterior edge of the sternocleidomastoid muscle.
- Inferior border: clavicle.
- *Contents:*
- Blood vessels: Subclavian artery and vein.
- Nerves: brachial plexus trunks.
- Lymphatics: supraclavicular lymph nodes.
- *Clinical Significance:* Virchow's node, the left-sided supraclavicular lymph node, should raise the suspicion of carcinomas originating from the abdomen. Troisier's sign (an enlarged, firm, non-tender Virchow's node) can indicate cancer arising from the stomach, ovaries, testicles, and kidneys.
- The right-sided supraclavicular lymph node drains lymphatic fluid from the thorax. A firm, enlarged, non-tender right-sided supraclavicular lymph node can indicate metastasis from lung or esophageal cancer and Hodgkin's lymphoma.

Lymphatic Drainage of the Head and Neck (Fig. 23.3)

Knowledge of the Lymphatic drainage of the Neck is of paramount importance in Clinical Examination both the drainage areas and Lymphatic groups:

The Head and Face can be divided into wedges:

- **The Central wedge:** The Chin, most of the Lower Lip, Filtrum and center of the upper Lip with underlying structures including Central incisors and Gum, anterior central wedge of the palate and Floor of the mouth as well as the tip of the tongue. They drain into the Submental Lymph Ns, which drains into the upper deep cervical LNs.
- **The Middle wedge:** which starts between two lines; a line anteriorly; at a point below made by the Facial artery on lower border of the mandible anterior to the masseter muscle and ends high at the inner canthus of the Eye. Posteriorly; a line

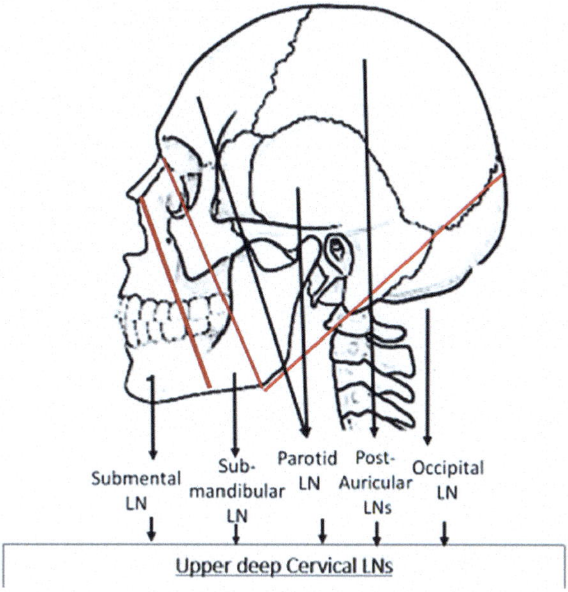

Fig. 23.3 Lymphatic drainage of the head and face

joining angle of the mandible to the external auditory meatus. It includes the angle of the mouth, outer parts of upper and lower lips, the cheeks and nose. It includes the wedge of the underlying tissues including the Canine teeth, Premolars and Molars with their gums, Sides of the tongue and Floor of the mouth, Sides of the palate as well as the Maxillary Sinus and Turbinate bones with their mucosa. They drain into the Submandibular LNs which drains into the upper deep Cervical Lymph nodes. Parotid gland, posterior face, anterior auricle, and anterior scalp can drain first to parotid lymph nodes then to upper deep cervical nodes.

- **The posterior (Outer) wedge:** the posterior scalp, posterior auricle and nape of the neck drain first to post auricular and occipital lymph nodes then to upper deep cervical lymph nodes.

The Lymphatic System of the Neck Is Arranged in Three Circles and Three Vertical Chains (Fig. 23.4)

Outer Circle: Submental, Submandibular, Parotid, Post auricular and Occipital LNs.

Inner Circle: Adenoids, Pharyngeal Tonsils, and Lingual Tonsils.
Middle Circle: Para-pharyngeal and Retropharyngeal LNs. (not clinically accessible).
Anterior Chain: Pre-Laryngeal, Pre-tracheal and Suprasternal LNs.
Posterior Chain: Accessory group of LNs.

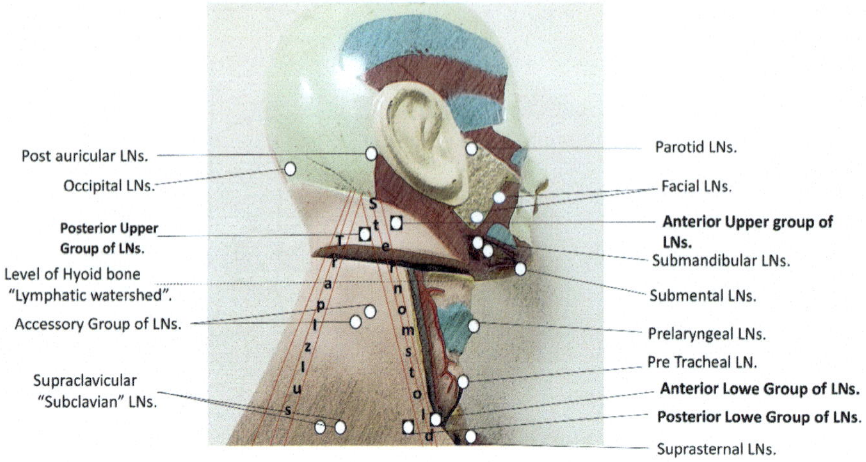

Fig. 23.4 Lymphatic drainage and cervical LNs

Middle Chain: which lies around the internal jugular vein and under the sternocleidomastoid muscle, dividing this chain of LNs into an anterior group and posterior groups. Also, divided at the level of the hyoid bone "C3" -not by the Omo-Hyoid muscle- into upper and lower groups. Thus four groups can be realized:

- Upper Anterior.
- Upper posterior.
- Lower anterior: DD is the Virchow LNs on the left side which is at the termination of the Thoracic duct before it drains into the Veins near the confluence of the Internal Jugular and Subclavian veins. This group of Lymph nodes can be the site of malignant infiltration by retrograde permeation from the thoracic duct after blockage of its termination by malignant cells which drains the Left Chest cavity and Lungs and drains the entire abdomen below the diaphragm "Except the bare area of the Liver which drains into the right thoracic duct through the diaphragm".
- Lower posterior: the outlying member of this group is the supraclavicular group on both sides.

- N.B. the Level of the hyoid bone is a *water-shed area* where Structure below this area e.g. the thyroid gland drains mainly in the Lower groups of LNs. Involvement of the upper groups of Lymph nodes occur by retrograde Lymphatic permeation after extensive metastases in the lower groups of Lymph Nodes. Isolated affection of the upper group of LNs with malignancy in the presence of a thyroid malignancy raises the possibility of Lymphoma "Not a metastatic affection from other types of thyroid Malignancy".

History and Clinical Examination

Personal History

Refer to the chapter of general sheath regarding *name, age, sex, residence, occupation, marital status and sexual relations and special habits of medical importance.* Special considerations are directed towards the age, sex, sexual relations and special habits as:

Neck masses affecting children are usually benign in contrary to those affecting adults (especially >35y) with higher incidence of malignancy.

Carcinomas are more common in male gender than females.

Malignant tumors are more common in HIV positive patients (risk factor). Also HPV predispose to oro-pharyngeal carcinomas. EPV is associated with lymphomas and nasopharyngeal carcinomas.

Tobacco smoking and Khat chewing predispose to lip, tongue, and oral mucosa and lung carcinomas. Also, alcohol intake increases risk of mouth, oro-naso-pharyngeal carcinoma and liver carcinoma.

Complaint

Neck **mass** is the most frequent presentation. Less frequently, the patient may present with **fistula, sinus, ulcer,** dysphagia (difficulty in swallowing), odynophagia (painful swallowing), or localized pain in the neck.

Present History

Analysis of the complaint (s) follows the general principles in the general sheath. Regarding a mass in the neck:

- *Onset*: Acute onset usually denotes acute inflammatory condition (e.g. acute abscess) or hematoma (following trauma) while gradual onset may be neoplastic.
- *Coarse*: Progressive coarse especially if rapid over short period of time is a character of malignancy. In contrary, regressive coarse denote resolving inflammatory condition.
- *Associated pain* denotes inflammatory condition e.g. acute lymphadenitis or acute sialadenitisdue to salivary duct stone (pain associated with mastication). Malignancy is painless, except late when infiltration of a nearby sensory nerve or adjacent structure occurs.
- *Associated lesions* in the scalp, face, ipsilateral upper limb, axilla, thorax and breast should be inquired about.

- *Local compression manifestations:* as dysphagia (compression on the esophagus), dyspnea (compression on the trachea), recent change of voice (infiltration of recurrent laryngeal nerve), ipsilateral otalgia (pain in the ear that may originate from an ear pathology or referred to it), facial edema (compression on jugular veins)
- *General systemic manifestation of inflammation or hyperfunctioning mass* e.g. fever, sweating and malaise. Night fever and sweating suggests TB, intermittent fever is common with IMN, thyrotoxic manifestations (intolerance to heat, loss of weight, insomnia, arrhythmias etc.),
- *Distant metastasis manifestations especially* those to lung, liver, bones and brain e.g. cough, hemoptysis, jaundice, bony pains or swellings.

Past and Family History

- Previous history of neck masses, irradiation or neck surgeries and HPV infection.
- Family history of neck masses or tuberculosis.
- Inquire about domestic animals, pets and birds (increase risk of toxoplasmosis and cat scratch disease).

General Examination

(Refer to general sheath.) Abdominal examination is particularly important as supraclavicular lymph nodes enlargement (Virchow's nodes) may occur due to metastasis from GIT tumors (Troisier's sign). Also enlargement of the liver or spleen may be found in cases of generalized lymphadenopathy.

Chest examination is also important as apical lung tumors may present in the supraclavicular region.

Local Examination

Inspection

The patient is examined while sitting on a chair in front of the examiner and exposed from head till middle of the chest. This includes:

- *Number*: Multiple swellings are usually lymph nodes.
- *Site*: The site oftentimes alludes to the diagnosis. Thorough knowledge of neck anatomical triangles helps approaching proper diagnosis. For instance, lymph node enlargement should be considered wherever aggregation of lymphatic tis-

sue exists. Dermoid cysts occur in the midline along lines of embryonic closure. Branchial cyst occurs at the junction of upper 1/3 and lower 2/3 of sternomastoid muscle partially covered by its anterior border. Thyroid gland enlargement (goiter) occupies lower part of front of the neck in the muscular triangle. Submandibular gland enlargement occurs at the submandibular triangle below lower border of the mandible. Lymphatic malformation (formerly known cystic hygroma) occurs at lateral neck in the posterior triangle.

- *Shape*: regular shape as rounded, oval, etc. or irregular. Benign masses tend to have regular shapes while malignant masses are usually irregular.
- *Size*: better described in centimeters
- *Overlying skin*: should be inspected for dimpling (suggests attachment of the mass to it), fistulae, sinuses (e.g. single in tuberculous caseating lymph node, multiple sinuses denote actinomycosis discharging sulphur granules), erythema due to increased vascularity (e.g. inflammation or sarcoma), scars of previous operation or trauma, and pigmentation (e.g. previous irradiation).
- *Surrounding areas:* refers to adjacent areas that may be the cause of neck swelling. This includes the **scalp** (for ulcers or masses), **face, nose, ears, lips, mouth and cheeks** including the **tongue** dorsum and undersurface, **oral mucosa, palate and tonsils** (pus from tonsillar crypts). Also the ipsilateral **hand, forearm, arm and axilla** should be inspected for ulcers, masses or wounds.
- *Special characters:*
  - Moving up and down with deglutition denotes that the swelling is enclosed within the pretracheal fascia, thus attached to the trachea and/ or the larynx (e.g. thyroid swelling, subhyoid bursa, tuberculous or malignant lymph node attached to the trachea).
  - Pulsation if the swelling is related to carotid or subclavian arteries. They are either true (e.g. aneurysm) or transmitted (e.g. lymph node superficial to the artery).
  - Impulse on cough (e.g. laryngocele).

Palpation

Includes tenderness, temperature, site, size, shape, surface, skin attachment, edge, consistency, mobility, lymph node assessment and special tests.

- *Tenderness*: inflammatory masses are tender (e.g. acute lymphadenitis, acute abscess). On the other hand, malignant masses are not tender except late when infiltration of a nearby nerve or adjacent structure occurs. Tender masses will preclude performing the rest of examination steps as it puts the patient under too much stress and makes it difficult to obtain reliable data. If so, other investigation tools should be done if needed.
- *Temperature:* swellings with increased vascularity (e.g. inflammation, sarcoma) may feel warmer than adjacent areas.

- *Site:* whether the mass is superficial or deep to related muscles. Swellings deep to a muscle tend to decrease in size while those superficial to a muscle will be more visible. Swellings arising from a muscle do not change their size with muscle contraction.
  - Platysma muscle: ask the patient to grimace and see if the mass becomes more or less visible. (e.g. Lipoma in a subcutaneous plane along the side of the neck will be more visible)
  - Sternomastoid muscle: to test a unilateral swelling, ask the patient to turn his chin to the opposite side against resistance. This will contract one muscle and its relation to that swelling can be identified. To test both muscles, ask the patient to push his chin downwards against resistance.
- *Shape:* should be described whether regular rounded, oval, …etc. (benign masses usually have regular shapes) or irregular in shape (malignant masses usually have irregular shapes)
- *Size:* the size is better described in numerical methods (e.g. centimeters) than descriptive methods. In case of irregular shapes, the largest two or three dimensions of the mass are recorded. This makes it easy for follow up of mass progression and for inter-physician communication.
- *Surface*: benign masses usually have smooth surface, while malignant masses usually have irregular surface.
- *Skin attachment:* is tested by gliding the skin over the underlying mass or pinching from it. Malignant tumors and tuberculous nodes become fixed to the superficial skin and may later ulcerate on the skin or develop a sinus discharging caseous material respectively.
- *Edge:* is well defined in benign lesions. Lipoma in specific has a characteristic slippery edge. In contrary, malignant and inflammatory lesions have ill-defined edges.
- *Consistency:* cystic swellings and lipomas feel soft. Benign and inflammatory lesions feel firm. Malignant neoplasms and malignant node metastasis feel hard.
- *Mobility:* Masses arising from longitudinal structures will move across but not along the coarse of that structure (e.g. carotid body tumor, sternomastoid tumors). Also, malignant masses and tuberculous nodes get attached to the surrounding structures e.g. muscles, trachea. So they may show restricted mobility when overlying muscle contracts.
- *Lymph nodal status:* all accessible neck nodes (external horizontal and vertical groups, tonsils and adenoids) should be evaluated for enlargement and signs of malignancy. They are suspicious of malignancy when they feel hard and get adherent to each other or adjacent structures and overlying skin. The lymph node group enlarged may give clue to primary area affected e.g.:
  - Submental nodes point to lesions of the chin, central lips, tongue tip.
  - Submandibular nodes point to lesions of floor of the mouth, cheeks and tongue.
  - Upper jugular nodes (jugulodigastric) point to lesion in the tonsils or nasopharynx.

  - Middle jugular nodes (jugulohyoid) point to lesions in the oropharynx, larynx, esophagus, and thyroid gland.
  - Supraclavicular nodes (Virchow's) point to lesions in the arms, axilla, breast, chest or the abdomen (Troisier's sign).

- *Special tests:*
  - *Compressibility*: either totally compressible as its content is displaced completely upon pressure (e.g. Venous malformation), or partially compressible when it does not empty completely as its contents move only to a communicating limited space (e.g. lymphatic malformation).
  - *Fluctuation test*: fluid filled cysts will show fluctuation e.g. Thyroglossal cyst, Branchial cyst, hyoid bursa and cold abscess. Beware of psuedofluctuation that occur with very soft large Lipoma.
  - *Transillumination*: clear fluid filled cyst will transilluminate (e.g. lymphatic malformation), while cysts filled with pus, caseous, proteinaceous, high lipid content or epithelial debris will not transilluminate (e.g. chronic abscess, cold abscess, dermoid cyst, Branchial cyst, Thyroglossal cyst).
  - *Valsalva's maneuver*: the mass will increase in size with blowing of the nose while the mouth and nostrils are closed e.g. laryngocele.

Percussion

Percussion directly over the manubrium is normally resonant, it may turn dull in huge goiters with retrosternal extension. Direct percussion over a swelling may elicit hyper-resonance in huge laryngocele.

Auscultation

A bruit may be heard over an aneurysm due to turbulence of blood flow or upper pole of thyroid gland in 1ry thyrotoxicosis due to increased vascularity.

Differential Diagnosis of Neck Masses (Table 23.1)

The etiology of neck masses can be generally be attributed to congenital, inflammatory and neoplastic causes. Although they are common presentation at all ages, the etiology of neck masses in children varies from those in adults. Most of neck masses in children are benign while those occurring in adults have a higher incidence of malignancy and should be considered malignant until proved otherwise.

Table 23.1 Common neck swellings according to site

	Benign	Malignant
Central masses	Ranula Thyroglossal cyst Thyroid adenoma, MNG Subcutaneous mesenchymal tumors e.g. Lipoma, fibroma	Thyroid carcinoma Metastatic carcinoma to lymph nodes Lymphomas
Lateral masses	Lymphadenitis Granulomatous diseases e.g. TB, sarcoidosis Branchial cyst Sialadenitis Neurofibroma, neuroma Paraganglioma Vascular malformations	Metastatic carcinoma Lymphomas Salivary gland tumors Sarcomas Malignant Fibrous histiocytoma

Congenital Anomalies

Vascular Origin

- Haemangioma: starts after birth, have three phases; progressive, stationary and finally regressive phases. 50% will disappear completely by 5 years.
- High flow vascular malformations e.g. arterial malformation and arteriovenous fistula
- Low flow vascular malformations e.g. venous malformations and lymphatic malformations

Non Vascular Origin

- **Thyroglossal cyst:** occurs in the midline in relation to the hyoid bone due to failure of complete closure of tract along which the thyroid gland descends from base of the tongue to its normal anatomic location in the neck. It moves up with protrusion of the tongue. Sudden enlargement may occur if infected and form an abscess. It may harbor thyroid tissue thus malignancy can occur.
- **Branchial cyst:** due to incomplete fusion of the 2nd brachial arch (95%) with the 5th arch. It presents as a cystic swelling in the lateral neck at the junction of upper 1/3 and lower 2/3 of sternomastoid muscle anterior border, lateral to internal carotid artery. It may grow rapidly in size if infected as its wall is rich in lymphatic tissue. It commonly presents in children but may present late.
- **Ranula:** is a retention cyst (Mucocele) due to obstruction of a sublingual salivary gland. It is usually asymptomatic found at one side of the midline at the upper neck. If large, it may interfere with swallowing or speech. When it occurs deep to mylohyoid muscle (plunging Ranula) it can be felt through the floor of the mouth.

- **Teratomas:** constitutes germ cell tumors containing all germ cell layers. Thus may contain fat, cysts, calcification and epithelial debris. They present as rapidly expanding neck mass that require rapid intubation. It may be associated with other anomalies e.g. cleft lip palate, heart anomalies, trisomy 13 or trisomy21.
- **Dermoid cyst:** contains only 2 germ cell layers (ectoderm and mesoderm). It occurs at the midline along lines of embryonic fusion.

Inflammatory and Infectious Lesions

- **Acute lymphadenitis:** is the most frequently encountered neck swelling as the neck is rich in lymphatic tissues that drain the scalp, face and upper aero-digestive tracts. They present as multiple tender mobile swellings in anatomical sites of lymph nodes. Symptoms of the primary lesion are usually present e.g. rhinorrhea, dysphagia, odynophagia, otalgia...etc. If necrosis within the lymph node occurs an abscess will develop and fluctuation can be elicited. Common organisms are bacteria (staphylococci and streptococci) and viruses (HPV; predisposes to oropharyngeal squamous cell carcinoma, and EPV predisposes to nasopharyngeal carcinoma).
- **Salivary gland sialadenitis:** presents with pain associated with mastication due to obstruction of a major salivary duct by a stone or decreased flow in cases of severe dehydration (especially in elderly). Note that carcinoma at floor of the mouth may compress and obstruct Wharton's duct and cause symptoms similar to stone obstruction.
- **Granulomatous diseases:** e.g. tuberculosis, sarcoidosis, cat scratch disease, Kawasaki disease. Other systemic manifestations are usually present and point to the disease.

Neoplasms

A. **Metastatic lymph node disease** from regional primary focus (in the head), distant primary focus (skin or viscera) or local primary in the neck (e.g. thyroid and salivary glands). They present as hard immobile nodes yet can be counted.
B. **Primary lymph node disease** e.g. Hodgkin and non-Hodgkin lymphomas. Systemic manifestations are usually present and many lymph node groups can be present at time of presentation.
C. **Thyroid gland neoplasms** present as anterior or lateral neck swellings.
D. **Salivary gland tumors** 80% of parotid gland tumors are benign, the commonest being pleomorphic adenoma. 50% of submandibular salivary gland tumors are malignant. The commonest malignant salivary gland tumor is mucoepidermoid carcinoma. Submandibular salivary gland mass cannot be rolled over the mandible while, a lymph node can be rolled over it.

E. **Neurogenic neoplasms**

- Schwannoma: arise from cranial, spinal nerves or sympathetic chain. In adults, usually found in parapharyngeal space.
- Neurofibroma: skin or subcutaneous nodule (s), may be associated with brownish pigmentation of the skin (café au lait patches).
- Tumors of neuroblastic origin e.g. neuroblastoma and ganglion neuroblastoma.
- Neuroma occurs from nerve injury during surgery or following trauma e.g. great auricular nerve injury during parotidectomy. Patient presents with small tender nodule with paraesthesia.
- Paraganglioma "carotid body tumor": it is neural crest in origin, arises in the carotid body and typically splays the internal and external carotids. It may secret catecholamines and leads to uncontrolled hypertension and needs special attention during surgical excision.

F. **Metastatic carcinoma with unknown primary** is a squamous cell carcinoma in 90% of the cases. Others include adenocarcinoma and melanoma. They need careful attention to hidden sites e.g. tonsils, nasopharynx, pyriform fossa and impalpable submucosal tumors.

Chapter 24
Examination of a Mass in the Head and Face

Ahmed Farag, Amr Kamel Elfeky, and Nicholas Johnson

Abstract Personal History: In the Pathology—Epidemiology section i.e. which type of patient can have this complaint. It should be interpreted after the complaint as a first Time-Out. Complaint: Swelling: painful or Painless. Ulcer or ulcerating mass. Site is the most important Item in interpreting the complaint.

Keywords Head · Face · Area · Parotid · Forehead · Scalp · Lymph · Node · Mass · Ulcer

Personal History

In the Pathology "Epidemiology section i.e. which type of patient can have this complaint" should be interpreted after the complaint as a first "Time-Out".

Complaint

1. Swelling "painful or Painless".
2. Ulcer or ulcerating mass.
3. **Site** is the Most important Item in interpreting the complaint:

- **Top and sides of the Head**:
    1. Common Swellings:

A. Farag (✉)
Kasr Alainy Hospital, Cairo University, Cairo, Egypt

A. K. Elfeky
Ain Shams University, Giza, Egypt

N. Johnson
SVUH, Dublin, Australia

A. Farag et al. (eds.), *Clinical Surgical Skills Made Easy*,
https://doi.org/10.1007/978-3-031-69158-4_24

Acute: Hematoma, Abscess and infected sebaceous cyst.
Chronic: Sebaceous cyst, Haemangioma, Lipoma, or Neurofibroma.

2. Less Common tumors:
   Bone Secondaries, Meningocele, Osteoma, Lymphoma and Multiple Myeloma, Encephalocele and hernia Cerebri.
3. Pulsating Tumors:
   Cersoid Aneurysm, Meningocele "Positive trans illumination", Encephalocele and Hernia Cerebri.
4. Ulcers or Ulcerating Masses:
   Ulcerating Sebaceous cyst "Cock's Peculiar Tumor", Malignant Ulcer including Squamous Cell Carcinoma, Basal Cell carcinoma or Rodent Ulcer, Sebaceous Carcinoma or Melanoma, Leishmanial ulcer, Lupus Vulgaris, and Keratoacanthoma.

The Forehead and Face

- Acute diffuse Swelling: Infections including osteomyelitis, and Allergies like Angioneurotic edema.
- Chronic diffuse Swelling: Diffuse Haemangioma and Plexiform neuroma "Pacchydermatocele".
- Chronic Localized: Sebaceous Cyst, dermoid cyst, Haemangioma, Lymphangioma, Neurofibroma, Lipoma, Melanoma, Keloid, Mucocele of the Nasolacrimal duct, mucous retention cyst from the buccal surface of the Cheek, Tumors of the Maxilla.
- Ulcer: Rodent Ulcer, Squamous Cell carcinoma, Molluscum Sebaceum and Keratoacanthoma. Lupus Vulgaris, Tuberculous Ulcer and Leishmanial Ulcer.

The Lips

- Diffuse Swellings: Lymphangioma, Lymphatic obstruction due to repeated infections and Diffuse Tertiary Syphilis "Rare nowadays".
- Localized Swelling: Mucous Cyst, Haemangioma, Lymphangioma Papilloma Squamous cell carcinoma.
- Ulcers: Central Cracks due to prolonged dryness of the Lips, Angular Cracks due to riboflavin deficiency, Squamous cell Carcinoma, Syphilis "Rare" and Dyspeptic ulcers "Mucous membranes:

- N.B. Dark muco-cutaneous pigmentations are indicative of peutz jeghers syndrome.

The Tongue

Swellings

- Localized: 1. Haemangioma. 2. Mixed salivary tumor. 3. Lingual Thyroid.
- Diffuse: 1. Haemangioma. 2. Lymphangioma. 3. Cretinism.
- Ulcers: 1. Traumatic. 2. Dental. 3. Dyspeptic ulcers.
- 4. Malignant. 5. Frenal ulcers. 6. Tuberculous.
- Fissures: 1. Congenital fissures. 2. Chronic superficial.
- Glossitis. 3. Median Rhomboid Glossitis.
- Pain: 1. Trauma "Biting the tongue". 2. Leukoplakia.
- 3. Superficial glossitis. 4. Cancer. 5. T.B. ulcers.

The Palate

Swellings: Mucous Cysts. Mixed salivary tumors.
Ulcers: Dyspeptic, Malignant and Syphilitic "rare".
Perforations: Congenital Cleft Palate, Traumatic and malignant.

Floor of the Mouth

Swellings: Ranula, Dermoid Cyst, Mucous retention cyst, Submandibular Salivary gland stone, Sialadenitis or tumor.
Ulcers: Dyspeptic or Malignant.

Cheek

Ulcers: Dyspeptic or Malignant ulcers.
Swellings: Mucous retention cyst, Mixed Salivary tumor, Haemangioma, Lymphangioma and Lipoma.

Swellings from the Jaw

Bone swellings:

- Acute inflammatory: Osteomyelitis: Dental caries, Periodontal abscess or post traumatic.
- Chronic inflammatory: From Carious tooth.
- Cysts and Neoplasms:

1. Dental Cyst.
2. Dentigerous Cyst.
3. Adamantinomas are locally invasive, highly destructive tumors of the jaw and commonly arise in the molar area. They are odontogenic tumors derived from tooth formation tissues.
4. Osteoclastoma: They are distinctive neoplasms characterized by a profuse multinucleate giant cells scattered throughout the stroma of mononuclear cells. These giant cells have some similarity with osteoclasts, and so are called Osteoclastoma
5. Benign tumors: Chondroma and Osteoma.
6. Carcinoma of the Maxillary Sinus.

Swellings from the Gum "Epulides':

1. Fibrous epulis.
2. Myeloid epulis.
3. Granulomatous epulis.
4. Carcinomatous epulis.
5. Sarcomatous epulis.

Swellings from the Parotid Area

Skin

- Benign tumors e.g. papilloma.
- Malignant tumors e.g. squamous cell carcinoma, basal cell carcinoma, malignant melanoma.
- Cyst e.g. sebaceous cyst.

Subcutaneous Tissue

- Benign tumors e.g. Lipoma, fibroma, Haemangioma, Neurofibroma.
- Malignant tumors e.g. sarcoma.
- Cyst e.g. dermoid cyst.

Parotid Lymph Node

- Chronic nonspecific lymphadenitis.
- Chronic specific lymphadenitis e.g. TB.
- Malignancy e.g. lymphoma

Parotid Gland

- Chronic parotitis.
- Parotid cyst.
- Tumors
  - Adenomas pleomorphic, Warthin tumor
  - Carcinomas Mucoepidermoid Carcinoma, Adenoid Cystic Carcinoma, Acinic cell carcinoma, Polymorphous low-grade adenocarcinoma
- Autoimmune diseases Mikulicz, Sjögren's syndromes.

Masseter Muscle

- Fibrosarcoma
- Rhabdomyosarcoma
- Myxoma
- Hypertrophid muscle

Ramus of the Mandible

- Osteomyelitis
- Osteoclastoma
- Secondaries
- Cyst
- Winged mandible

Mucosa of the Cheek

- Squamous cell carcinoma.

Others

- Branchial cyst.
- Neuroma.
- Fascial vein thrombosis.
- Temporal artery aneurysm.
- Mastoiditis.

Clinical Classification

A swelling in the parotid area in history either acute or chronic, on examination it is either glandular origin or extraglandular.

Acute Swelling

- **Parotid**

Septic parotitis, mumps.

- **Extra parotid**

Hematoma, abscess, acute lymphadenitis or osteomyelitis.

Chronic Swelling

- Parotid
  - Unilateral

    A. Cystic:
    Parotid cyst or Adenolymphoma.

    B. Solid:
    Chronic parotitis, tumors.
  - Bilateral
  - Adenolymphoma, autoimmune disease
- Extraparotid
- Skin, SC tissue, masseter, etc.

Acute Swellings

Mumps

Young child, usually bilateral, influenza like symptoms, low grade fever, painful, tender, edema in the face, difficult mastication, self-limited.

Acute Parotitis

Middle age, unilateral, fever, painful, tender, pus emerged through the duct, enlarged tender and hot cervical lymph nodes.

Chronic Swellings

Parotid Cyst

Translucent, aspiration clear, duct examination shows stone.

Adenolymphoma (WARTHIN TUMOR)

Men more than women, bilateral in 10–15%- soft or cystic- usually at lower part of the parotid, spherical, smooth surface, well defined edge-mobile.

In pathology has true capsule- full of B lymphocytes.

Pleomorphic Adenoma

75% of parotid tumors, unilateral, equal male to female ratio, ant. & sup to the jaw angle, spherical when small and lobulated when large, it is smooth and mobile "not attached to skin or deeper structures" and firm in consistency. Don't forget parotid tumors mostly raises lobule of the ear.

Pathology incomplete capsule- mixed cellularity.

Malignant Parotid Tumors

- Criteria of malignancy
  - Rapid growth (short history)
  - Hard in consistency
  - Fixation may attached to skin or deeper structures
  - Fascial nerve affection (mouth angel deviation- eye incomplete closure)
  - Pain in 30% may referred to ear (auriculotemporal nerve affection)
  - Enlarged regional lymph nodes

Autoimmune Diseases

- MIKULIKZ syndrome

- Bilateral enlargement of all salivary glands and lacrimal glands- dryness of the eye and mouth
- SJOGRIN syndrome
- Same as Miculikz in addition to keratoconjunctivitis, polyarthritis, other manifestations of Systemic lupus erythematosus (SLE).

Present History

- **Onset**: Acute onset associated with pain suggest inflammatory pathology and if associated with trauma it may indicate traumatic pathology. Insidious pathology indicates benign or malignant tumors.
- **Course:** In cases with insidious onset a rapid progression "Weeks or months" indicates benign pathology, while slow progression indicates benign pathology. And regressive course indicates inflammatory lesion and intermittent course indicates an autoimmune disease and salivary gland stone.
- **Duration:** As mentioned above.
- **Analysis of the complaint:**

Pain:

- Type "A submandibular salivary stone may cause a colicky like pain during meal or immediately after it especially after Citrus fluids (Lemon Test)".
- Site: indicates the site of pathology.
- Radiation: may refer to the tip of the tongue "Submandibular sialadenitis" or the Tempro mandibular Joint "Parotitis"
- What brings pain: Eating especially citrus fruits.
- What relieves pain: Sometimes by milking of the parotid by the palm of the hand towards the mouth.

Associated Symptoms

- Enlargement of the lacrimal glands with or without Xerostomia and Dry eye "Mikulicz Syndrome or Sjögren syndrome".
- Bilateral affection of the salivary glands: Mumps, Autoimmune parotitis, Whartin's Tumor.

Past Medical history: For:

- Diseases of Medical importance.
- Previous history of the same condition.
- Surgical History.
- Allergies.

Family History

Past Medical History of importance.

General Examination

- Associated diseases of medical importance.
- Stage of the disease in cases of malignant tumors of the Head and Face.
- Stigmata of autoimmune disease such as SLE.

Local Examination

See the Sheet of Swelling and sheet of Ulcers according to the affected site as mentioned above.

Trauma Examination Sheet

Nicholas Johnson

The trauma examinations are a reproducible, reliable, and systematic set of clinical examinations of a patient separated into three distinct phases: primary survey, secondary survey, and tertiary survey.

The primary survey is used to identify and correct immediate life-threatening complications from trauma and is therefore a combination of assessment and treatment to stabilize the patient.

The secondary survey is a methodical head to toe examination of the stable patient in the acute setting, combined with radiology as indicated, to accurately define prioritize and direct management of the patient.

The tertiary survey is a complete re-examination of the patient following treatment and is usually completed 24 to 48 h after injury. It is designed to pick up missed injuries following initial assessment and management or those which have developed as part of a progressive evolution of injury.

These examinations while simple, need to be protocolized and planed as a team orientated activity. Ideally in a trauma setting, you will have separate clinicians performing the various parts of the primary and secondary survey simultaneously, with a team leader overseeing the process and not getting task focused on any specific part of the examination itself.

A good trauma examination however involves more than just a head to toe examination of the patient. It begins by gathering as much information as possible before the patient arrives so planning can be activated, the team assembled, and tasks prioritized. While this is not always possible, information from the first responders about the nature of the incident, injuries identified what has been done and the response to these actions is invaluable in planning reception. If this information is not available, understanding the mechanism of the injury, the patient's potential fragility (frailty score) and the result of the primary survey and response to critical interventions directs a good trauma clinician to identify patterns of injury, and expected outcome. Combined with the secondary survey this will identify injuries and direct on-going management. Sudden unexpected deterioration should initiate a return to a primary survey.

History

An understanding of the mechanism of injury and patient comorbidities is essential for an effective and thorough clinical examination. Unlike most clinical histories that a physician takes, a trauma history is focused only on pertinent information relating to the trauma the patient has experienced and the relevant medical conditions that may impact the patient's imminent clinical course or surgical needs. There are several acronyms which aid in gathering this information.

Mechanism of Injury

All trauma involves a transfer of energy, resulting in tissue damage and injury. In low velocity blunt and penetrating injuries, the trauma is localized to the path of transit of the knife or projectile or to the site where the trauma was sustained. However, in high velocity penetrating trauma and in blast injuries the injury is unpredictable and atypical. This is important information when determining what injuries, it is expected that a patient may have. While information may be elicited from the patient's themselves, often the information is relayed from first responders as patients may be incapacitated on arrival or under the influence of drugs (alcohol, opiates).

Blunt Trauma

Blunt trauma has a wide range of potential mechanisms (fall from height, being hit by a car or bat). What struck the patient, at what speed, where on their body and how many times is what determines their injuries.

**Trauma Pearl: Patients who have had a delayed arrival to hospital can self-select out some major injuries (major cardiac or vessel transections have a high fatality rate even when immediately transferred to hospital) but also include new unexpected injuries (a patient who has fallen at home, and been left lying for 24 h has a high likelihood of rhabdomyolysis and dehydration).

Falls

When assessing a fall: knowledge of the height they fell from, what they landed on (concrete or a car cushioning their landing, and water introduces the consideration of a drowning and what body part sustained the impact will greatly change the injury pattern you are looking at (a 2 m fall onto their feet may result in a broken ankle, whereas a fall onto the head can result in death.

Motor Vehicle Accidents

In a motor vehicle accident knowing what speed the vehicle was travelling at, where the patient was in the vehicle, how it was hit (a driver hit from behind is different to being impacted on the passenger side which is different to an impact on the driver side or head on), if the patient was restrained/ejected (which changes the profile of the mechanism of injury), and if any other occupants were injured or killed is useful information when considering what injuries the patient may have. A lower speed accident will have less energy transfer and therefore usually less significant injuries. High speed accidents can have large forces exerted on the body, and more catastrophic injuries for example a transected thoracic aorta in a high speed head on collision with a restrained driver.

For pedestrians struck by a vehicle, knowing the speed of the vehicle, whether the windscreen damaged and how far they were thrown is essential. Patients are often hit in the legs (which can fracture), land on the bonnet (often with their head onto or through the windscreen resulting in cranial and spinal injuries) and are thrown to the ground (traumatizing the torso and long bones further). This mechanism is seldom trivial.

Alleged Assault

In the setting of assaults, knowing what the patient was hit with and how many times will direct you to where you are expecting to find injuries, knowing if it was witnessed or unwitnessed can give important information regarding secondary possible injuries (such as a hidden stab wound, or head strike when falling or the development of rhabdomyolysis if the patient has been left unconscious for hours or days).

Penetrating Trauma

The two key factors for determining what injuries a patient may have in a penetrating trauma are the velocity of the projectile and where the patient was hit.

High Velocity vs Low Velocity

A low velocity weapon is defined as those travelling at <2000 fps (609 mps). These include stab wounds and small caliber pistols and rifles. In these types of injuries, the damage that occurs is in the line of the projectiles path. There is no cavitation and while a bullet may bounce off bone or move within tissue planes, the damage is in the line of the projectile. When examining these patients, always look for both entrance and exit wounds from the projectile, particularly in penetrating injury to the intestine where there can be some distance between entry and exit wound. A stab wound to the abdomen will have a predictable course, should management proceed to a laparotomy, damaged organs are typically in line with what was stabbed or path of the bullet, but not always, beware of dismissing as "tangential" a single identified wound.

High velocity weapons have a different and more devastating pattern of injury. Beyond 2000 fps, (690 mps) bullets cause a large area of cavitation due to pressure transmission, they become unstable and tumble, resulting in extensive tissue damage much greater than the diameter of the projectile. They will often have small entry wounds and large exit wounds. High velocity projectiles can result in traumatic amputation of limbs and devastating intra-abdominal and intra-thoracic events, they were designed to cause maximum injury.

Blast Injuries

Blast injuries from explosions are unique and have 4 phases of injury to be considered:

1. The percussion phase: this results in a combination of blunt trauma from the shockwave and potential burn injuries to the patient from any combustible element.

2. Projectile phase: most explosions result in debris being thrown at various speeds into patients, resulting in potential penetrating or multiple penetrating injuries of varying velocities that need to be assessed.
3. Blunt injury phase: as a patient is thrown from the explosion, they will eventually impact something that stops them moving, being it a wall or the ground. From this, they may have patterns of injury that mimic blunt trauma.
4. Barotrauma phase: this is a unique form of injury that is linked to the percussion phase and predominately affects air filled organs (lungs, ears, gastrointestinal tract) but can also effect fluid filled structures such as the eyes. With the sudden compression and decompression of any air-filled or fluid filled organ, barotrauma will occur. The significance of this may not be evident for days, as the tissue necrosis that is associated will not be immediately apparent. These patients may deteriorate days after their initial trauma from the explosion due to intestinal ischemia, or blast related lung injuries.

Patient Frailty Index

Understating the patient's frailty guides how significant their injuries will be from the causative trauma. It also helps determine how much reserve a patient will have before they decompensate and eventually succumb to their injuries. An elderly osteoporotic patient can sustain significant trauma from even a minor event, whereas a young fit patient can sustain far greater forces on their body without injury (a fall from 2 meters will have a substantially different injury pattern in a 95 year old compared with a 15 year old). Similarly to this, the frail patient will decompensate early from more minor injuries (lower blood volume, less cardiac and respiratory reserve), whereas more robust patients will compensate for far longer. This can be an important trap for managing younger trauma patients however, as they have the ability to mask more severe injuries and lull the clinician into a false sense of security.

Expected and Patterns of Injury

Putting the above factors from the patient's mechanism of injury together allows a good clinician to determine what they expect a patient to have, even before they have seen them.

A pedestrian who has been hit by a car, is expected to have long bone injuries where the car hit them, and if they were thrown into the air: truncal injuries from where they went over the car and head/neck injuries from the windscreen and ground. Therefore these are the areas of special focus in the trauma examination but are still only part of the whole examination.

A patient who has been stabbed in the arm, provided they have not been assaulted anywhere else, should not have injuries outside of this anticipated area. Knowledge of the expected pattern of injury must not stop a full clinical examination of the patient essential in all trauma patients.

Patients Medical History

While a standard medical history is necessary, in the setting of trauma, the essential part of the history relates to what will immediately impact patient resuscitation and potential immediate surgical intervention. The AMPLE acronym is useful for this.

Allergies: specifically but not only to antibiotics and analgesic medication. In the setting of trauma these are often readily delivered and knowledge of potential anaphylaxis is essential to prevent complicating the patient's resuscitation.

Medication: A thorough medication review is not needed in the acute trauma setting. Medications that will immediately change clinical management are crucial, these include: anticoagulants, steroid use and insulin dependence. Similarly use of beta blockers can alter a patient's observations and prevent or mask detection of decompensation.

Past medical history: cardiac and respiratory function are critical as they can determine a patient's reserve, as well as be important for their resuscitation (a patient with known cardiac failure is important when resuscitating the patient).

Last oral intake guides planning, precautions and timing of surgical intervention. If immediate surgery is required, then this information is vital. If a patient is not fasted and requires a less urgent procedure, it may be more prudent to wait until gastric emptying has occurred to prevent potential aspiration.

Environment: was the patient exposed to the elements for a prolonged time. Was there a delay to presentation?

Trauma Examination

The trauma examination is a protocolized, therefore a consistent and reproducible assessment of the patient's injuries divided into primary survey, secondary survey and tertiary survey. It focuses on identifying and correcting issues in a stepwise manner prioritizing those that present the most immediate threat to life and function. The structured nature allows for it to be reproducible and interpreted between clinicians, allowing for deterioration to be rapidly identified and acted upon.

Primary Survey

The primary survey in the trauma bay is the same as the first responders' primary survey (DRSABC), with the addition of more advanced treatment measures. The treating doctor should not proceed to the next phase of the primary survey until they have completed the step they are performing. Ideally in the major trauma setting, a team approach is utilized allowing different operators to be performing different jobs simultaneously, overseen by the team leader directing the resuscitation. The allocation of tasks ideally should be planned following discussion with the primary responders before arrival of the patient or patients.

C: Correction of Life Threatening in Bleeding

Any catastrophic bleeding must be stopped in a fast and efficient manner. This does not need to be the definitive treatment for the traumatic injury, but a temporizing measure to allow for the rest of the primary survey to be conducted, and ideally proceed to secondary survey and investigation of the stable patient. It includes tourniquets for traumatically amputated limbs, splinting of femoral fractures, manual pressure to acute arterial bleeding, pelvic binders for pelvic fractures. If these issues are not immediately addressed, it is not possible to proceed effectively with further resuscitation.

A: Airway

Confirming a patent airway is the first step in a resuscitation scenario. It may be obvious from the outset at either end of the patency spectrum (a patient who is able to talk to you has a patent airway, an obtunded patient, or patient with severe facial injuries [gunshot wound, severe facial fractures] heaving and unable to move air does not). The assessment and management go hand in hand.

Examination of the Airway

Look and listen check the patient's mouth for debris or dislodged dentures. If present, remove them. Snoring and other upper airway sounds demonstrate an unprotected airway.

Obviously Patent Airway

These patients often present talking or are breathing on their own in the trauma bay, make sure there are no transmitted upper airway sounds.

Partially Obstructed Airway

These patients often are often obtunded or have debris or foreign material in their mouth on arrival. Assessment of their oropharyngeal area to remove debris may be required (such as false teeth or blood). Typically, simple airway maneuvers are enacted to allow for appropriate ventilation of the patient, either spontaneously or with bag and mask ventilation, (jaw thrust and chin lift, insertion of an oropharyngeal airway). Nasopharyngeal airways should be avoided as base of skull fractures or cribriform plate fractures may result in mal positioning. Start with the simple maneuvers before moving onto more advanced ones.

It is important to note that while a patient may have a patent airway now, that may not be the case in the immediate future. Bag-mask ventilation of a patient is resource intensive and tiring, if this is the only way then a definite airway is required. Similarly, in patients with facial burns, those who are shocked and those who are going to require immediate lifesaving interventions are often best served with early intubation (chest tube placement, major trauma surgical interventions).

Obstructed Airway

Intubation or a surgical airway may be required. Patients who obviously have an obstructed airway require either intubation or a surgical airway. In the absence of severe facial trauma, intubation is preferable, however if this is not achievable then a surgical airway should be obtained. Other reasons a patient may require a surgical airway may become obvious as you proceed through the primary survey (patients whose airways are currently patient but this is unlikely to last [GCS < 8, facial burns], inability to ventilate due to severe thoracic trauma, circulatory collapse due to multi system trauma).

Once you are confident the patient has a safe and established airway, you proceed to assessing the patients breathing effort.

**Trauma Pearl: It is at this stage that you should be considering putting on a C Spine collar or sandbagging the patients head. If in doubt, or you have no clinical history, one should be placed. Major trauma patients should be treated in full spinal precautions until the spine is cleared, which is an early but not emergency priority.

Breathing

Assessment of ventilation of the patient involves the look, listen, and feel while measuring the patient's ability to ventilate.

Look: with the patient completely exposed, look for rise and fall of the chest wall bilaterally. It should be symmetrical and regular. If intubated or being bag mask ventilated, fogging of the tube or mask is a sign of air movement. At this point, you are also looking for evidence of thoracic trauma that may need to be immediately addressed (open sucking chest wounds, clinical tension pneumothorax). Bruising and abrasions may also suggest underlying rib fractures. Paradoxical chest wall movement is a sign of a flail chest segment, and if present should be splinted to decrease both pain and work of breathing when appropriate.

Listen: bilateral lung auscultation is required for all patients. Symmetrical breath sounds are normal and what is expected. Absence of breath sounds may either suggest a pneumothorax or haemothorax or both, which need to be addressed immediately if causing hemodynamic compromise.

Feel: during this part of the exam, you are assessing for signs of tension pneumothorax (contra lateral tracheal deviation with ipsilateral barreling and hyper-resonant percussion of the chest wall), subcutaneous emphysema (considered synonymous with a pneumothorax in the trauma setting. Be wary of this sign, as these patients may go on to develop a tension pneumothorax as they are decompressing into their soft tissues) and may have unidentified penetrating thoracic injuries.

Measure: check the patients' respiratory rate and saturations, use pulse oximetry. If hypoxic they require greater oxygenation (nasal prongs, Hudson mask, high flow respirator, increased oxygen delivery on the ventilator). The aim in the trauma setting should be 95–100% in this primary survey phase.

**unilateral barreling of the chest, absent breath sounds, distended neck veins and tracheal deviation may all be signs of a tension pneumothorax that requires immediate decompression (needle thoracostomy or chest tube placement).

**trauma pearl: supplemental oxygen is considered free in the trauma setting. Have no hesitation to give it.

Circulation

Assessment of the circulation involves measuring the patient's heart rate and blood pressure, capillary refill and if they are peripherally shut down.

Looking: check the patient's general pallor and color. Are they pale, diaphoretic clammy and cold? These suggest circulatory collapse and aggressive resuscitation is often required.

Measuring: check the heart rate and blood pressure. Tachycardia is the first response to hypovolemia. Patients becoming hypotensive is a later sign particularly in the young and is suggestive of circulatory collapse. While there are many causes for tachycardia in the trauma setting (pain, stress), it should be assumed it is due to blood loss until proven otherwise.

**trauma pearl: 2 large bore cannulas should be inserted at this point in the trauma assessment.

**traumatic resuscitation is best performed with blood products (they have lost blood, so replace it). Crystalloids can be used sparingly as required, but take care as they can cause hypothermia, electrolyte derangement, third space fluid overload and coagulopathy in large volumes.

Disability: Measure and document the patients Glasgow Coma Scale (GCS). This is a guide to potential head trauma, and also to those patients who will be unable to protect their own airway in the trauma setting (a GCS < 8 typically requires intubation in the trauma setting).

AVPU is a quick useful assessment (Alert, Verbal, Pain Response, and Unresponsive).

Exposure: ensure that the patient is completely exposed. All clothing should be removed, as should bandages and dressings placed pre-trauma to ensure adequate immediate hemorrhage control is being achieved. It is vitally important however to avoid the patient becoming hypothermic in the trauma assessment area as resuscitation fluids may be cold, and the triad of hypothermia, coagulopathy and acidosis needs to be prevented.

Adjuncts to the Primary Survey

The primary survey is not complete without additional bedside adjuncts being performed. These include F.A.S.T. Scanning (assessing intra-abdominal free fluid, pericardial effusions, pneumothoraxes', pleural adhesions and pleural fluid), chest X-ray and pelvic X-ray. These can be performed at the bedside and provide vital information in guiding the patients resuscitation.

The primary assessment can be performed very quickly (less than 10 s in a well patient) or be a difficult long process in the severe trauma patient. It is important to note during this time that patients who have refractory shock may have critical intra-thoracic or intra-abdominal bleeding, and resuscitative thoracotomies or laparotomy with packing may be required as part of the immediate resuscitative process.

Secondary Survey

The secondary survey should be performed when the primary survey and resuscitation has the patient stabilized, or as stable as they are going to be become in the trauma setting (it may not be possible to achieve normal physiology while the patient is internally bleeding). It involves a full examination of the fully exposed torso with exposure of covered wounds, assessing and documenting all traumatic injuries in a systematic way. Often pre-filled trauma assessment documents will make this easier to document and ultimately make you more methodical and efficient in your assessment.

General Inspection

Take a moment to look at the patient from the end of the bed. Do they look well, or unwell? This may seem redundant in many trauma situations; however it is vitally important to prepare yourself for the pathology you expect to find. A patient who looks well may have something wrong with them, but a patient who looks unwell definitely will.

Head

Look: look at their head for obvious lacerations and open fractures. Check for raccoon eyes and bruising behind the ears which may suggest a base of skull fracture. Check to see if there is blood or fluid leaking from their ears or nose. Examine inside their mouth for injuries and missing teeth CXR to exclude inhalation.

Feel: examine the patients' whole head. You are examining for obvious soft tissue injuries (lacerations on the face and in the hair line) and evidence of skull fractures (depressed areas, boggy areas, obvious open cranial fractures). Palpate the patients' orbital margins, cheek bones, and mandible for tenderness. Check their tympanic membranes for hemotympanum or any obvious inner ear trauma.

**asking if it feels normal when the patient bites their teeth together is a very sensitive way to detect mandibular fractures or damage to the patients teeth.

Neurological: perform an abbreviated cranial nerve examination. Ask if they can see your finger in front of their eyes (CN2). Then check all eye movements (CN3/4/6). Check pupillary size and reflexes, ask them to raise their eyebrows, squeeze their eyes shut, blow their cheeks out (CN7), poke their tongue forward (CN12), shrug their shoulders (CN11) and assess for sensation in the regions of CN5. Check their hearing (CN8). While this is in not a complete cranial nerve exam, it is a quick and reliable baseline to document and compare to in the future.

Neck

Look: Look for bruising, swelling (both soft tissue and venous) and lacerations to the neck. Remove the patient's C spine collar safely while doing so. Swellings and bruising of the neck are ominous features in the trauma setting, as carotid dissections and tracheo/laryngeal injuries are often difficult to examine for. Have a low threshold for getting CT imaging of these areas in the setting of trauma.

Feel: Examine for tracheal deviation (again) and assess for any C Spine or soft tissue tenderness which may mandate further imaging.

***Pearl:* neck swelling is an ominous sign in the trauma setting. These patients may have contained hematoma and are at risk of losing their airway.

Chest

Look: like the assessment during the primary survey, reassess for any new bruising or injuries that may have been missed initially. The trauma setting is dynamic and often new injuries will be identified.

Feel: Palpate the clavicles bilaterally, ballot the patient's sternum for tenderness (sternal fractures signify a high impact trauma) and spring the patients ribs bilaterally assessing for any fractures. Reassess for any penetrating injuries or new subcutaneous emphysema which may have developed in the interim.

Abdomen

Look: look for penetrating wounds, lacerations, abrasions and bruising of the patient's abdomen. Penetrating wounds from knives are often multiple, and their location should be clearly documented. If a gunshot wound is identified, always assess for the presence of an exit wound. Always remember penetrating wounds are often angulated, so it is not just the organs immediately deep to where the wound is that may have been injured (an epigastric stab wound can range from the heart to the aortic bifurcation, with the same range laterally). It is also essential to document bruising around the abdomen. Obvious areas (such as under seatbelts) may have associated fat fracturing and pain, however atypical bruising (such as bilateral flank bruising) can suggest retroperitoneal organ injury and hematoma formation.

Feel: examine the patient's abdomen in all 4 quadrants. Document any local tenderness or abdominal masses.

Is patient peritonitic or not? This is the most important question in the abdominal trauma examination. Peritonitic patients require surgical intervention, with or without further imaging (based upon patient hemodynamic stability). All patients will have local tenderness around bruises, but if a patient has peritonitis after an abdominal trauma, they will require surgical intervention.

Pelvis

Look: bruising, lacerations and penetrating wounds should be identified and documented, as with the abdomen.

Feel: palpate the pubic symphysis for tenderness. Gently spring the patient's pelvis for mobility. If there is a suggestion of pelvic instability, a pelvic binder should be immediately placed. Assess their femoral pulses for presence and character. The patients' genitals and perineum should be examined at this point.

Upper Limb and Lower Limbs

Look: assess for any obvious bony deformity (angulation, shortening, and swelling) and associated open wounds. An open wound over a fracture should be considered to be communicating unless clearly otherwise. Document any bruising and lacerations that require treatment.

Feel: examine the entire limb for tenderness:

Arm: acromioclavicular joint, humerus, radius, ulnar, carpal bones including the anatomical snuff box, and hands.

Leg: femur, patella, tibia and fibulae in their entirety and metatarsals. Any bony tenderness should be imaged. Any obvious fracture should be reduced, immobilized and should have the joint above and below imaged.

All peripheral pulses should be checked to make sure symmetrical and present. If not the case, it must be assumed this is from the trauma and urgently managed (compartment syndrome, traumatic dissections or transactions are surgical emergencies).

Neurological: assess for tone, power and sensation of the limbs. (This can be done quickly and bilaterally).

In the upper limb: Get the patient to abduct their arms against resistance, flex and extend the elbow against resistance, flex and extend the wrist against resistance, cross their fingers, give a "thumbs up" and check their thumb and index finger opposition strength). Then assess sensation bilaterally in all dermatomes.

In the lower limb: get the patient to raise their leg against resistance, push their leg into the bed, bend their knee against resistance, straighten it against resistance, Dorsiflex and plantarflex their angle against resistance, extend and flex their great toe against resistance. This will often need to be done one leg at a time, then compared with the opposite.

Any abnormality will require a full formal neurological assessment, and further consideration of spinal or plexus injuries. However if these are grossly normal in the secondary setting, this should be documented and is reassuring.

Log Roll

This require several people to help with spinal stabilization, injuries through the back are important and easily missed parts of the trauma assessment. With the patient rolled, you must.

Look: assess for any penetrating, lacerations, or bruises to the back of the chest and abdomen. Have a scribe handy documenting your findings as you dictate your findings as this step is often painful for the patient and should be done quickly and thoroughly.

Feel: palpate the patient's entire spine for tenderness and document any areas of pain. Ensure sensation of their back is intact, and finally check their perianal sensation and ask them to squeeze their buttocks together.

**a convenient time to do this is when transferring a patient between beds (from ambulance trolley to the trauma bed or similar).

Special Examinations

Spinal injuries: in the setting of a suspected spinal injury: a full upper and lower neurological examination is required (assessing tone, power, sensation, reflexes and coordination). Documentation of this is often protocolized depending on your hospital and spinal service.

Pelvic injuries: If a pelvic injury is suspected then the patient requires a PR exam, PV exam and retrograde urethrogram.

In all severe trauma a whole of body contrast CT scan is an essential part of the examination but is directed by clinical examination.

Tertiary Survey

The tertiary survey essential and as important as the primary and secondary survey. It is performed at least 24 to 48 h after the trauma admission, when the patient is stable, or has had their definitive trauma imaging and emergency primary surgery performed. It involves 2 phases.

First Phase: Examination

This examination is identical to the secondary survey, but in more detail. Without distracting injuries (pain from long bone fractures, shock from the initial accident), other injuries will often be identified. Typically missed injuries are non-displaced fractures, however in the authors experience craino-cervical dislocations and open book pelvic fractures have been identified at this stage, especially when the patient was intubated or non-communicative on arrival. Any bony tenderness should be considered fractured and imaged unless already performed. If the patient's examination is incongruous with their imaging, look harder at it! Tibial plateau fractures can be subtle, as can hairline fractures. Trust the patient's examination more than X-rays, and be kind to your radiologist because the answer is not always obvious.

Second Phase: Imaging

Any new injuries need to be imaged appropriately. Additionally all the patients imaging up to this point should be re-reviewed and documented. All traumatic injuries should be documented, along with the plans for that injury. Ideally all imaging should be formally reported at this stage to ensure nothing is missed.

Tips in Management of Trauma Patient

- Consider the position of the victim during the injury specially the bullet injuries "Like bending forwards for example", which can make the bullet move in the body in an unexpected path. An example is an entry point of bullet injury just above the iliac crest caused an injury in the mid-rectum which had been missed during the initial and second operation.
- Inspect the neck veins at early examination of trauma patient if distended we have to suspect intra-Thoracic cause of Shock e.g. Tension pneumothorax or Pericardial tamponade which will need immediate confirmation by auscultation and urgent intervention.
- All major trauma patient should be suspected to have a cervical spine injury and stabilization of the neck in relation to the body should be done through all the stages of transportation or examination. The use of Cervical collar may be advised or alternatively, the so called longboard, on which the patient is laid and then attached by the straps, until confirmation or exclusion of Cervical spine injury by X-ray.
- The contour of the abdomen when abnormally distended, after a major injury in a shocked patient who failed to be resuscitated using the initial 2 liters of initial resuscitation has to lead to an aspiration bedside examination of the abdomen with or without FAST "Focused Abdominal sonography for trauma", for suggested massive intra-abdominal exploration as a part of resuscitation to stop a massive intra-abdominal bleeding from a major vessel to allow for resuscitation.
- A scaphoid abdomen after a major blunt trauma like compression injury of the abdomen between a car and the wall has to raise the possibility of a ruptured

diaphragm and herniated intra-abdominal viscera "mainly stomach and Colon into the left thoracic cavity. A misinterpretation of a plain X-ray chest as a Pneumo-Hemothorax may lead to a mistake of insertion of A Chest tube into those viscera.

- **Bed-side Diagnostic Procedure** such as needle aspiration from the chest or abdomen or DPL "Diagnostic Abdominal Lavage" can be considered as a Clinical skill or an investigation among radiology.

Chapter 25
Clinical Examination of Thoracic Surgery

Sandhya Chalasani

Abstract Aims of clinical exam: to identify disease, to plan surgery and to identify problems that may delay recovery. Surface Anatomy includes Bony landmarks: The first rib is not palpable. Second rib joins the manubrium just above the sternal angle. The first rib space is just above and lateral to the sternal angle. Costal margin is formed by the 7–10 ribs along with 11 and 12.

Keywords Chest · Lung · Thoracic · Pleura · Heart · Examination · Sheet · Anatomy · Landmarks · Auscultation

Aims of clinical exam: to identify disease, to plan surgery and to identify problems that may delay recovery.

Surface Anatomy (Table 25.1)

Bony landmarks: The first rib is not palpable. Second rib joins the manubrium just above the sternal angle. The first rib space is just above and lateral to the sternal angle. Costal margin is formed by the 7–10 ribs along with 11 and 12.

Incisions

- Median sternotomy—gold standard midline incision used for most cardiac procedures and for heart-lung transplant.
- Anterior mediastinotomy—This incision is a transverse incision along 2nd intercostal space laterally from parasternal edge. Its often used to perform a Chamberlain procedure and care should be taken to avoid damaging the internal mammary artery.

S. Chalasani (✉)
General Surgery, SVUH, Dublin, Ireland

A. Farag et al. (eds.), *Clinical Surgical Skills Made Easy*,
https://doi.org/10.1007/978-3-031-69158-4_25

Table 25.1 Landmark structure

Landmark	Structure
C6	Cricoid cartilage
T2	Suprasternal notch
T4/5	Sternal angle of Louis and bifurcation of trachea
T9	Xiphisternal joint
T8	Inferior angle of scapula
T3	Spine of scapula posteriorly
T3—6th costal cartilage	Oblique fissure
5th Rib	Horizontal fissure
1 cm lateral to sternal edge	Internal thoracic arteries
Second and 3rd right costal cartilages	SVC origin from Innominate veins
Upper right 5th rib at midclavicular line	Right hemi-diaphragm
Lower left 5th rib at midclavicular line	Left hemi-diaphragm

- Anterior thoracotomy—transverse incision from parasternal edge along the inframammary crease to the anterior axillary line in the 4th interspace. The pectoralis major muscle can be elevated off the chest.
- Thoraco-sternotomy ('clamshell')—incision from anterior axillary line along inframammary crease bilaterally elevating in the midline to the level of the nipple. The pectoralis major is raised as a flap and the sternum is divided transversely.
- Lateral 'muscle-sparing' thoracotomy—lazy 'S' incision along the submammary crease starting below nipple passing upwards towards the axilla.
- Lateral thoracotomy—curvilinear incision passing from the anterior axillary line to 2 cm below the tip of scapula.
- Posterolateral thoracotomy—curvilinear incision from anterior axillary line passing 3–4 cm below tip of scapula and continuing superiorly halfway between medial border of scapula and spinous processes of vertebral column. This incision involves dividing the latissimus dorsi and serratus anterior.
- Thoracoabdominal incision—oblique incision similar to the posterolateral incision but extending anteriorly across the costal margin at the level of the 7th intercostal space towards the midline.

Physiology of Breathing

Breathing is stimulated by the rising levels of carbon dioxide in the blood. When the diaphragm descends there is an increase in the intra-thoracic pressure. The intrapulmonary pressure decreases drawing air into the lungs as the pressure outside of the lungs is greater than the pressure inside. Lungs are elastic and naturally tend to recoil with pleura. The elasticity creates a negative pressure and causes the lungs to inflate.

Lungs are surrounded by pleura which have a thin layers of fluid between them. The Intra-pleural pressure is always negative (−4 cm H_2O) but during inspiration is more negative (−8 cm H_2O). On expiration its less negative (−4 cm H_2O). Loss of the intra-pleural pressure due to penetrating trauma can cause the lung to collapse and a chest drain with an underwater seal may be required to restore the correct pressures.

Examination

General Inspection

- Medications and bedside paraphernalia of lung
- Disease (spirometers/inhalers)
- Cyanosis
- Dyspnea
- Signs of COPD (barrel chest, use of accessory muscles of respiration—"pink puffers" or "blue bloaters").
- Cough—nature of cough (productive or dry).
- Sputum—color of sputum (whitish, yellow, green, bloody).
- Stridor.
- Wheezes.
- Hoarseness.

Hands

(a) Clubbing—Hypertrophic Pulmonary
(b) Osteoarthropathy (lung cancer)
(c) Nails (nicotine staining)
(d) Pallor (anemia)
(e) Flapping tremor/asterixis (CO_2 retention)
(f) Pulse—rate/bounding pulse (CO_2 retention)
(g) Wasting and weakness—T1 nerve compression from Tumors e.g. Pancoast's tumor.

Face

(a) Plethora—SVC syndrome
(b) Leathery skin and wrinkled—smoker
(c) Horner's syndrome—Pancoast's tumor (ptosis, miosis and facial anhidrosis)—C8/T1 compression of nerve root due to tumor
(d) Tongue for central cyanosis
(e) Puffiness—central cyanosis

Neck

(a) Trachea displacement.
    - Towards Lung collapse, fibrosis, pneumonectomy.
    - Away Tension pneumothorax, Massive effusion Retrosternal goitre.
(b) Lymph nodes.
(c) JVP—raised JVP—Venous hypertension—caused by pulmonary hypertension, Heart failure, pericardial Tamponade. In an acute situation it may indicate a pericardial hematoma or Tension Pneumothorax.
(d) Use of accessory muscles of respiration such as the Sternomastoid, Pectoral muscles and Latissimus Dorsi.

Chest

Patient should be positioned at 45 degrees at the edge of the bed and appropriately exposed.

Inspection

Deformities

- Barrel chest (COPD).
- Kyphoscoliosis.
- Pectus Carinatum.
- Pectus Excavatum.
- Poland syndrome .
- Cleft Sternum—rare genetic disorder due to failure of fusion of sternum.

- Thoracic Ectopic Cordis—complete or partial Displacement of the heart outside the thoracic Cavity.
- Asphyxiating thoracic dystrophy (Jeune syndrome)
- Spondylothoracic dysplasia (Jarcho Levin Syndrome)

Tumors

- Primary chest wall tumors: Benign/malignant - Sarcoma, Desmoid tumors.
- Secondary chest wall tumors—breast, lung and Thyroid cancer" Follicular type".

Thoracic Outlet Syndrome

- Adson test—Loss of the radial pulse in the arm by rotating head to the ipsilateral side with neck extended on deep inspiration.
- Halsted test—loss of radial pulse when arm is abducted to 45 degrees and should extended at 45 degrees and externally rotated upward extremity while applying a downward distraction to the arm.
- Wright test—Loss of radial pulse with arm.
- Hyperabducted and externally rotated.
- Roos test—patient flex their arms and elbows to 90 degrees with their elbows braced somewhat posteriorly. Have the patient open and close their fists at a moderate speed for 3 min.

Chest Trauma

- Paradoxical movement of chest wall—Flail chest/diaphragmatic paralysis secondary to trauma or nerve damage.
- Bleeding.
- Foreign body impaled.
- Open pneumothorax.
- Unequal sides of the chest as a sign of tension Haemothorax, Pneumothorax, or Haemo-Pneumothorax.
- Tracheal shift and or Laryngeal tilt.

Palpation

- Tenderness (fractures pathological or trauma, tumors invasion, shingles).
- Tactile fremitus.

- Chest expansion normal being 5 cm—Hoover sign in Over-expanded COPD." I.e. lung hyperinflation leading to a flattened diaphragm which causes the lower rib cage to move paradoxically during inhalation, in an inward direction rather than normally outwards".

Percussion

- Dullness—effusion (transudative or exudative) or haemothorax or pneumonia.
- Hyper resonance—COPD.
- Traub's area.

Auscultation

- Intensity of breath sounds—reduced in collapse, pleural effusion, neoplasm, COPD, pneumothorax.
- Bronchial breath sounds—pneumonia, fibrosis, effusion, lung collapse.
- Added sounds:
    - Wheeze (Expiratory).
    - high pitched with Asthma.
    - Low pitched with COPD.
    - Stridor (both inspiratory and expiratory)—obstruction.
    - Early inspiratory crackles—COPD.
    - Late inspiratory crackles.
    - Fine crackles—ILD.
    - Medium crackles—left ventricular heart failure.
    - Coarse crackles—bronchiectasis.
    - Vocal resonance—Pulmonary consolidation.
    - Whispered pectoriloquy refers to an increased loudness of whispering noted during auscultation with a stethoscope on the lung fields.
    - Despine sign: It is a bronchial breathing heard over the vertebral spines (on the back) below the level of tracheal bifurcation; below the fourth thoracic spine in adults if there is subcarinal (Mediastinal) lymphadenopathy.

Chest Drains

Principles of Underwater Seal Drainage

The main aim of a chest drain is the remove air/fluid from the intrapleural space and preventing it from re-entry. Negative pressure during inspiration causes the water level in the tube to rise and positive pressure during expiration pushes the fluid out. Air bubbles out of the tube into the underwater seal. Fluid drains via gravity mixing with water and raising the fluid level.

How to Insert a Chest Drain—Step Wise Approach (Fig. 25.1)

Relevant anatomy—Triangle of safety: posteriorly is the anterior border of latissimus dorsi, anteriorly is the lateral border of the pectoralis major, and inferiorly is the fifth intercostal space and apex below the axilla.

British Thoracic Society guidelines for insertion of surgical chest drain

1. Position—patient at 45 degrees and arm elevated above head.
2. Ensure all required materials are opened in a sterile fashion and ready to use.
3. Identify landmarks—palpate 5th intercostal space and identify triangle of safety. It often helps to draw out the triangle of safety in patients.
4. Surgically prepare the area.
5. Administer local anaesthetic layer by layer.
6. Incise skin parallel to the upper border of the chosen rib.
7. Blunt dissect using a Roberts forceps until you feel a give into pleural cavity.
8. Widen the hole and place finger into the cavity and do a finger sweep.
9. Stay sutures/closing suture are generally place in a horizontal mattress suture format to help swift tying off the skin when chest drain is removed at a later stage once its served its desired purpose (Fig. 25.2).
10. Hold the tube with the clamp and direct it superiorly for pneumothorax or inferiorly for pleural effusions while ensuring the other end of the tube is clamped off using non crushing chest drain clamps so that air doesn't enter chest cavity. Ensure the sentinel eye is well within the chest. The black dots should (usually two of them on wide bore surgical drains) must not be visible.
11. Holding suture placed onto tube. Ensure that this suture is not pulling on the skin - a thick bite but not tight should be taken using 1 ethilon or heavy silk suture.
12. Drain is connected to the under-water seal and one should look for "swinging" of the fluid. If there is no swing as soon as the tube is inserted it often means that the tube is misplaced or kinked and this needs to be looked into immediately.

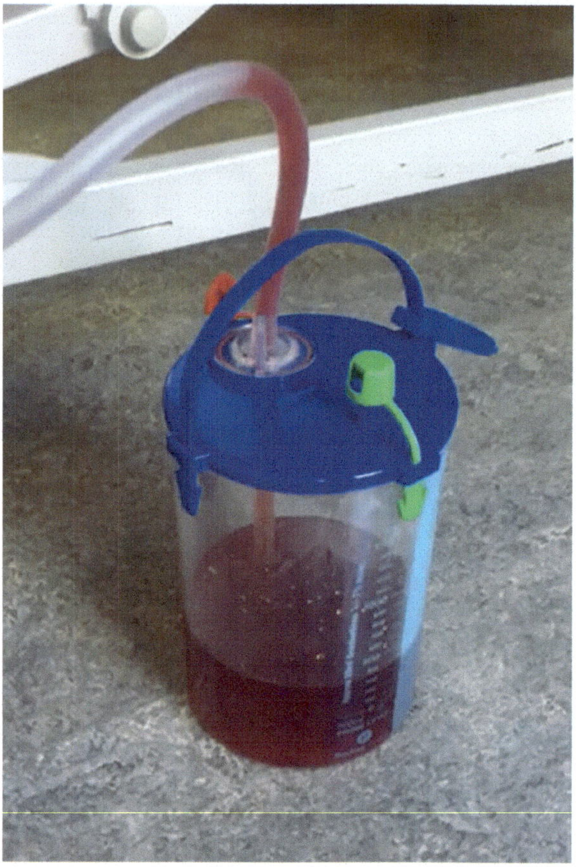

Fig. 25.1 Underwater seal

Assessment of Chest Drains

When one is called to assess a chest drain these are the features one needs to look into to understand what could be the underlying pathology.

1. Location—Is this an apical chest drain placed for pneumothorax or a basal chest drain placed for draining fluid (blood/pus, etc.). It is also important to note which side the chest drain is.
2. Pain—Larger surgical chest drains are often associated with increased amounts of pain as they press on the intercostal nerves. There is a huge variation in the analgesia pattern prescribed for these patients but most of them include: regular paracetamol, regular NSAIDs (PO/PR) along with a PPI, regular long acting opiates (titrated based on their renal function and weight), neuropathic pain killer (e.g. pregabalin) and prn short acting opiates. Some patients may need more analgesia and often a paravertebral block with catheter where continuous

Fig. 25.2 Stay suture

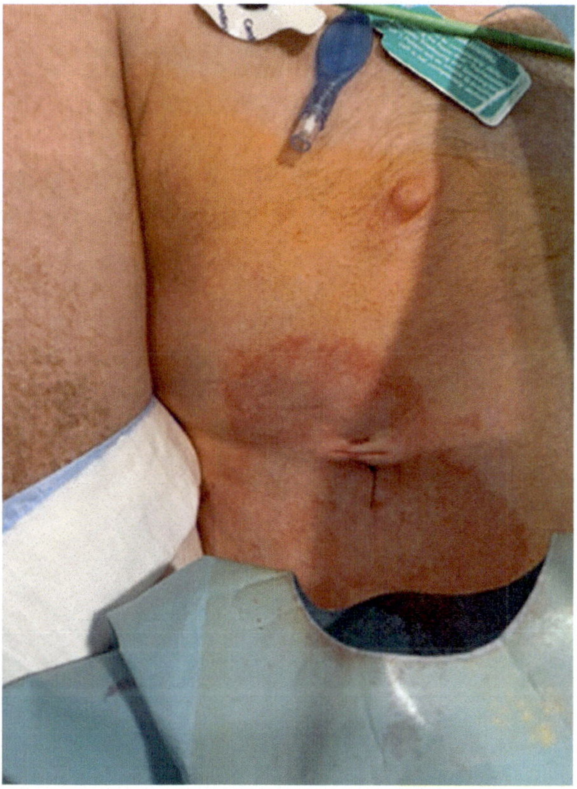

infusion of local anesthetic can be delivered can prove very useful while the chest drain is in position.

3. Subcutaneous emphysema—If there is crepitus in the skin it often signifies that the chest drain is blocked or there could be an air leak in the pulmonary ventilation. Placing the drain on suction often reduces the emphysema. Rarely upsizing of the chest drain may be required.
4. Swinging—If the drain does not swing as soon as it is placed it usually needs attention and is often due to the drain being kinked or misplaced (in the wrong layer). If the drain does not swing after a few days or gradually then it usually signifies that lung is fully expanded. If the drain has been placed on suction it could stop the swinging. In this scenario turn off the suction and see if the drain swings.
5. Bubbling—Bubbling of a chest drain signifies air leak. If the patient coughs once and there are bubbles it usually is not significant but recurrent bubbling after few coughs signifies air leak. Post robotic thoracic surgery sometime one could see air leaks for a prolonged periods of more than 24 h. In this scenario one should leave the drain in for an extra day or so for the air leak.
6. Drain level—amount of blood or serous fluid or pus. Quantity is recorded over 24 h period.

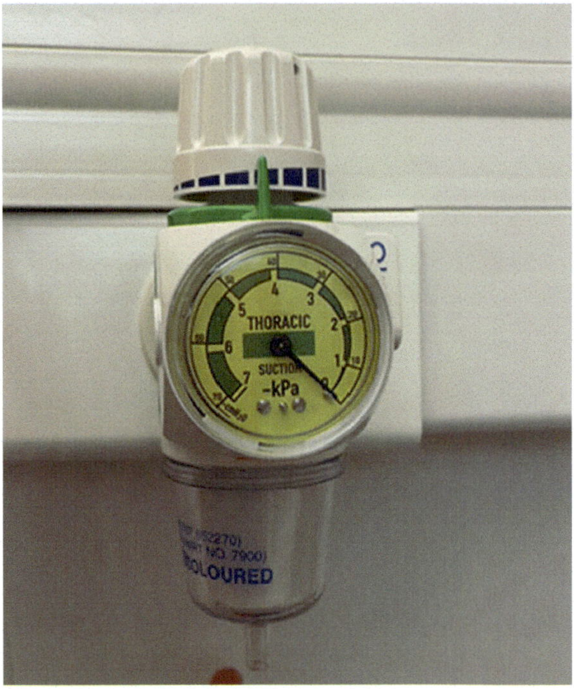

Fig. 25.3 The thoracic wall suction adapter

7. Suction—This is important in patients who have had pleurodesis procedure where we aim to obliterate the space quickly. Post thoracic surgery patients will often be placed on thoracic suction of 3–5 kPa generally. It is very important to familiarize oneself with the thoracic suction adaptor in your place of work. Wall suction that is used regularly on the wards is much higher and is different from the thoracic wall suction parameters. The thoracic wall suction adapter looks like this (Fig. 25.3).
8. CXR—any patient with a chest drain should have a chest x-ray on a daily basis.

Handling of Chest Drains

How to handle chest drains is as important as knowing how to insert them.

- One should familiarize themselves with the location of clamps in case of accidental disconnection. The nurses usually ensure clamps are placed by the patient's bedside.
- Under-water drains have to always be placed/held at a level lower than the insertion site.
- Drains should never be clamped unless its ready to be removed or while changing the underwater seal bottle if its full/damaged.

- If the chest drain is passed over the patient fluid from the bottle can traverse back into patients cavity. If this needs to be done during transfer etc. then the drain should be clamped very briefly.
- If there is accidental disconnection of chest drain from the underwater seal, clamp the drain and call for help immediately.
- If the tube falls out of chest cavity or sentinel eye is out then place some Vaseline soaked dressing and gauze and place pressure over the drain site. If the tube is half out take it out fully and place pressure (as above) over drain site and call for help.

When to remove a chest drain

- If the drain output is less than 100 ml in 24 h.
- If there is minimal swing in 24 h.
- There is no bubbling or air leak passively or on coughing.
- CXR confirms re-expansion.

Chapter 26
Peripheral Nerve and Hand Examination

Husam Hosny

Abstracts The hand is a complex organ composed of skin, subcutaneous tissue, neurovascular elements and musculoskeletal elements i.e. bones, joints, muscles and tendons. Those elements work in an integrated manner so that any lesion affecting one of them may have detrimental effects on hand function if left untreated. Thus assessment of the hand is never complete unless all these elements have been examined. Nerve lesions of surgical importance include nerve injuries, compression and tumours. Both sensory and motor functions should be evaluated. moreover, special and provocative tests are important for accurate diagnosis and follow up.

Keywords Hand · Nerves · Examination · Tests · Function · Deformity · Contracture · Injury

Introduction

The hand is a complex organ composed of skin, subcutaneous tissue, neurovascular elements and musculoskeletal elements i.e. bones, joints, muscles and tendons. Those elements work in an integrated manner so that any lesion affecting one of them may have detrimental effects on hand function if left untreated. Thus assessment of the hand is never complete unless all these elements have been examined.

Nerve pathologies of surgical importance include nerve injury, compression and tumors.

Nerve injury due to trauma is seldom isolated and commonly associated with other injuries e.g. bony fractures, tendon injuries, vascular injuries and muscle tear. Moreover, multiple nerves may be injured e.g. median and ulnar nerve injuries by wounds near the wrist. Thus examination of all these structures is essential in every

H. Hosny (✉)
Cairo University, Cairo, Egypt
e-mail: husamhosny@kasralainy.edu.eg

A. Farag et al. (eds.), *Clinical Surgical Skills Made Easy*,
https://doi.org/10.1007/978-3-031-69158-4_26

case of suspected nerve injury similar to examination of all abdominal organs and viscera in cases of abdominal trauma or disease.

Compression can affect multiple sites along the affected nerve coarse, thus examination of all sites of possible entrapment is paramount. Moreover, nerve compression at particular site decreases the threshold along other sites of compression of the same nerve due to changes in the interior environment of circulating substances and neurotransmitters within the affected nerve giving rise to additional symptoms of proximal compression in cases of distal compression and vice versa.

In cases of nerve compression, motor affection is a late sign, while sensory abnormalities start early even before electro-physiologic changes are detected, thus sensory examination and provocative tests are needed to early diagnose these cases before irreversible histo-pathologic changes occur.

Sensory receptors include slowly adapting receptors; concerned with static touch and quickly adapting receptors; concerned with moving touch. Clinical evaluation of sensory receptors includes assessment of sensory threshold (minimum stimulus needed to elicit a response) and innervation density (number of innervated receptors).

The aim of history and physical examination is to identify the level of the lesion, documentation of improvement or decline in motor and sensory functions and determination of treatment options.

History

Personal history: As usual with special emphasis on occupation and hand dominance.

Complaint:

- Altered sensation: complete loss of sensation (anesthesia) or abnormal sensation e.g. tingling, pricking, compression (paresthesia).
- Inability to perform a previous movement/ function.
- Deformity.

Present history: (How?—When?—Sequelae?)

- **Spontaneous** (nerve compression) or **related to trauma** (cut/lacerated wounds, crush injuries, fractures).
- **Time of injury** is crucial as denervated muscles for more than 12 months will pass into an irreversible degeneration and regain of function is unlikely even after nerve repair. This fact will determine the treatment options whether nerve repair or other options as proximal nerve transfer or tendon transfer may be needed.
- *Effect of the pathology on patient's quality of life* and psychological state. Patients may lose their job or change their career and psychological instability may occur.

Past history:

- Previous trauma or surgical intervention within the affected limb and its outcome.
- Exposure to neurotoxic substances e.g. lead or arsenic metals.
- Any chronic disease especially diabetes and leprosy, or comorbidities.

Examination

(See, feel & move).

- I - Inspection (see)
  (scars- swelling- wasting- deformity-trophic changes)

Posture: the patient is examined while sitting in front of the examiner resting his/her forearm and hand on a table or pillow. Both hands, forearms, arms, shoulders and neck should be exposed to compare both sides.

Start in a systematic way, from distal to proximal i.e. dorsum of fingers, hands, wrist, forearm, elbow and arm then ask the patient to turn his hands to inspect volar aspect of the whole limb and finally the neck.

1. Scars/wounds especially those over the course of the nerve or at sites of surgical decompression should be reported including its length, width, direction, and type of healing.
2. Swelling over the course of a nerve may arise from the nerve itself (neuroma or nerve tumor) or others compressing the nerve.
3. Wasting (compare both sides) at the areas of muscles supplied by the affected nerve will develop due to muscle atrophy in long standing cases. For instance, wasting of the medial aspect of the hand, 1st web space and guttering of hand dorsum occur due to atrophy of Hypothenar muscles, adductor pollicus and interossei muscles in cases of ulnar nerve injury (Fig. 26.1). In higher level ulnar

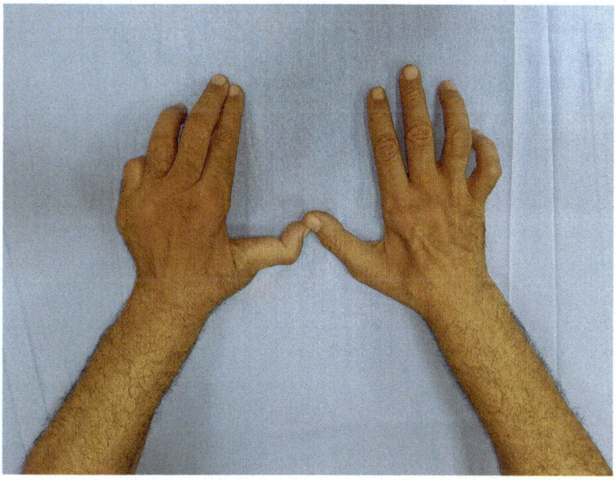

Fig. 26.1 Wasting of 1st web space, guttering at the hand dorsum and wasting at medial side of the right hand in ulnar nerve injury

nerve injury, wasting of the medial aspect of the forearm will occur due to atrophy of flexor carpi ulnaris.

Wasting of thenar area occurs in median nerve injury.

4. Deformity: the deformity is usually characteristic and reveals underlying nerve injury.

   Wrist drop and finger drop (due to paralysis of wrist and fingers extensors) occur in radial nerve injury (Fig. 26.2).

   Finger drop alone occurs in posterior interossei nerve injury.

   Partial claw hand (extension at 4th & 5th MP joints and flexion of interphalangeal joints of little and ring fingers) occur in distal ulnar nerve injury due to paralysis of interossei and medial two lumbricals muscles while finger flexors (FDS & FDP) and extensors action are unopposed (Fig. 26.3)

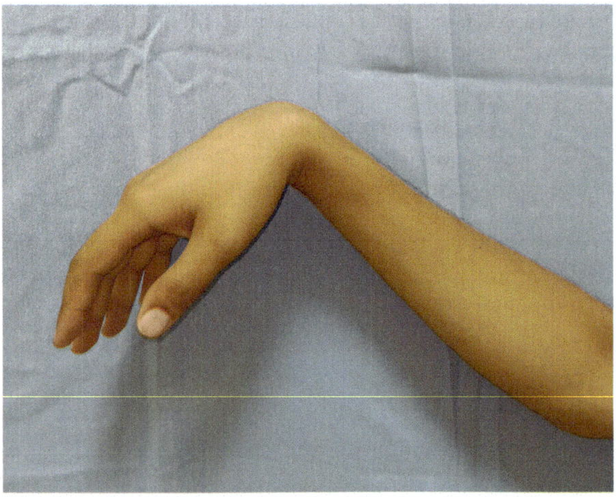

Fig. 26.2 Inability to extend the wrist "wrist drop" in case of radial nerve injury

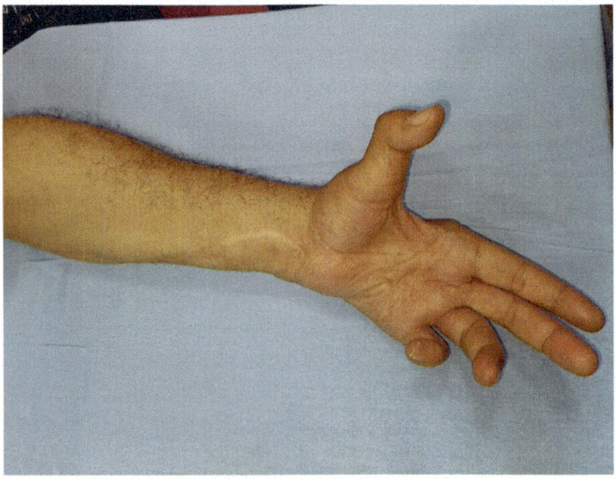

Fig. 26.3 "*Partial claw hand*" extension of 4th and 5th metacarpo-phalangeal joints while the interphalangeal joints are flexed in ulnar nerve injury

N.B. *Ulnar paradox* describes less deformity in cases of higher level ulnar nerve injury as paralysis of flexor carpi ulnaris (FCU) and flexor digitorum profundus (FDP) to the little and ring fingers results in less flexion deformity at interphalangeal joints.

Complete claw hand affecting all medial 4 fingers occurs in T1 lesions or combined ulnar and median nerves injury (Figure).

Ape hand deformity (flat hand at thenar eminence) occurs in median nerve injury due to atrophy of thenar muscles and loss of opposition.

Policeman tip deformity (shoulder adducted& internally rotated and elbow extended and pronated) occurs in upper brachial plexus injury due to paralysis of abductors and lateral rotators of the shoulder (deltoid, supra and infraspinatus muscles), and paralysis of elbow flexors and supinators (biceps, brachialis, brachioradialis and supinator muscles) (Fig. 26.4).

Any other deformity due to fractures malunion or soft tissue contractures e.g. Duputryn's contracture (Fig. 26.5) or post burn deformities should be recorded.

5. Trophic changes at the tips and nails of affected fingers may be present due to frequent trauma or burns that pass unnoticed.

II-Palpation: (feel)

- Assess hand vascularity by feeling both radial and ulnar arteries at the wrist.
- Capillary pulsation or/refill at each finger especially in cases of recent trauma.

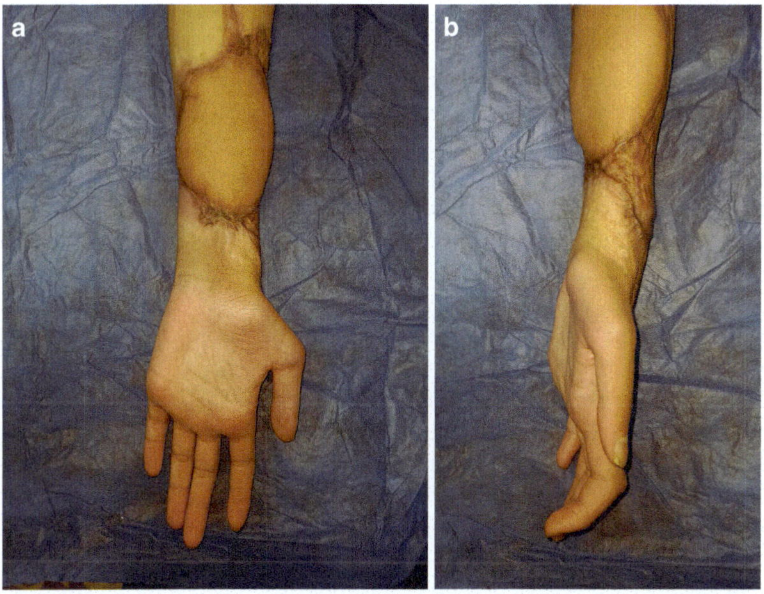

Fig. 26.4 Antero-posterior view (**a**), and lateral view (**b**) of the right hand; showing wasting and flattening of the thenar eminence due to median nerve injury. *Note a fasciocutaneous flap and skin graft reconstruction of the traumatic soft tissue defect at the anterior aspect of the forearm*

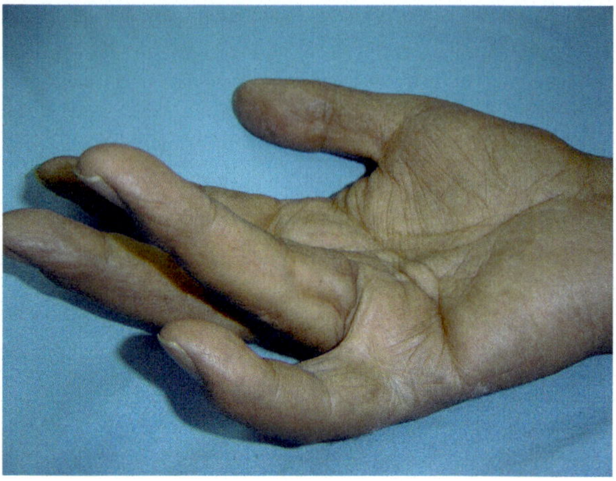

Fig. 26.5 Abnormal thickening of the skin and palmar fascia to form cord like structure and nodules pulling the ring finger towards the palm in *Dupuytren's disease*

- Feel (on the dorsum of the hand) along each finger and related metacarpal to elicit tenderness e.g. Fractures or abnormality e.g. nodules that are not visible.
- Feel (on the volar aspect) along the course of ulnar, median, superficial radial nerves for any tender swelling e.g. Neuroma.
- Examine the joints DIP, PIP & MP joints by pressing each joint mildly between your thumb and index fingers to elicit tenderness due to intra-articular fracture or joint disease e.g. Rheumatoid arthritis.

III-Move

A. Passive movements of each joint (DIP, PIP, MP, wrist, elbow, and shoulder) through its whole range of movement (ROM) to reveal limitation, stiffness or tenderness.
B. Active movements (without resistance then against resistance) for assessment of intrinsic and extrinsic muscle of the hand.
   Fingers abduction and adduction (spread fingers apart then bring them back together) to test interossei muscles (ulnar nerve).
   Little finger abduction (ulnar nerve).
   Bring thumb tip against index tip (Ok sign) or the little finger to test opponens pollicus (median nerve).
C. Sensory assessment (Light moving touch) -by the examiner index tip- of both sides of all digits is a simple and rapid test for sensation (as unilateral digital nerve pathology will result in sensory loss along the border of affected finger).
   Test sensation on the lateral aspect of the palm (median n.), then the medial aspect; both ventrally and dorsally (Ulnar n.) and finally, at the dorsal aspect of the thumb base (Radial n.).
   N.B. Detailed assessment of sensory threshold and innervation density of slowly and rapidly adapting receptors is provided within the special tests (Table 26.1).

Table 26.1 Assessment of sensory threshold and innervation density of slowly and rapidly adapting receptors

	Threshold	Density
Quickly adapting	Vibration tests	Moving 2-point discrimination
Slowly adapting	Cutaneous pressure test	Static 2-point discrimination

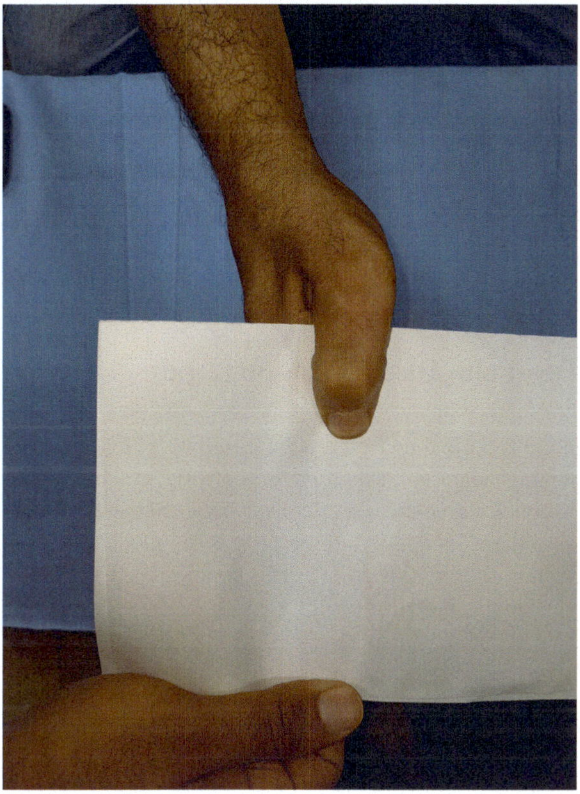

Fig. 26.6 The patient is unable to hold the card in the 1st web space while the thumb is extended. *Note the patient has to flex the thumb interphalangeal joint to hold the card* "+*ve Froment's test*"

Special Tests

Allen's test to ensure good anastomosis between both arteries through palmer arches should any vessel is needed for soft tissue coverage.

Card (Froment's test): ask the patient to hold a card between extended thumb and index. In case of ulnar nerve injury, the patient will hold the card by flexing thumb interphalangeal joint (positive test) (Fig. 26.6).

N.B. the same test can be applied by asking the patient to hold the card between the extended fingers in the 2nd, 3rd, and 4th web spaces while the examiner is pulling the card away.

Vibration Threshold Assessment

Tuning fork applied to the bulb of index and little fingers will test threshold level of rapidly adapting receptors. Loss of sensation at high frequency (e.g. 256 cps) can be the only manifestation at early stage of nerve compression and even precedes electrophysiologic abnormalities. While regain of sensation to low frequency vibration (e.g. 30 cps) can be detected early after nerve repair before regain of light touch.

Cutaneous Pressure Threshold

Using Semmes-Weinstein monofilament apparatus; consisted of many monofilaments of different diameters, the smallest diameter the patient can feel is recorded as the pressure threshold.

Two-Point Discrimination (2-pd)

Static and moving 2-pd tests are used to evaluate the density of slowly adapting and quickly adapting receptors respectively. An instrument having one and multiple 2-probes with increasing distance between the 2-probes is used (e.g. Disk-criminator instrument) is applied to the pulp of fingers and the patient is asked to tell if he is feeling one or two points. The smallest gap the 2-probes the patient can feel is recorded as 2-pd test result.

Provocation Tests

Used over sites of nerve compression. It is also of value after nerve repair to detect level of nerve regeneration. They include:

- **Tinel sign:** 4–6 digital taps are applied over sites of possible nerve compression. Positive test is recorded if tapping produces electric shock symptoms along sensory distribution of tested nerve.
  Median nerve: tap just proximal to the wrist (+ve test suggest carpal tunnel). Also tap at proximal forearm (area of pronator teres).
  Ulnar nerve: tap from above the medial epicondyle then along the course of the nerve on the medial aspect of the forearm till distal to the wrist (Guyon's canal).
  Brachial plexus: tap on the supraclavicular area over scalene muscles.
- Positional and/ or direct pressure tests: applying direct pressure or stretch of the nerve for one minute will produce symptoms along sensory distribution of the affected nerve.

Median nerve is tested by flexion of both wrists against each other, or flexion of the wrist by the examiner and applying direct pressure over the carpal tunnel.
Apply direct pressure over pronator teres muscle in the proximal forearm.
Ulnar nerve: extension of the elbow (positive if Cubital tunnel).
Superficial radial nerve: wrist extension with ulnar deviation.
Brachial plexus: to test for thoracic outlet syndrome (TOS).
Adson test: The arm is slightly abducted and externally rotated, and the radial pulse is felt on the wrist. Then the patient is asked to extend the neck, turn it towards the tested shoulder and ask the patient to take deep breath and hold it for a while, test is considered positive if the patent feels symptoms or radial pulse diminishes.
Wright's test: the arm is abducted to 90° and externally rotated and the radial pulse is felt. Then the arm is raised up (hyperabduction) to narrow the costoclavicular space, if symptoms develop or radial pulse diminishes this indicates TOS.

Chapter 27
Neurological Examination

Ahmed Adel Mohamed Ezzat and Hazem Abdel Badie Ahmed Gouda

Abstract Neurologic examination is a standardized Clinical examination which is done in a well-structured steps. The mental status evaluation consists of a series of questions and tasks, such as naming objects, recalling short lists, writing sentences, and copying shapes observed during interview with the patient.

Keywords Neurologic · Examination · Sheet · Cranial · Peripheral · Consciousness · Gait · Nerves

Neurologic examination is a standardized Clinical examination which is done in a well-structured steps.

A) **Mental state**
B) **Speech**
C) **Cranial nerves examination**
D) **Motor system examination**
E) **Sensory system examination**
F) **Tests for coordination**
G) **Gait assessment**
H) **Others**

A) **Mental state**:

- Level of consciousness.
- Orientation to time place and persons.
- Memory.
- Mood and affect.
- Intelligence.
- Behavior.

A. A. M. Ezzat (✉) · Hazem Abdel Badie Ahmed Gouda
Cairo University, Cairo, Egypt
e-mail: aadel.ezzat@kasralainy.edu.eg

A. Farag et al. (eds.), *Clinical Surgical Skills Made Easy*,
https://doi.org/10.1007/978-3-031-69158-4_27

The mental status evaluation consists of a series of questions and tasks, such as naming objects, recalling short lists, writing sentences, and copying shapes observed during interview with the patient.

Glasgow's coma scale (Table 27.1):

A normal patient is fully conscious, cooperative, oriented to time place and persons, and has average memory, mood and mentality.

B) **Speech**

Disorders of speech:

- Aphasia (dysphasia): a problem in understanding, thoughts or word finding.
- Dysphonia: a problem in voice production.
- Dysarthria: a problem in articulation in spite of good communication.
- Aphasia: (Inability to formulate speech):

Sensory aphasia:

- Auditory agnosia. (Area 22).
- Visual agnosia (18–19).
- Alexia (39—angular gyrus).
- Jargon's aphasia i.e., word salad (40—supramarginal gyrus).
- Motor aphasia.
- Verbal aphasia (44).
- Writing aphasia i.e., agraphia (45).

Dysarthria (Inability to articulate speech):

- Staccato speech: "Cerebellum".
- Monotonous speech: "Parkinsonism".
- Slurred speech: "UMNL and LMNL affecting speech muscles".

Table 27.1 The Glasgow coma scale

Domain	Response	Scale
Best eye response (4)	No eye opening	1
	Eye opening to pain	2
	Eye opening to sound	3
	Eyes open spontaneously	4
Best verbal response (5)	No verbal response	1
	Incomprehensible sounds	2
	Inappropriate words	3
	Confused	4
	Orientated	5
Best motor response (6)	No motor response	1
	Abnormal extension to pain	2
	Abnormal flexion to pain	3
	Withdrawal from pain	4
	Localizing pain	5
	Obeys commands	6
Total score	Deep Coma	3
	Normal	15

- Scanning speech (slurred staccato): "Cerebellum".

C) <u>**Cranial nerves examination**</u>

There are 12 pairs of cranial nerves, which connect the brain with the eyes, ears, nose, face, tongue, throat, neck, upper shoulders, and some internal organs.

A cranial nerve may be damaged anywhere along its length as a result of any of the following:

- An injury.
- Impaired blood flow.
- An autoimmune disorder.
- A tumor.
- An infection.

Increased pressure in the skull (intracranial pressure).

The exact site of the damage can often be identified by testing the functions of a particular cranial nerve.

A) **Olfactory nerve I**: Bed side test.

- Use common odors.
- Avoid irritating substances.
- Examine each nostril alone.

Unilateral <u>Anosmia</u>:

(a) Skull base fracture.
(b) Basal meningitis.
(c) Foster Kennedy Syndrome (Triad): optic atrophy, contralateral papilledema, and anosmia, caused by an olfactory groove meningioma or large frontal lobe tumors.

Bilateral Anosmia

(a) Nasal causes.
(b) Hysterical.

B) **Optic nerve II**: Examine each eye alone then compare both eyes.

- Visual acuity.
- Chart down to 1 m.
- Counting fingers 30–60 cm.
- Hand movement at 30 cm.
- Light perception (with good or bad projection).
- Pin hole test.
- Visual field.
- Bedside confrontation test.
- Perimeter.
- Color vision.
- Fundus examination.

C) **Oculomotor III, Trochlear IV and Abduces VI nerves**:

- Pupillary reaction (light and near).
- Ocular motility and conjugate eye movement.
- Ptosis (Oculomotor palsy vs. Horner syndrome vs. myasthenia gravis) (Table 27.2).
- Nystagmus.

D) **Trigeminal nerve V**

1. Motor: Temporalis, masseter and pterygoids.
2. Sensory: Facial sensations.
3. Reflexes: Jaw reflex and corneal reflex (afferent).

E) **Facial nerve VII**

- Motor: Frontalis, orbicularis oris, orbicularis oculi and retractor anguli muscles.
- Sensory: Chorda tympani supplies taste sensation to anterior 2/3 of the tongue.
- Reflexes: Glabellar reflex and corneal reflex (efferent).

F) **Vestibulo-cochlear nerve VIII**

Examination of cranial **nerve** VIII should cover both cochlear and vestibular function:

- Hearing can be assessed by whispering a number into each ear separately, making a distracting noise with your fingers in the contralateral ear, and asking the patient to repeat.
- If any hearing loss suspected, perform Rinne's and Weber's test.
- Balance has no truly satisfactory test for assessment.
- Formal vestibular testing can be performed.

G) **Glossopharyngeal IX and Vagus X Nerves**

CN IX and CN X nerves can be assessed together:

- Ask the patient to cough (assessing CN X).

Table 27.2 DD of ptosis

Diagnosis	Eyelids	Extraocular motility	Pupils
CN III Palsy	Unilateral ptosis.	Limited adduction, Supraduction and Infraductions	Normal or dilated. When present anisocoria worse in dim illumination
Horner's Syndrome	Mild Unilateral ptosis Reverse ptosis.	Normal unless concurrent pathology is present	Constricted and Anisocoria is worse in bright illumination
Myasthenia Gravis	Variable ptosis. Unilateral or Bilateral	Variable deficit. Any pattern of limitation may be seen	Normal

- Ask the patient to open the mouth wide and say 'ah', using a tongue depressor to visual the palate and posterior pharyngeal wall (assessing CN IX and X). The soft palate should move upwards centrally.
- Testing of the gag reflex should not be performed unless bulbar impairment is suspected, as it is uncomfortable to the patient.

H) **Accessory Nerve XI**

The accessory nerve is a **purely** motor branch to the trapezius "Shrugging of Shoulders" and sternocleidomastoid muscles "Flexion of the head to one side".

I) **Hypoglossal nerve XII**

The hypoglossal nerve **is** a purely motor branch to the muscles of the tongue.

D) **Motor system examination**

A. **Inspection**

- Morphology
- Abnormal movements
- Apparent deformities
- Trophic changes
- Involuntary movements

Interpretation:

- Wasting: LMNL, Disuse atrophy, Ischemia and/ or Aging,
- Hypertrophy: True or pseudo (check power). Pseudo-
- Hypertrophy is associated with weakness"
- Abnormal movements: Anterior Horn cell "AHCs" pathology.
- Trophic changes: Ischemia.

B. **Tone** (Table 27.3):

- Upper limb: Shaking, Passive movements, and Gower's method.
- Lower limb: Shaking, Passive movements, and Rolling.

Interpretation**:**

C. **Power** (Table 27.4):

D. **Reflexes** (Table 27.5):

- Physiological: Superficial (Abdominal, plantar and cremastric) and deep (Biceps, brachioradialis, triceps, knee and ankle)
- Pathological: Hoffman, supraspinatus, patellar and adductor.

Table 27.3 Assessment of muscle tone

Hypotonia	Normal	Hypertonia

• Flaccidity
• Causes:
  • LMNL
  • Cerebellar Lesion
  • Posterior Column Lesion
		• Spasticity or rigidity
		• Causes:
		  • Pyramidal or extrapyramidal Lesions
		  • Meningeal Irritation
		  • Hysterical

Table 27.4 Assessment of muscle power

MRC research council grade	
Grade	Muscle state
0	No Contraction
1	Flicker or trace of Contraction
2	Active Movement with gravity eliminated
3	Active Movement against gravity
4	Active movement against gravity and resistance
5	Normal power

Table 27.5 Assessment of reflexes

Reflexes
• 0 = absent
• 1+ = Reduced
• 2+ = Normal
• 3+ = increase (Hyperactive) Brisk
• 4+ = Clonus

Interpretation:

- Abdominal reflex: Normally the umbilicus moves towards the stimulus. Absent reflex: UMNL above the level of the segmental supply.
- Plantar reflex:
  - Normal: Flexion of the toes
  - Babinski sign "Extensor response" Positive plantar response: Pyramidal tract lesion, Deep sleep or coma, Infants.
  - Absent (equivocal): Thick or cold skin, LMNL or peripheral neuritis "PN".

- Causes of hyper-reflexia: UMNL or Hysterical.
- Causes of hypo-reflexia: LMNL or Posterior column affection.
- If there is hyper-reflexia, proceed to perform pathological reflexes and clonus.
- Clonus: (Wrist, patellar, ankle) rapid regular rhythmic contraction due to sudden sustained stretch of the muscle which stops on release of stretch (in contrast to hysterical which continue without stretch).

E) **Sensory system examination**

- Superficial: Pain, touch and temperature.
- Deep: Vibration sense, joint muscle and nerve.
- Cortical: Tactile localization, 2 point discrimination, stereognosis, graphesthesia, perceptual riverly.
- Interpretation:
  - Stock and glove: PN.
  - Radicular sensory affection: Root.
  - Saddle area affection: Cauda equine syndrome.
  - Jacket sensory loss: Intramedullary lesion.

- Hemihyposthesia: Capsular and brain stem lesion.
- Cortical sensory loss: Area 3, 2, 1 of parietal lobe.

F) **Tests for coordination**

1. Coordination: finger to nose, finger to finger, heel to knee
2. Equilibrium: walking along a straight line, Romberg test
   Tests of coordination are not done in limbs showing paralysis
   - **Romberg test**: The Romberg test is a test that measures your sense of balance. It's typically used to diagnose problems with your balance, which is composed of your visual, vestibular (inner ear), and proprioceptive (positional sense) systems during a neurological exam.

Interpretation:

- Normal
- Normal with open eyes, but fall when eyes are closed: loss of proprioception: Sensory ataxia (PN or Posterior column fracture)
- Fall with eyes open: Unsteadiness: (Cerebellar or Vestibular pathology)
- Rocking forth and back with eyes closed: Cerebellar pathology.

Tremors (Table 27.6):

G) **Gait assessment** (Table 27.7):
Approach to a gait **abnormality**:
A) Symmetrical:

- Small paces = short Steppage: (Parkinsonism: No arm swing or NPH: Normal arm swing).
- N.B. NPH is associated with a classic triad of dementia, gait disturbance, and urinary incontinence. Because this clinical syndrome is potentially reversible by the placement of a ventriculoperitoneal (VP) shunt, it is important to recognize and diagnose accurately.

Table 27.6 Causes and DD of tremors

Tremors	Clinical Features
Essential	• Bilateral action tremors of the hands, usually without leg involvement • Possible isolated head tremors without dystonia • Usually no other neurologic signs • Relieved with alcohol in many cases
Parkinson's Disease	• Resting tremors (4–6 HZ) that decreases with voluntary movements • Usually involves Legs and hands • Fascial involvement is less common
Cerebellar	• Usually associated with Ataxia, dysmetria and gait disorders • Tremors increase steadily as the hand reaches its target
Physiologic	• Low amplitude (10–12 HZ) not visible under normal conditions • Acute onset with increased Sympathetic activity (e.g. Drugs, anxiety, Hyperthyroidism and caffeine • Usually worse with movement and can involve the face and extremities

Table 27.7 Gait assessment

Lesion	Cause	Gait
UMNL	Unilateral hemiplegia Bilateral paraplegia	Circumduction Scissoring
LMNL	Peripheral neuropathy	High Steppage
Cerebellar	Archicerebellum Neocerebellum	Drunken Wide base deviation/Zigzag
Extrapyramidal	Parkinsonism chorea	Short Steppage or Dancing gate

- Feet separation = Wide base: (High Steppage gait: sensory ataxia. No high Steppage gait: Cerebellar ataxia).
- Others: Waddling: Myopathy.

B) Asymmetrical:

- Foot drop: Radiculopathy L5/Common peroneal nerve injury: Pyramidal tract lesion.
- Pain Trauma: Arthritis.
- Bone deformity: Short limb or after surgery.
- Hemiplegia.

H) **Others**

- Inspect for deformities: Scars, Scoliosis or Kyphosis.
- Examine the back and palpate spinous processes, any abnormal swelling, any tender points.
- Examine range of movement of the neck and lumbar vertebrae.

Chapter 28
Examination of the Spine

Khaled Saoud

Abstract With the presence of advanced investigations nowadays, no single diagnostic modality can replace a careful history tacking and thorough examination of the spine on reaching exact diagnosis of patient condition. Since clinical picture varies according to the affected spine level, we divided local examination into cervical and dorsolumber spine examination.

Keywords Spine · Nerves · Clinical · Examination · Sheet · Neurovascular · Psycho-social · Gait

With the presence of advanced investigations nowadays, no single diagnostic modality can replace a careful history tacking and thorough examination of the spine on reaching exact diagnosis of patient condition.

Since clinical picture varies according to the affected spine level, we divided local examination into cervical and dorsolumber spine examination.

Neck and back pain are common presentations in primary care. Many cases of neck and back pain are due to benign functional or postural causes, but a thorough history and examination is essential to assess the cause, any associated psychological difficulties (e.g. depression, anxiety or somatization disorder), and any functional impairment, including restrictions with work, leisure and domestic activities.

General Examination of the Spine

The examination should begin as soon as you first see the patient and continues with careful observation during the whole consultation.

It is essential to observe the patient's gait and posture. Inconsistency between observed function and performance during specific tests may help to differentiate between physical and functional causes for the patient's symptoms.

K. Saoud (✉)
Faculty of Medicine, Ain Shams University, Cairo, Egypt

A. Farag et al. (eds.), *Clinical Surgical Skills Made Easy*,
https://doi.org/10.1007/978-3-031-69158-4_28

Inspection

Examination of any localized spinal disorder requires inspection of the entire spine. The patient should therefore undress to their underwear.

Look for any obvious swellings or surgical scars.

Assess for deformity: scoliosis, kyphosis, loss of lumbar lordosis or hyperlordosis of the lumbar spine. Look for shoulder asymmetry and pelvic tilt.

Observe the patient walking to assess for any abnormalities of gait.

Palpation

Palpate for tenderness over bone and soft tissues.

Perform an abdominal examination to identify any masses and consider a rectal examination (cauda equina syndrome may present with low back pain, pain in the legs and unilateral or bilateral lower limb motor and/or sensory abnormality, bowel and/or bladder dysfunction with saddle and perineal anesthesia, urinary dysfunction and bowel disturbances, and rectal examination may reveal loss of anal tone and sensation).

Movement

The normal range of movements are outlined in the relevant sections below.

Examination of the spine must also include examination of the shoulders and examination of the hips to exclude these joints as a cause of the symptoms.

Neurovascular Examination

A thorough examination of sensation, tone, power and reflexes should be performed.

Always consider the possibility of acute spinal cord compression, which is a neurosurgical emergency.

All peripheral pulses should also be checked as vascular claudication in the upper and lower limbs can mimic symptoms of radiculopathy or canal stenosis (see articles on Cardiovascular History and Examination and Examining the Pulse).

Psychosocial Factors (Table 28.1)

The assessment should include psychological, occupational and socio-economic factors, which may either play a role in the cause of back problems, or adversely affected as a result of back problems.

Table 28.1 The 5 categories and 8 nonorganic signs of Waddell score

Categories	Nonorganic tests	Nonorganic signs
Tenderness	Superficial	Tenderness not related to a particular skeletal or neuromuscular structure; may be either superficial or nonanatomic Superficial The skin in the lumbar region is tender to light pinch over a wide area not associated with the distribution of a posterior primary ramus
	Nonanatornic	Deep tenderness, which is not localized to one structure, is felt over a wide area and often extends to the thoracic spine, sacrum, or pelvis These tests give the patient the impression that a particular examination is being carried out when in fact it is not Low back pain is reported when the examiner presses down on the top of the patient's head; neck pain is common and should not be considered indicative of a nonorganic sign
Simulation test	Axial loading	Back pain is reported when the shoulders and pelvis are passively rotated in the same plane as the patient stands relaxed with the feet together; in the presence of root irritation, leg pain may be produced and should not be considered indicative of a nonorganic sign
	Rotation	A positive physical finding is demonstrated in the routine manner, and this finding is then checked while the patient's attention is distracted; a nonorganic component may be present if the finding disappears when the patient is distracted
Distraction tests	Straight leg raising	The examiner lifts the patient's foot as when testing the plantar reflex in the sitting position; a nonorganic component may be present if the leg is lifted higher than when tested in the supine position Dysfunction (e.g., sensory, motor) involving a widespread region of body parts in a manner that cannot be explained based on anatomy; care must be taken to distinguish from multiple nerve root involvement
Regional disturbances	Weakness	Demonstrated on testing by a partial cogwheel "giving way" of many muscle groups that cannot be explained on a localized neurologic basis
Overreaction	Sensory	Include diminished sensation to light touch, pinprick or other neurologic tests fitting a "stocking" rather than a dermatomal pattern May take the form of disproportionate verbalization, facial expression, muscle tension and tremor, collapsing, or sweating; judgments should be made with caution, minimizing the examiner's own emotional reaction

Neck Examination

Examination of the neck is important in the events of trauma (poly-trauma or isolated neck trauma as whiplash injury). Also, in cases of neck pain due to cervical spondylosis.

Examination would always include full neurological examination of upper and lower limbs, gait as well as bladder and bowel disturbances "As mentioned before".

Inspection

- Deformity: may be seen in cervical spondylosis or acute torticollis.
- Instability of the cervical spine: while the patient is sitting check that the patient can support their head in neutral position.
- Asymmetry, fullness of the supraclavicular fossa in cases of Pancoast tumor, Torticollis (affected side and chin often tilted to opposite side) or sternomastoid 'tumor' in infants.
- Arms and hands: for wasting, fasciculation, motor abnormalities (tone, power), sensory deficits and any indication of thoracic outlet syndrome.
- Lower limb motor or sensory deficits may be caused by cervical spinal cord compression.

Palpation

- Palpate for tenderness, masses or any scars: Posterior in the midline, Lateral, Supraclavicular - cervical rib, lymph glands, tumors, Anterior - including thyroid examination.
- Midline tenderness in the cervical spine: may be due to supraspinous damage following whiplash injuries or may also indicate more major neck trauma.
- Palpate lateral aspects of vertebrae for masses and tenderness (the most prominent spinous process is T1).
- Paraspinal tenderness radiating into trapezius is common in cervical spondylosis.
- Crepitation: facet joint crepitus may be detectable with flexion and extension of the neck by either palpation or auscultation on either side of cervical spine; facet joint crepitus is common in cervical spondylosis.

Cervical Movement

- Flexion: normal range is 80° with chin able to touch region of sternoclavicular joint.
- Extension: normal range 50°, so normal for full flexion to full extension is 130°, primarily involves the atlanto-axial and atlanto-occipital joints.
- Lateral flexion: normal range is 45° to both sides; restriction of lateral flexion is common in cervical spondylosis. Inability of lateral flexion without forward flexion at same time suggests atlanto-axial and atlanto-occipital joint abnormalities.
- Lateral rotation: normal range is 80° to both sides; normally just short of plane of shoulders at full rotation. Rotation is restricted and painful in cervical spondylosis.

Neurological Involvement

Neurological features associated with cervical radiculopathy:

- C5 nerve root:
- Muscle weakness: shoulder abduction and flexion/elbow flexion. Reflex changes: biceps.
- Sensory changes: lateral arm.
- C6 nerve root:
- Muscle weakness: elbow flexion/wrist extension. Reflex changes: biceps/supinator.
- Sensory changes: lateral forearm, thumb, index finger.
- C7 nerve root:
- Muscle weakness: elbow extension, wrist flexion, finger extension. Reflex changes: triceps.
- Sensory changes: middle finger.
- C8 nerve root:
- Muscle weakness: finger flexion.
- Sensory changes: medial side lower forearm, ring and little finger.
- T1 nerve root:
- Muscle weakness: finger abduction and adduction. Reflex changes: none.
- Sensory changes: medial side upper arm/lower arm.

Thoraco-Lumbar Spine Examination

Low back pain is a very common presentation in general practice. Common causes include spine pathology, trauma, muscle diseases. Rare caused may include hidden malignancy or aortic aneurysm. A thorough examination of the spine and lower limbs are essential.

Inspection

Observe for abnormal gait and posture, which may provide clues as to the nature and severity of the problem.

Superficial landmarks include:

- T1 is the most prominent spinous process at the base of the neck.
- T7/T8: lower border of scapulae.
- L4: iliac crests.
- S2: dimples at posterior superior iliac spines.

Assess curvature: kyphosis, scoliosis.

- Ask the patient to bend forwards: postural scoliosis resolves; a structural scoliosis does not disappear and therefore needs further assessment. A lumber scoliosis may be associated with a prolapsed intervertebral disc. Disappearance of a scoliosis when sitting suggests that the scoliosis may be secondary to shortening of a leg. Idiopathic scoliosis leads to short stature with the trunk short in proportion to the limbs.
- Ask the patient to extend their lower back. An increased kyphosis which is regular, and mobile is found in postural kyphosis. Common causes of a fixed regular kyphosis are senile kyphosis, and ankylosing spondylitis.
- Lumbar curvature: flattening or reversal of the normal lumbar lordosis as in a prolapsed intervertebral disc, osteoarthritis of the spine and ankylosing spondylitis. An increase in the lumbar curvature may be normal or due to spondylolisthesis, or secondary to an increased thoracic curvature or a flexion deformity of the hip.

Skin examination is essential: Cafe-au-lait patches, a sign neurofibromatosis is important finding. Tuft of hair over the pelvis may indicate spina bifida.

Palpation

Check for bone tenderness of the spine: tenderness may indicate serious pathology such as infection, fracture or malignancy.

- Ask the patient to lean forwards and palpate the spines and spaces in between. This would give you clue on alignment. Step may indicate spondylolisthesis. Tenderness between the spines of the lumbar vertebrae and at the lumbosacral junction and over the lumbar muscles may occur with prolapsed intervertebral disc and mechanical back pain.
- Check for tenderness over the sacroiliac joints (sacroileitis and sero-negative rheumatoid arthritis are common causes).

Percussion

Ask the patient to bend forward. Lightly percuss the spine from the root of the neck to the sacrum. Significant pain is a feature of infections, fractures and neoplasms.

An exaggerated response may be a feature of a non-organic problem.

Movements

Flexion, extension rotation and lateral bending should be examined.

- Flexion: Most normal people can reach within 7 Cm from the floor when flexed. Limitation of flexion may be due to muscle spasm or advanced spondylosis or ankylosing spondylitis.
- Restricted extension occurs in prolapsed lumber disc, lumber spondylosis or facet joint diseases.
- Rotation is tested while the patient is seated. Normally around 40° can be reached.
- Lateral bending is tested by asking the patient to slide their hands down the side of each leg in turn, and record the point reached from the position that the fingers reach on the legs.

The contributions of the thoracic and lumbar spine are usually equal.

Specific Tests

- Straight leg raising: Passively flex thigh with extended leg while patient is supine. Dorsiflexion of foot helps to elicit pain. Stop when the patient complains of back or leg pain. The test is negative if there is no pain. Paresthesia or pain in root distribution is very significant, indicating nerve root irritation.
- The angle of pain elicited should be recorded.

- Back pain suggests a central disc prolapse, and leg pain suggests a lateral protrusion.
- Crossed straight leg raising positive test indicate more significant disease (raising the asymptomatic leg causes pain in the symptomatic side).
- It is positive in cases of L5 and S1 root compression.
- Femoral stretch test: With the patient prone and the anterior thigh fixed to the couch, flex each knee in turn. This causes pain in the appropriate distributions by stretching the femoral nerve roots in L2-L4.
- The pain produced is normally aggravated by extension of the hip.
- The test is positive if pain is felt in the anterior compartment of thigh.

Neurological Involvement

Test the patellar (L3, L4) and Achilles (L5, S1) reflexes.

Root pressure from a disc may affect myotomes and dermatomes in a selective fashion; record any muscle wasting (compare girths of calf and thigh muscles):

Myotomes:

- L2, L3: hip flexion and internal rotation
- L4, L5: hip extension and external rotation.
- L3, L4: knee extension
- L5, S1: knee flexion
- L4, L5: ankle dorsiflexion
- S1, S2: ankle plantar flexion L4: ankle inversion
- L5, S1: ankle eversion

Dermatomes:

- L2: upper thigh
- L3: knee
- L4: medial aspect of the leg
- L5: lateral aspect of the leg, medial side of the dorsum of the foot
- S1: lateral aspect of the foot, the heel and most of the sole
- S2: posterior aspect of the thigh
- S3-S5: concentric rings around the anus, the outermost of which is S3Umbilical reflex

The reflex is absent in cases with upper motor neurons lesion above the level of thoracic spine. We use blunt object to stroke the skin in each paraumbilical quadrant of the skin. Normally the umbilicus twitches to the direction of stimulated quadrant. The muscles of the upper quadrants are supplied by T7-T10, and the lower quadrants by T10-L1.

Chest expansion

- Check the patient's chest expansion at the level of the 4th interspace.
- The normal range for an adult of average build is at least 6 cm.
- Less than 2.5 cm is considered abnormal.it is affected in cases with cervical cord injury and in diseases with affection of the movement of rib joints as ankylosing spondylitis.

Abdominal examination is important especially with non-spine causes of back pain such as aortic aneurysm and gynecological tumors.

Peripheral pulses should be palpated to rule out vascular claudication.

Hip and sacroiliac joint examination

Check the hip joints for range of movement and for pain or limitation. Hip problems may present with predominantly back and buttock pain as well as pain in the groin. A loss of range on internal rotation of the hip is often the earliest sign of hip disease.

Osteoarthritis of the hip may be clinically confused with low back pain, particularly prolapsed intervertebral disc.

Sacroiliac joints

The most commonly used is FABER test, **F**lexion, Abduction and **E**xternal **R**otation of the leg applies pressure on the SI joint of the affected side.

Compression on the pelvis with the patient lying lateral position with the affected side away from examiner hand. The joint commonly affected with degenerative scoliosis and rheumatological disorders.

N.B. FABER or Patrick's test is used to identify the presence of hip pathology by attempting to reproduce pain in the hip, lumbar spine or sacroiliac region.

Chapter 29
Orthopedic Examination

Mahmoud Massoud and Ashraf Mohey

Abstract History taking, Examination scheme, Spine Examination, Shoulder Examination, Elbow Examination, Hand & Wrist Examination, Hip Examination, Knee Examination, Ankle & Foot Examination, Pediatric Examination, Brachial plexus Examination, Check list OSCE, Orthopedic imaging, Relevant Orthopedic History Taking. Personal history NAME/AGE/SEX/JOB/ADDRESS/SPECIAL HABITS/DOMINANT HAND. Past history of Disease: DM/HTN—TB/Tumor—Operations/Drugs.

Keywords Orthopedic · Bone · Joints · Examination · Deformity · Gait · Movement · History

- History taking
- Examination scheme
- Spine Examination
- Shoulder Examination
- Elbow Examination
- Hand & Wrist Examination
- Hip Examination
- Knee Examination
- Ankle & Foot Examination
- Pediatric Examination
- Brachial plexus Examination
- Check list OSCE
- Orthopedic imaging

M. Massoud (✉) · A. Mohey
AFCM, Cairo, Egypt

A. Farag et al. (eds.), *Clinical Surgical Skills Made Easy*,
https://doi.org/10.1007/978-3-031-69158-4_29

Relevant Orthopedic History Taking

Personal history

NAME/AGE/SEX/JOB/ADDRESS/SPECIAL HABITS/DOMINANT HAND

Past History

Disease: DM/HTN—TB/Tumor—Operations/Drugs

Family history

DISEASES/DEFORMITIES

Obstetric history (FOR LADIES)

DURING PREGNANCY: DM/HTN/DURING DELIVARY/POST PARTUM

Develop history (PEDIATRICS)

Menarche age

C/O

Onset/course/duration

Abnormal Look

1. Swelling: (site, size, shape, surface, consistency).
2. Deformity.

Abnormal Feel

1. Pain: site, type, course, nature, radiation.
2. Deformity.

Abnormal Move

1. Tingling/Numbness: e.g.
   Acute with activity ≈ structural abnormality After activity ≈ inflammatory Chronic/aching ≈ degenerative Night ≈ TB/Tumor.
2. Instability//Giving away *(how many times)*.
3. Stiff//Locking

Others Affecting ADL (activity daily living)

Snap/click/clunk (non-significant if not with one of chief c/o).

feed/WC—sleep/sex— work/driving.

GAIT:

- GENERAL: Rhythm, speed, limp, turning.
- PHASES: Heel-strike, stance, push-off, and swing.

Examination

General Rules of Examination

- Greetings
- Introduce yourself

- Ask for consent of examination
- Necessary exposure one joint above and one joint below
- Thank the Patient at end

Should do Examination on 4 Os

- Open (bared limb)
- Order

    (standing-sitting- lying)
    (superficial to deep) (proximal to distal)

- Opponent (MCL = LCL)
- Other side (The other limb) Comfort & easy

Rapid Screening Tests

The Shoulder Joint

Put the hand on the head, other shoulder and behind the shoulder (Fig. 29.1a–c).

The Elbow Joint

Supination, Pronation, Flexion, extension (Fig. 29.2a–c).

The Wrist Joint & the Hand

Grasp, flexion, extension of the fingers and the wrist.

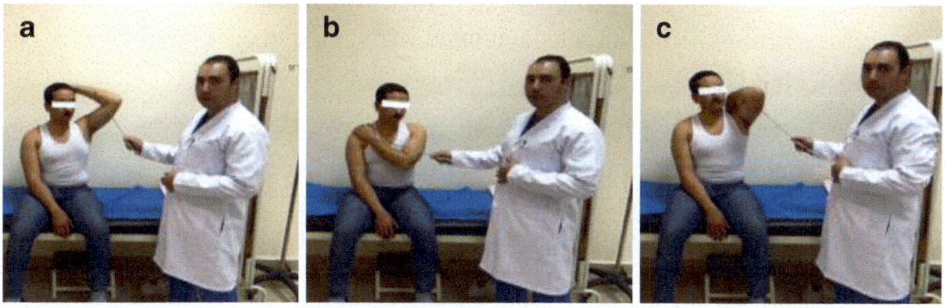

Fig. 29.1 (**a**–**c**) Screening for the shoulder joint

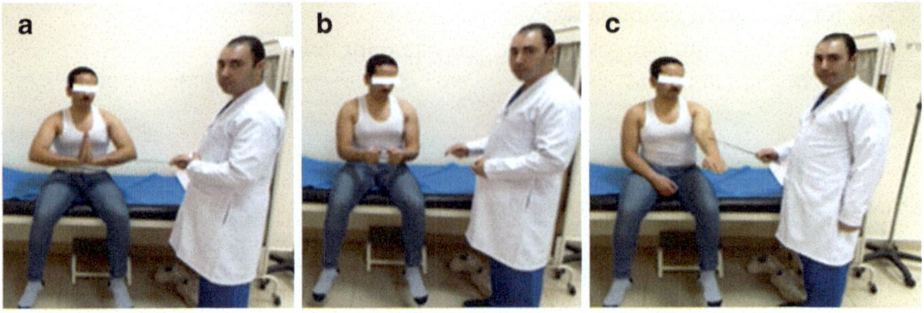

Fig. 29.2 (a–c) Screening for the elbow joint

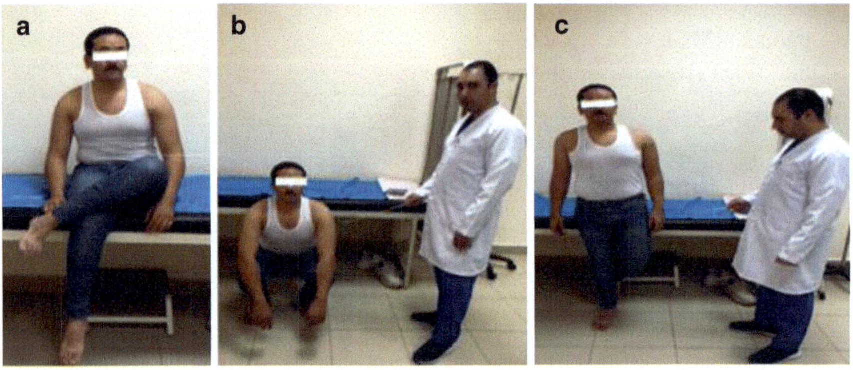

Fig. 29.3 (a–c) Screening for the hip and knee joint

The Hip & Knee Joints

Squat, stand on one limb, cross leg position (Fig. 29.3a–c).

Ankle Joint

Gait, stand on heels, stand on tip toeing (Fig. 29.4a–c).

Hyper Laxity

Beighton score, is a system used to assess joint hypermobility. It involves a series of maneuvers to test the flexibility of various joints in the body, such as bending the thumb backward to touch the forearm or hyperextending the knees and elbows. Each maneuver is assigned a point, and a total score is calculated. Higher scores indicate greater joint hypermobility (Fig. 29.5a–c).

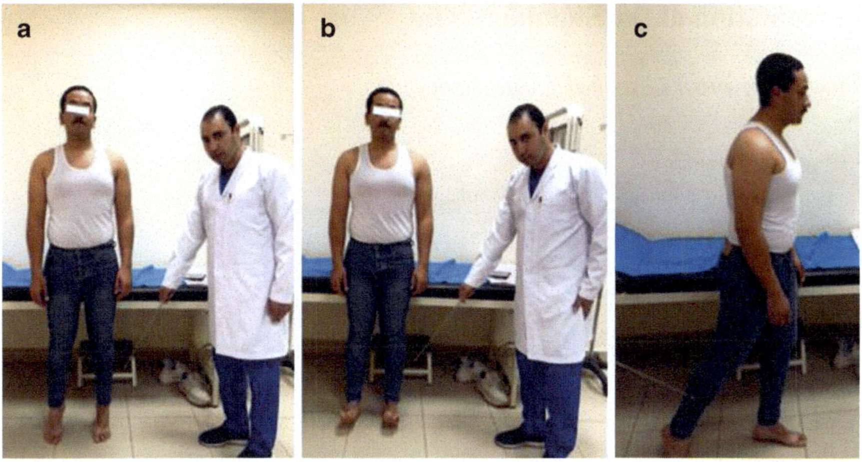

Fig. 29.4 (a–c) Screening for ankle joint

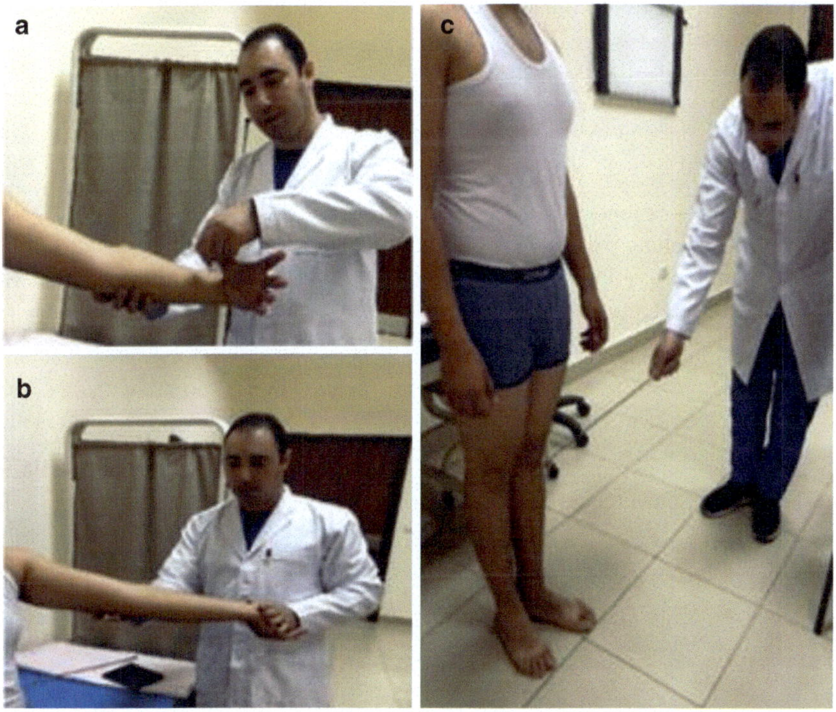

Fig. 29.5 (a–c) Examination for laxity of the joints

Examination of the Shoulder Joint

Most Common Clinical Conditions

- Frozen shoulder.
- Recurrent or acute dislocation shoulder.
- Rotator cuff tear.
- Bicipital tendonitis.
- Rupture of the long head of biceps.
- Osteoarthritis.
- Referred pain from near or far lesions.

Mechanism of Injury

Certain mechanisms of injury result in characteristic patterns of structural damage.

E.g. Fall on outstretched hand → anterior dislocation of shoulder → Fracture of proximal humerus

General: SCHEME + Cx spine

Hyperlaxity: SCHEME

Gait: as before and we will examine cervical spine

Type of Pain:

* Aching pain → degenerative changes
* Sharp pain/catching pain → ACJ pathology → subacromial impingement
* Pain after activity → inflammatory arthropathy → tendinosis Night pain → rotator cuff lesion → glenohumeral arthritis → adhesive capsulitis → infection**Look**

A: alignment (shoulder drop).
S: symmetricity/muscle wasting (supra-infraspinatus) injury suprascapular. N.
S: skin (Fig. 29.6a, b).**Move:**

Active (flexion extension/Abduction, Adduction/internal, external rotation)
The range of movement of the shoulder joint in degrees is as follows:

- Flexion: 0–180 degrees
- Extension: 0–60 degrees
- Abduction: 0–180 degrees
- Adduction: 0–45 degrees
- Internal rotation: 0–70 degrees
- External rotation: 0–90 degrees (Fig. 29.7a–d).

Muscle Power

Medical Research Council Scale Grade Description:

0 no contraction

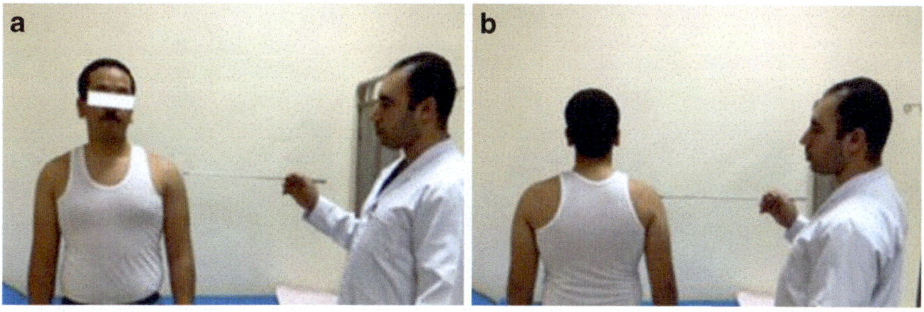

Fig. 29.6 (**a**, **b**) Inspection of the shoulder joint

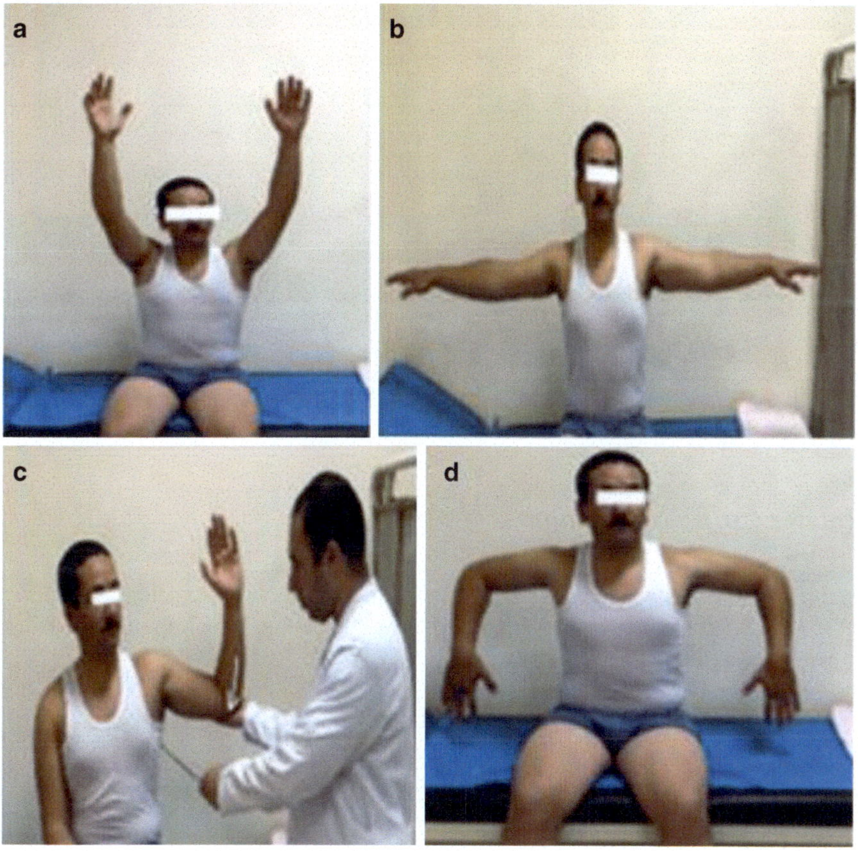

Fig. 29.7 (**a**–**d**) Inspection for movement of the shoulder joint

1 flicker or trace of contraction
2 active movement with gravity eliminated
3 active movement against gravity
4 active movement against gravity and resistance
5 normal power

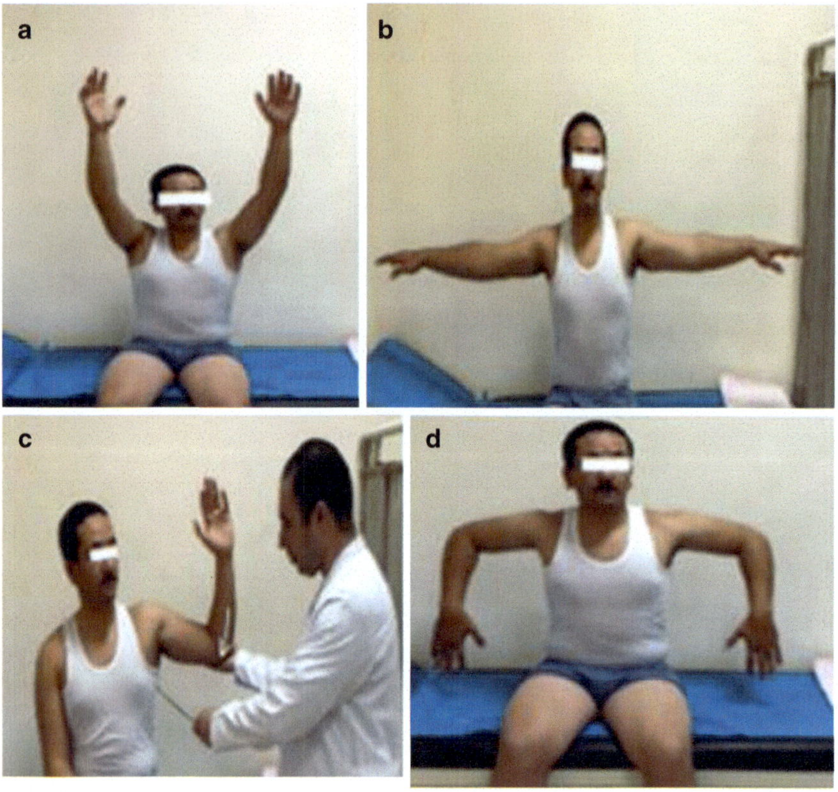

Fig. 29.8 (**a**–**d**) Lift off test

Rotator Cuff Examination

Active against resistance Passive (lag test) Drop arm tests supraspinatus (Abduction 0/90^{0}) IS (external rotation in Adduction) T minor (external rotation in Abduction) subscapularis (left off test).

Lift off Test

The patient stands and places the dorsum of the hand against mid-lumbar spine. The patient then lifts his hand away from the back. An inability to perform this action indicates a lesion of the Subscapularis muscle (Fig. 29.8a–d)

Special Test: Specific to c/o (Passive)

Impingement Neer's sign: While the patient is sitting or standing, the examiner passively elevates the patient's internally rotated arm in the plane of the scapula (about 30° from the coronal plane) (Fig. 29.9a, b).

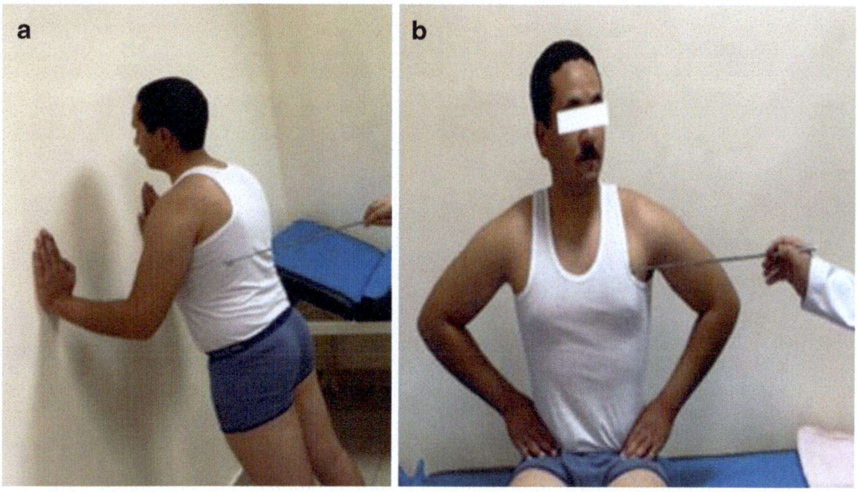

Fig. 29.9 (**a**, **b**) Serratus and Pectoralis major tests

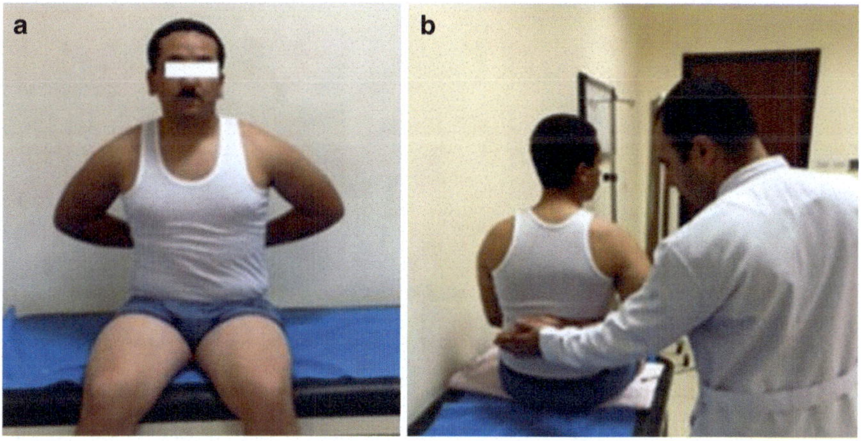

Fig. 29.10 (**a**, **b**) Left off test

Drawer tests: for subluxation and dislocation: These are performed to quantify the amount of anterior and posterior laxity.

While standing behind the patient, use one hand to stabilize the shoulder girdle by holding on to the scapula with your thumb and coracoid with your index finger and, with the other hand, hold on to the humeral head (Fig. 29.10a, b).

The SLAP TEST: patient is positioned in 90° of shoulder abduction, and 65–70° of elbow flexion and the forearm in a neutral position

Biceps Tendon Hold the arm in 10° of internal rotation and run your thumb just distal to the anterior edge of the acromion (Fig. 29.11a)

Acromio-Clavicular joint: Follow the clavicle laterally to its end. Usually, one can feel the articulation between the acromion and clavicle (Fig. 29.11b).

Serratus Anterior (Long Thoracic Nerve C5, 6, 7) Stand behind the patient and ask him to push against the wall with arms at the level of the shoulder. If weak or

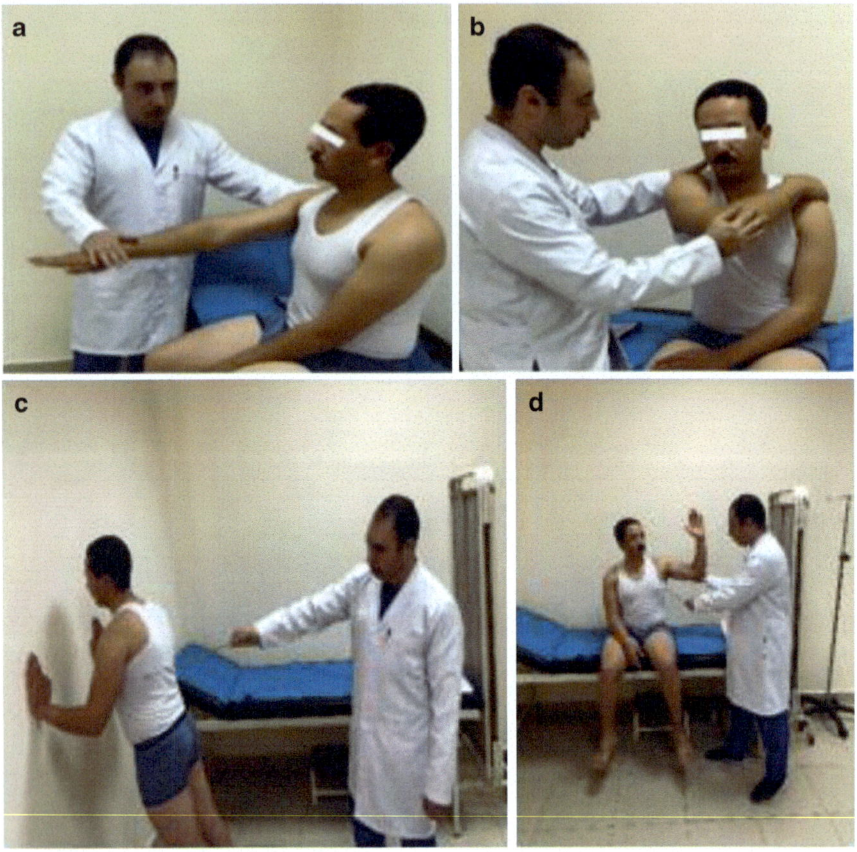

Fig. 29.11 Tests for Biceps tendon "**a**", Acromioclavicular joint "**b**", Serratus anterior muscle "**c**" and Latissimus Dorsi muscle "**d**"

paralyzed, the medial border of the scapula moves away from the chest wall "scapular winging" (Fig. 29.11c).

Latissimus Dorsi (Thoracodorsal Nerve C6, 7, 8).

Ask the patient to abduct the arm to 90°. The examiner applies resistance to the point of the elbow and asks the patient to pull the elbow down to the side. The other hand feels for the contracting muscle (Fig. 29.11d).

Trapezius Tenderness and trigger points may be elicited, which are usually associated with cervical spine pathology.

Deltoid (Axillary Nerve C5, 6) Ask the patient to abduct the shoulder to 90° and hold the position. The anterior, middle, and posterior fibers are now palpable.

Rhomboid (Dorsal Scapular Nerve C5).

The patient is asked to pull the shoulders back, while the examiner applies resistance to the spine of the scapula (Fig. 1.17).

Pectoralis major (Lateral Pectoral Nerve C5, 6).

Stand facing the patient, who is instructed to place the hands on the hips and press firmly.

Rotator Cuff: consists of the tendons of four muscles: subscapularis, supraspinatus, infraspinatus and teres minor.

Subscapularis muscle: (Suprascapular Nerve C5, 6) Stand behind the patient. The patient is asked to place the back of his hand into the small of the back (to eliminate the action of pectoralis major).

Hawkins/Kennedy Impingement

Patient's arm shoulder in 90 degrees of shoulder flexion with the elbow flexed to 90 degrees and then internally rotates the arm.

Vascular:

- Pulsations "see vascular Sheet".
- Venous disease.
- Edema.
- Whole limb Duplex.**Neuro:**

  Sensory/motor/reflexes (axillary N → patch area).

Examination of the Elbow Joint

Most Common Clinical Conditions

- Osteoarthritis
- Fractures and Dislocation
- Olecranon bursitis
- Rheumatoid arthritis
- Tennis elbow
- Golfer's elbow

General: SCHEME + Cervical spine.

Hyperlaxity: SCHEME.

Gait: as before and we will examine cx spine.

Look **A: Alignment** static (cubitus varus/valgus) carrying angle.

S: Symmetricity/wasting (girth of arm).

S: Skin/Swelling (olecranon bursitis) (Fig. 29.12a, b).

Feel **T:** temperature (bursa/septic/gout).

T: tender points (bone/soft tissue).

Move Flexion/extension/Pronation/supination (90/90).

Muscle power: against resistance.

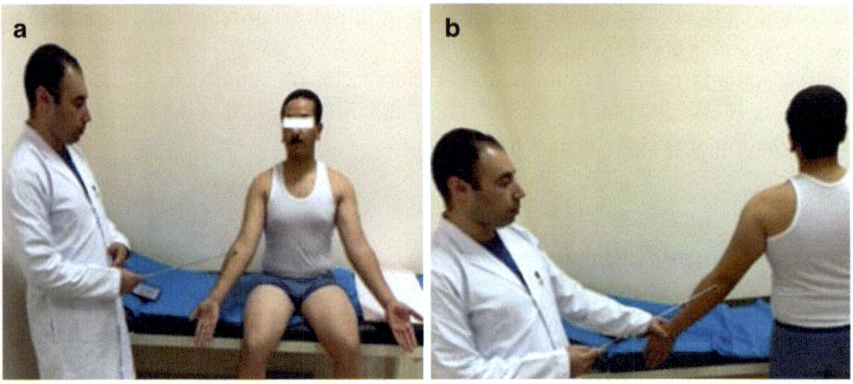

Fig. 29.12 (**a**, **b**) Inspection of the elbow joint

Elbow pivot shift

Valgus stress to the elbow while flexing and extending it, feeling for a subluxation or reduction of the radial head.

Tennis elbow:

Is characterized by the presence of pain and functional disability associated with tendon dysfunction of the lateral epicondyle musculature.

Golfer elbow

Patients report medial elbow and proximal forearm pain with activities requiring wrist flexion and forearm pronation. The doctor may rest the arm on a table, palm side up, and ask the person to raise the hand by bending the wrist against resistance.

Examination of the Hand & Wrist Joint

Most Common Clinical Conditions

- Dorsal Ganglion and trigger fingers
- Osteoarthritis .
- Psoriatic arthritis:
- median, radial, or ulnar nerves lesions
- De Quervain's tenosynovitis
- Madelung's deformity.
- Dinner Fork Deformity and Dupuytren's disease
- Volkmann's ischemia contracture.
- Wrist drop.
- Rheumatoid arthritis and gout.

General: SCHEME.

Hyperlaxity: SCHEME.

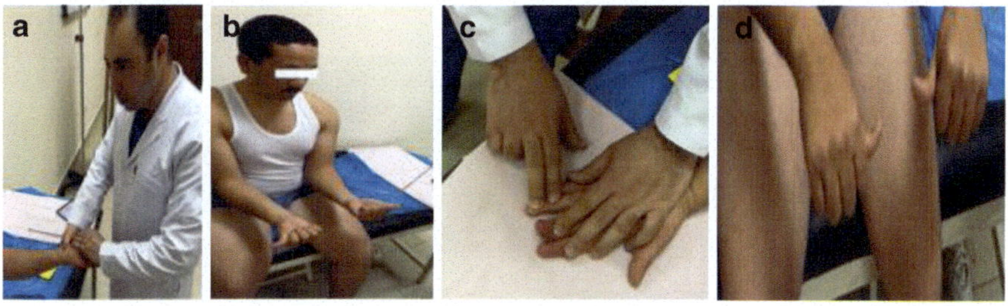

Fig. 29.13 (**a–d**) Tests for hand grips

Gait: SCHEME + Cervical spine.
Look:

A: Alignment static (arcade pattern—nail parallel/dynamic).
(Point finger at flexion to scaphoid).
Congenital finger: Macrodactly/Microdactly/Syndactly/Clinodactly/Campotodactly.
Abnormal. Flexion/extension.
S: symmetricity/muscle wasting (nerve injury).
S: skin and/or swelling (ganglion or cord -Dupuytren's contracture).**Feel:**

T: temperature (bursa/septic/gout).
T: tender points (bone/soft) and/or Truck "crepitus".**Move**

Wrist: Flexion –extension, ulnar-radial deviation and Pronation-supination.
Hand (5 grips): Fist (flexors). Hook (extrinsic), hold pen, pinch (intrinsic).
Muscle and key or coin holding test (Flexor polices longus + Flexor digitorum profundus) (Fig. 29.13a–d).

Special Test

Specific to the Complaint

1st Done as Screening

- **T:** temperature (bursa/septic/gout).
- **T:** tender points (bone/soft)/Truck: crepitus.
- Carpal tunnel tests: Try to elicit *Tinnel's sign* by extending the hand and tapping on the median nerve in the carpal tunnel.
- Flexor profundus: by holding the finger extended at the proximal interphalangeal joint and ask the patient to flex the distal interphalangeal joint of that same finger.
- Bunnell test is a physical examination maneuver used to assess the integrity of the intrinsic muscles and the tightness of the intrinsic and extrinsic finger flexors.

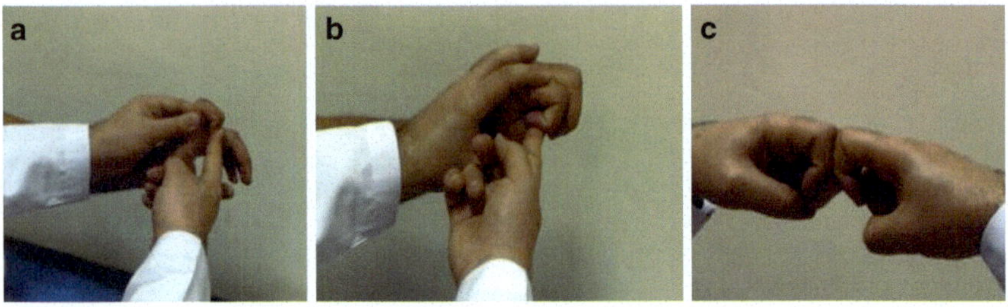

Fig. 29.14 Bunnel test "**a, b**", and The Elson Test "**c**"

It helps diagnose conditions such as intrinsic muscle tightness, intrinsic-plus finger deformity, and assess joint mobility in the fingers (Fig. 29.14a, b) During the test, the examiner stabilizes the metacarpophalangeal (MCP) joint while passively flexing the proximal interphalangeal (PIP) joint. If the PIP joint cannot be flexed when the MCP joint is held in extension, it suggests intrinsic tightness. Conversely, if the PIP joint can be flexed when the MCP joint is held in extension, it indicates extrinsic tightness. This test assists in determining the appropriate treatment plan for conditions affecting finger mobility and function.

- for Central Band Disruption in fingers is used to diagnose injuries to the central slip of the extensor tendon in the fingers, particularly in cases of mallet finger or central band injuries. The test involves assessing the ability to extend the distal interphalangeal joint (DIP joint) against resistance with the proximal interphalangeal (PIP) joint held in flexion. If the DIP joint cannot be extended while the PIP joint is flexed, it suggests a disruption in the central band of the extensor tendon. This test helps clinicians diagnose and determine the severity of finger injuries, guiding appropriate treatment plans (Fig. 29.14c).
- Tenodesis effect tendon: involves passive flexion or extension of the wrist causing passive movement in the fingers.

Never miss **Neurologic:** sensory/motor/reflexes
Above wrist (Dynamic).
Vascular examination: Distal pulse, Veins and edema.

Hip Joint Examination

Common Clinical Hip Joint Conditions

- Fracture or fracture dislocation of the Hip
- Osteoarthritis.
- Congenital hip dysplasia.
- Avascular necrosis of the Head of the Femur.
- Slipped upper femoral epiphysis.

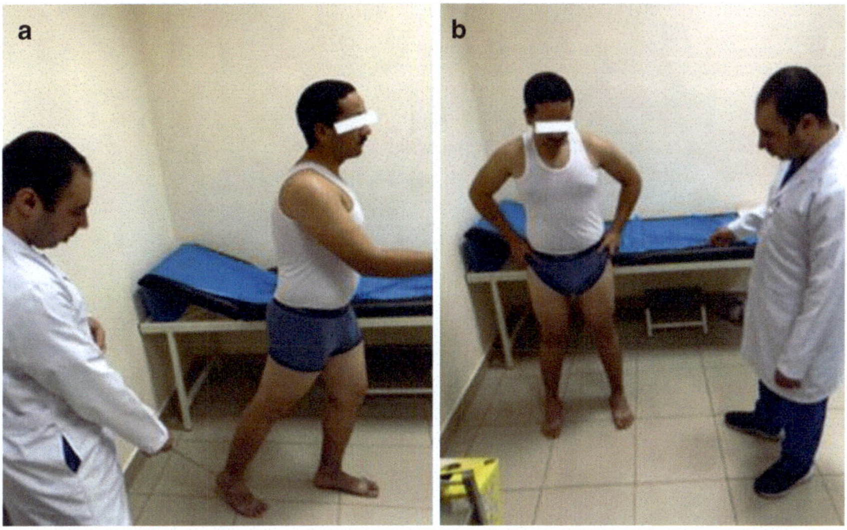

Fig. 29.15 (**a**, **b**) Trendelenburg gait

- Trendelenburg gait.
- Antalgic gait.

General: Screening SCHEME "Above".

Gait: Trendelenburg Short limb excessive lateral trunk sway or leaning toward the stance limb during the stance phase of walking. This occurs due to weakness or dysfunction of the hip abductor muscles, particularly the gluteus medius muscle (Fig. 29.15a, b).

Hyperlaxity: SCHEME "above".

Look in Standing and Sitting Position

Trendelenburg Test (Injury Gluteus Muscle)

Patient stands on one leg while the examiner observes the position of the pelvis. If the hip abductors are weak or dysfunctional, the pelvis on the unsupported side will drop or tilt downward instead of remaining level (Fig. 29.16a–d).

Feel **T:** temperature.

T: tender points (bone/soft)/Truck: crepitus.

Leg length discrepancy (Fig. 29.17a–d):

Limb length discrepancy (supra/infra trochanteric)

1. **Visual Inspection**: The examiner visually compares the lengths of the lower extremities while the patient lies supine on an examination table. They observe the relative positions of the feet and ankles.

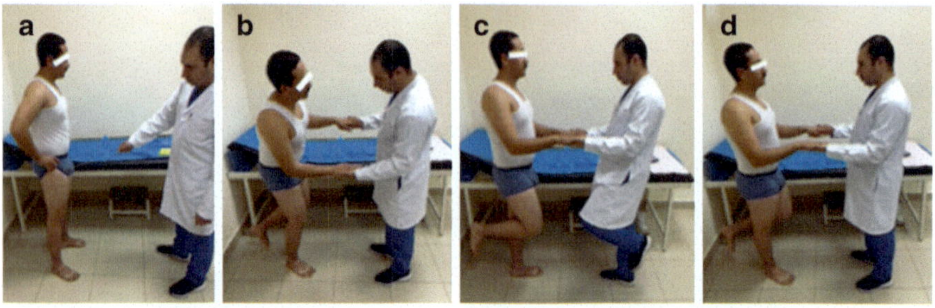

Fig. 29.16 (**a**–**d**) Trendelenburg test

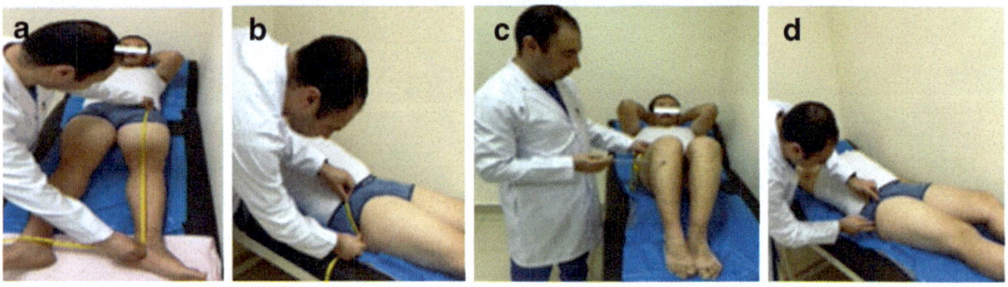

Fig. 29.17 (**a**–**d**) Leg length discrepancy

2. **Measuring Tape**: With the patient lying supine, the examiner measures the distance from the anterior superior iliac spine (ASIS) to the medial malleolus on each leg using a measuring tape. Any difference in these measurements indicates leg length inequality.
3. **Block Test**: The patient stands barefoot, and wooden blocks of varying heights are placed under the shorter limb until the pelvis becomes level. The difference in height between the blocks indicates the leg length inequality.
4. **Functional Assessment**: The patient walks or runs, and the examiner observes any compensatory movements or gait abnormalities that may be indicative of leg length discrepancy.

Move: SCHEME "Above"

Limb length discrepancy (supra/infra trochanteric)

Special test (supine):

Test Specific to complaint

Flexion abduction external rotation:(FABER)

Fig. 29.18 A: Pain posterior: Sacroiliac pathology

Flexion, adduction, internal, rotation (FADIR) (Fig. 29.18b).

Pain anterior: Hip pathology.

Thomas Test + Flexion ROM (Fig. 29.18c–e).

Lying flat on your back while bringing one knee to your chest. The angle of the other leg hanging off the edge of the table or bed can indicate the tightness of the hip flexors.

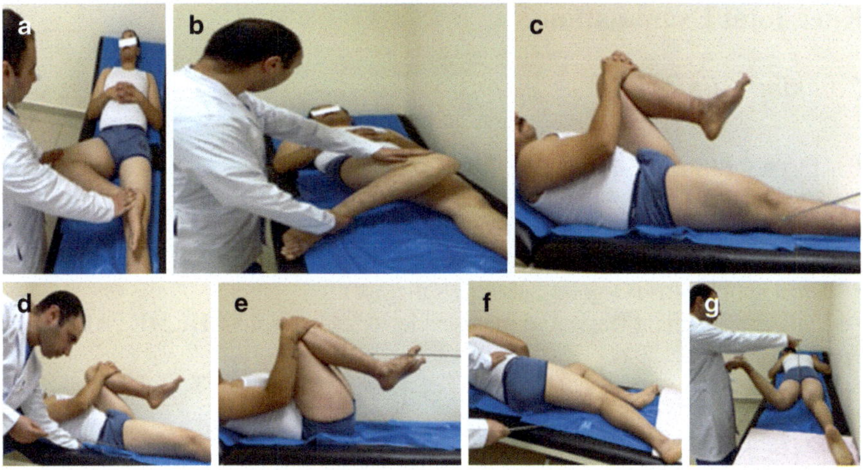

Fig. 29.18 (**a–g**) Thomas Test + Flexion ROM

Movements:

- Flexion: 0–120 degrees
- Extension: 0–30 degrees
- Abduction: 0–45 degrees
- Adduction: 0–30 degrees
- Internal rotation: 0–45 degrees
- External rotation: 0–45 degrees**On side**

Ober test (contracture iliotibial tract): the patient lies on their side with the bottom leg stability, while the examiner passively extends and abducts the upper leg (Fig. 29.18f).

Prone Craig test

On prone position internal rotation of hip joint till greater tubercle is maximum then measure angle with vertical (Fig. 29.18g). **The patient lies prone while the examiner palpates the greater trochanter of the femur. The hip is then flexed and internally and externally rotated until the greater trochanter is felt to be at its most prominent point. The angle of the thigh relative to the examining table or bed indicates the degree of femoral anteversion or retroversion.**

Trendelenburg gait:

It is a type of abnormal gait pattern characterized by a dropping of the pelvis on the side of the unsupported leg during the stance phase of walking.

Antalgic gait: It is a type of abnormal gait pattern that is characterized by a shortened stance phase on the affected side due to pain

- **Never miss: Neurologic:** sensory/motor/reflexes "SCHEME"
- **Vascular: arteries.** Whole limb, capillaries Refill, duplex Femoral A./popliteal A., Dorsalis Pedis A., Post. Tibial A. and ABI (ankle brachial index). BP leg/Arm >0.9 normal.

Knee Joint Examination

Common Clinical Knee Lesions

- Osteoarthritis and Rheumatoid arthritis.
- Baker's (popliteal) cyst.
- Prepatellar and infrapatellar bursitis.
- Chondromalacia and subluxation patellae.
- Tibial apophysitis (Osgood-Schlätter's disease).
- Collateral ligament tears. And meniscal lesions.**General SCHEME "Above"**

Pain:

Localized pain e.g. meniscus injury

Generalized pain → degenerative changes → patellofemoral joint

Gait **Thrust gait:** (G. varum, valgum or recurvatum)

Crouch: (hamstring spasm hip/knee) + pseudoequinus.

Hyperlaxity: SCHEME "above".

Look in standing and sitting position

A: Alignment static: (Genu. Varum, valgum or recurvatum)

S: Symmetricity: m. wasting (muscle girth thigh and/or calf) Localized swellings:

Anterior aspect of the knee Prepatellar bursitis, Infrapatellar bursitis Lateral aspect of the knee, Lateral meniscal cyst Postero-medially Semimembranosus bursitis, Posteriorly Baker's cyst Popliteal aneurysm (rare cause).

Other causes for swelling Ganglion Osteophytes Osgood–Schlätter's disease Swelling.

Q Angle: The quadriceps angle or, in short, the "Q angle" is the angle between the longitudinal axis of quadriceps muscle and the patellar tendon and reflect the angle of quadriceps muscle force.

Feel: Effusion: Effusion is assessed by "milking" fluid distally from the suprapatellar pouch and palpating the area adjacent to the patellar tendon for fluid accumulation. A ballotable patella may be palpated after similar effusion milking.

Move:

- Flexion: 0–135 degrees
- Extension: 0–0 degrees (fully extended).
- Medial rotation: 0–10 degrees.
- Lateral rotation: 0–30 degrees.**SCHEME**

Special test: Specific to complaint

Patella: look. site (Baja/Alta) size(brave/magna) shape(osteophytes/bipartite)

Move. Track flexion/extension, Lateral Push and Feel.

Ligaments injury: Grade (I/II/III)-

End point: (firm → intact ligament/soft→ partial tear, and

If no end point → complete tear)

- **Varus Stress Test (for LCL)**: This test involves applying a varus force (outward stress) to the knee (Fig. 29.19a).
- **Valgus Stress Test (for MCL)**: This test involves applying a valgus force (inward stress) to the knee while it is slightly flexed (Fig. 29.19b).
- **Apley's Compression Test**: This test involves applying downward pressure on the foot while rotating the tibia to assess for pain and clicking, which may indicate a meniscal injury (Fig. 29.19c).**ACL specific anterior drawer test:**

The patient lies supine with the knee flexed at about 90 degrees. The examiner stabilizes the lower leg with one hand while grasping the upper tibia with the other hand and pulls the tibia forward. Excessive anterior translation of the tibia relative to the femur, (Fig. 29.19d), compared to the unaffected side, can indicate a tear or laxity in the ACL.

PCL posterior drawer test

The patient lies supine with the knee flexed at about 90 degrees. The examiner stabilizes the lower leg with one hand while grasping the upper tibia with the other hand and pushes the tibia backward. Excessive posterior translation of the tibia relative to the femur, compared to the unaffected side, can indicate a tear or laxity in the PCL.

PLC dial test:

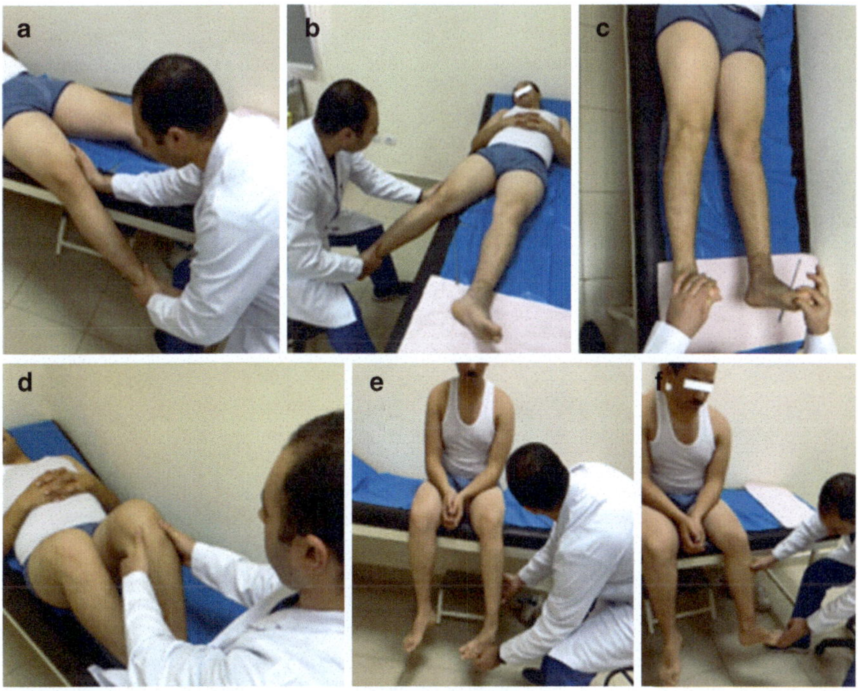

Fig. 29.19 (**a–f**) Tests for the knee injuries

The patient lies prone with the knees flexed at 30 degrees and the feet hanging off the edge of the table. The examiner externally rotates both feet and compares the degree of external rotation between the injured and uninjured knee. Excessive external rotation or asymmetry between the knees suggests a posterolateral corner injury (Fig. 29.19c).

OCD Wilson test;

The patient is seated with the knee flexed at 90 degrees. The examiner internally and externally rotates the tibia while also applying a valgus and varus stress to the knee (Fig. 29.19e, f).

McMurray's test (Fig. 29.20):

- To test the medial meniscus, palpate the posteromedial margin of the joint. Then hold the leg in external rotation and extend the knee.
- To test the lateral meniscus, palpate the posterolateral margin of the joint. Then hold the leg in internal rotation and extend the knee.**Never miss**

Neurologic: sensory, motor and reflexes.

Vascular: Arteries, veins and edema.

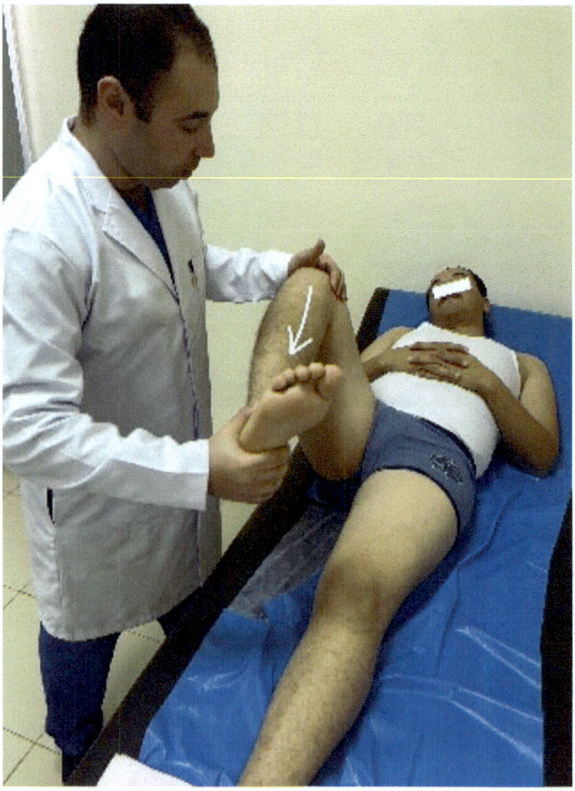

Fig. 29.20 McMurray's test

Ankle & Foot Examination

Common Clinical Conditions

- Sprain and tear of the ligaments
- Rheumatoid arthritis
- Ankle injuries e.g. fractures and dislocations
- Deformities of the foot and hallux valgus
- Plantar fasciitis & gouty lesions.**General: Scheme**

  Gait:
  Range of motions of the ankle joint and the foot:

- Dorsiflexion: 0–20 degrees
- Plantarflexion: 0–50 degrees
- Inversion: 0–35 degrees
- Eversion (turning the sole of the foot outward): 0–15 degrees
- **Hindfoot (Equines/calcaneus) (varus/valgus)**
- **Forefoot (Adduction/Abduction) (supination/ pronation)Hyperlaxity: SCHEME**

  Look in standing and sitting position

A: Alignment. (Congenital dactely, abnormal flexed fingers: Hummer, claw, Mallet toes) and forefoot.
S: Symmetricity: Muscle. Wasting and Calf girth.
S: Skin: SCHEME

Feel T: temperature.**T:** tender points (bone/soft tissue) or Truck: crepitus.
Move: Active and passive muscle power.

- Ankle: dorsal/planter flexion.
- Subtalar: inversion/eversion.

Special Test: Specific to Complaint

- **Jack test and tip toeing:** The patient stands on their tiptoes, and the examiner observes the arch of the foot. If the arch reappears or becomes more pronounced, it suggests that there is flexibility in the arch and that the patient may have a flexible flatfoot. If the arch remains flattened, it may indicate a rigid flatfoot.
- **Hindfoot Coleman block test:** The examiner observes the arch of the foot. If the arch height increases or partially restores when weight-bearing is shifted onto the forefoot, it suggests a flexible flatfoot. Conversely, if the arch height remains low or unchanged, it may indicate a rigid flatfoot.
- **Ankle:**

- **Squeeze test:** the examiner applies pressure to the tibia and fibula just above the ankle joint. If there is pain elicited with this maneuver, it suggests possible syndesmotic injury. The test helps clinicians diagnose and differentiate between various types of ankle injuries, guiding appropriate treatment and management strategies (Fig. 29.21a).

N.B. A syndesmotic, or 'high' ankle sprain is one that involves the ligaments binding the distal tibia and fibula at the Distal Tibiofibular Syndesmosis. Injuries can occur with any ankle motion, but the most common motions are extreme external rotation or dorsiflexion of the Talus.

- **Tinel test:** The examiner taps or lightly percusses along the course of the posterior tibial nerve, typically just behind the medial malleolus (inner ankle bone). A positive test is indicated by tingling or electric shock-like sensations radiating into the foot, which can suggest nerve irritation or compression in the tarsal tunnel (Fig. 29.21b).
- **Anterior drawer test**: The patient is usually lying on their back with the knee flexed and the foot resting on the examination table. The examiner stabilizes the lower leg with one hand while grasping the heel with the other hand. Then, the examiner pulls the heel forward (anteriorly) while stabilizing the lower leg. Excessive anterior movement of the talus bone under the tibia compared to the uninjured side or the presence of pain may indicate an injury to the ATFL, often associated with ankle sprains (Fig. 29.21c)
- **Achilles' tightness: Gastrocnemius, Soleus, Silverskoiled test:**
- Ankle dorsi flexion increases with knee Flexion due to cause in gastrocnemius (Fig. 29.21d).
- **Mulder (Morton neuroma):**

The examiner uses one hand to apply pressure to the metatarsal heads while using the other hand to squeeze the foot transversely. This maneuver compresses the forefoot and can elicit pain or a clicking sensation in the area of the neuroma, typically between the third and fourth metatarsal heads. If pain or a click is reproduced during this maneuver, it is considered a positive Mulder Test and may suggest the presence of Morton's neuroma.
Never miss **Neuroloic:** sensory/motor/reflexes.
Vascular: whole limb/capillary Refill and duplex.

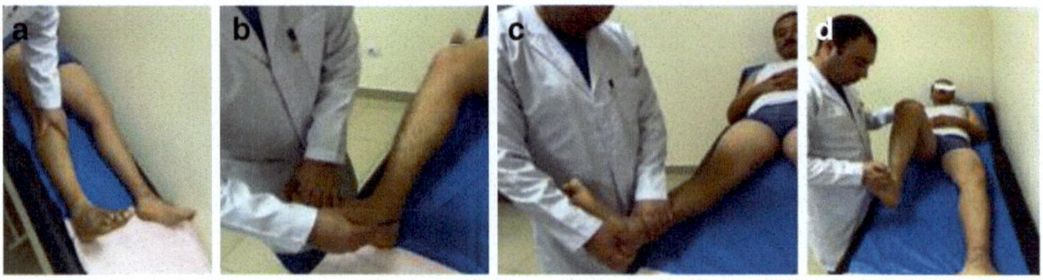

Fig. 29.21 (**a–d**) Tests for ankle and foot injuries

Chapter 30
Sheet for of a Swelling from the Bone

Ashraf Mohey and Ahmed Hassan Amin

Abstract Boney Swelling is a part of General rules of examination including History and Clinical examination to be followed by investigations. And as a part of Limb examination with its rules mentioned earlier in this book and Examination of swelling with DD according to the area of presentation of the Swelling.

Keywords Bone · Swelling · Examination · Sheet · General · History · Benign · Malignant · Inflammation

Boney Swelling is a part of General rules of examination including History and Clinical examination to be followed by investigations. And as a part of Limb examination with its rules mentioned earlier in this book and Examination of swelling with DD according to the area of presentation of the Swelling this will include:

- From the General sheet:
- Area to be examined including examination of the other areas e.g. in a LL swelling examination. The examination has to include all areas below the diaphragm namely, the other lower Limb "For comparison or for bilateral swelling", Abdomen "Front, back and perineum" for a source of Secondaries and a minimum of the Virchow's L.N. While a swelling in the upper Limb, the areas to be examined are the other Limb, The head, Neck and mouth, The Chest front and back and breast and at least the Liver from the organs below the diaphragm.
- Complete General examination which may lead to assessment of the general condition of the patient, Assessment of the stage of the disease e.g. in Primary malignant bone tumors. Assessment of the stage or cause of the swelling "Signs of systemic inflammation may suggest the cause of the boney swelling in osteomyelitis including Acute, T.B. or rarely nowadays Syphilis. It may also be the only Clue for diagnosis in multiple exostosis for example or multiple enchondromas "Ollier's disease".

A. Mohey
AFCM, Cairo, Egypt

A. H. Amin (✉)
Faculty of Medicine, Ain Shams University, Cairo, Egypt

A. Farag et al. (eds.), *Clinical Surgical Skills Made Easy*,
https://doi.org/10.1007/978-3-031-69158-4_30

- From the Limb sheet: The Limb should be examined distally arteries, veins and nerves including edema deformity and gait.
- From the swelling sheet: Multiplicity and DD between solid and Cystic lesions.

Personal History

Age

In **children**, bony swellings can be caused by a variety of conditions. Some common causes of bony swellings in children include:

1. Growth plate injuries: Children's bones are still growing, and injuries to the growth plates (epiphyseal plates) can lead to bony swellings. These injuries can occur due to trauma or overuse.
2. Bone infections: Conditions like osteomyelitis (bone infection) can cause bony swellings in children. These infections can be bacterial or fungal in nature and may require antibiotic treatment.
3. Benign bone tumors: Osteochondromas are the most common benign bone tumors in children. These tumors typically arise near the growth plates and can cause bony swellings.
4. Bone cysts: Simple bone cysts or aneurysmal bone cysts can also lead to bony swellings in children. These cysts are fluid-filled cavities within the bone.
5. Osteoid osteoma: This is a benign bone tumor that can cause bony swellings and is more common in children and young adults. It typically presents with localized pain that worsens at night.
6. Fibrous dysplasia: This is a rare bone disorder where normal bone is replaced with fibrous tissue, leading to bony swellings and deformities.

In **adolescent** patients, bony swellings can also be caused by a variety of conditions. Some common causes of bony swellings in adolescents include:

1. **Osteochondritis dissecans:** This condition occurs when a piece of bone and cartilage separates from the end of a bone due to a lack of blood supply. It can lead to bony swellings and joint pain, typically in the knee, elbow, or ankle.
2. **Osteosarcoma:** Osteosarcoma is a type of bone cancer that primarily affects adolescents and young adults. It can cause bony swellings, bone pain, and fractures.
3. **Enchondroma:** Enchondromas are benign cartilage tumors that can develop in the bones of adolescents. They can cause bony swellings and may be associated with fractures or deformities.
4. **Ewing sarcoma:** Ewing sarcoma is a rare type of bone cancer that can occur in adolescents. It can cause bony swellings, bone pain, and may be associated with fever and weight loss.

5. **Giant cell tumor of bone:** This is a benign but locally aggressive tumor that can occur in the bones of adolescents. It can cause bony swellings and may be associated with pain and limited range of motion.
6. Paget's disease of bone: Paget's disease is a chronic bone disorder that can affect adolescents. It leads to abnormal bone remodeling, resulting in bony swellings, bone pain, and deformities.

In **adults**, bony swellings can also be caused by a variety of conditions. Some common causes of bony swellings in adults include:

1. **Osteoarthritis:** Osteoarthritis is a degenerative joint disease that can lead to bony swellings, known as osteophytes or bone spurs, at the edges of affected joints. These swellings can cause pain, stiffness, and limited range of motion.
2. **Rheumatoid arthritis:** Rheumatoid arthritis is an autoimmune disease that primarily affects the joints. It can cause bony swellings, called rheumatoid nodules, around the affected joints. These nodules are typically firm and non-tender.
3. **Gout:** Gout is a type of arthritis caused by the buildup of uric acid crystals in the joints. It can lead to bony swellings, known as tophi, in the joints and soft tissues. Tophi are typically visible as lumps under the skin.
4. **Bone tumors:** Various types of bone tumors, both benign and malignant, can cause bony swellings in adults. Examples include osteochondromas, chondrosarcomas, and metastatic bone tumors.
5. **Paget's disease of bone:** Paget's disease is a chronic bone disorder that primarily affects older adults. It can lead to bony swellings, bone pain, and deformities due to abnormal bone remodeling.
6. **Osteomyelitis:** Osteomyelitis is a bone infection that can cause bony swellings, localized pain, and tenderness. It is typically caused by bacteria entering the bone through a wound or bloodstream.
7. **Hyperparathyroidism:** Hyperparathyroidism is a condition characterized by excessive production of parathyroid hormone, leading to elevated calcium levels in the blood. This can cause bony swellings, bone pain, and fractures.

Site in Relation to the Long Bone and Other Types of the Bones

Swelling at the **epiphysis of long bones** can be a sign of various conditions, including:

1. **Osteomyelitis:** This is an infection of the bone that can cause swelling, redness, and pain at the affected site.
2. **Osteochondritis dissecans:** This is a condition where a piece of bone and cartilage becomes detached from the end of a bone, leading to swelling and pain.
3. **Growth plate injuries:** Injuries to the growth plate, which is located at the epiphysis of long bones, can cause swelling and pain.

4. **Osteoarthritis:** This is a degenerative joint disease that can affect the epiphysis of long bones, leading to swelling and stiffness.
5. **Bone tumors:** Tumors that develop in the bone can cause swelling at the epiphysis.

Swelling at the **diaphysis of long bones** can also be a sign of various conditions, including:

1. **Fractures:** A fracture in the diaphysis of a long bone can cause swelling, pain, and deformity at the site of the injury.
2. **Osteomyelitis:** Infections can also affect the diaphysis of long bones, leading to swelling, redness, and pain.
3. **Osteosarcoma:** This is a type of bone cancer that can develop in the diaphysis of long bones, causing swelling and pain.
4. **Stress fractures:** Overuse or repetitive stress on a bone can lead to stress fractures in the diaphysis, resulting in swelling and pain.

Swelling of the **flat bones** can also be a sign of various conditions, including:

1. **Osteomyelitis:** Infections can affect flat bones like the skull, ribs, and pelvis, leading to swelling, redness, and pain.
2. **Bone tumors:** Tumors can develop in flat bones, causing swelling and pain. These tumors can be benign or malignant.
3. **Paget's disease:** This is a chronic bone disorder that can affect flat bones, leading to swelling, deformity, and pain.
4. **Fibrous dysplasia:** This condition can cause abnormal growths in flat bones, resulting in swelling and pain.

Swelling in the **short bones** can also be a sign of various conditions, including:

1. **Fractures:** Short bones like those in the hands and feet can be fractured due to trauma or repetitive stress, leading to swelling, pain, and limited range of motion.
2. **Arthritis:** Conditions like osteoarthritis or rheumatoid arthritis can affect short bones, causing inflammation, swelling, and stiffness.
3. **Osteomyelitis:** Infections can also affect short bones, leading to swelling, redness, and pain.
4. **Bone tumors:** Tumors can develop in short bones, causing swelling, pain, and potential deformity.
5. **Osteochondroma:** This is a benign bone tumor that can develop in short bones, leading to swelling and pain.

Complaint

Mass which may be painful or painless.

Present History

Onset: Acute Onset in acute osteomyelitis, insidious onset in tumors as osteochondromas.

Course: Progressive increase in Size raises the possibility of bone tumor "A rapid increase in Size in Sarcoma and a slow increase in size in giant cell tumor of bone (Osteoclastoma) "Benign tumors show a very slow increase in size which may stop increasing in size at a certain age and become stationary".

An Acute appearance with a rapid increase in Size and later regressive course suggests an inflammatory Lesion "Osteomyelitis".

Duration: A short durations weeks or a month suggests Osteomyelitis DD. Ewing's sarcoma "Both presents with systemic inflammatory manifestations in young age". And a long duration more than a year suggests benign lesions like osteoma, Chondroma or bone cysts.

Associated Symptoms

- Relation of Pain to the swelling: Benign tumors are usually painless, in Osteosarcoma pain precedes the swelling in contrast to Osteoclastoma where the swelling precedes pain which is a late presentation. Secondaries may present with pathologic fracture associated with pain which precedes the appearance of the swelling. In Osteomyelitis pain, Swelling and inflammation appear simultaneously. Swelling after a history of fracture may indicate a Callus, Ununited or Malunited fractures.
- Deformities from pathologic fracture, Gait abnormalities and Loss of function distally after pathologic fracture or due to pain or muscle and/or tendon infiltration".
- Systemic manifestations of acute inflammation, T.B., stigmata of Syphilis, other symptoms of metastases "Liver, lung or brain".

Other swelling: Bone metastases, multiple exostosis and encondomatosis.

Past History

- Diseases of medical importance "DM, HTN, Cardiac, Chest, liver, kidney …etc.'
- Diseases which may affect Bone such as T.B.
- Previous operations or fracture.
- Allergies.
- Medications including Anticoagulants.

Family History: of diseases of medical importance.

General examination: For;

- Assessment of the General condition of the patient including his/her fitness for an operation, and discovery of any associated disease of medical importance not reported by the patient "arrhythmias, hyperthyroidism …etc."
- Assessment of the stage of the disease in cases of malignant tumors.
- The only Clue for diagnosis may be in the General examination e.g. multiple bone swellings "D.D.", Systemic manifestations of acute inflammation, T.B., Stigmata of tertiary stage of Syphilis "rare" and osteogenesis imperfecta as examples".

Local Examination

Important points to bear in mind while examining a Bony swelling:

Bony swelling are:

- Deep to muscles. If it invades the muscle some difficulty in DD from a soft tissue sarcoma invading the bone "D.D. if the tumor can be felt from other sides of the bone it is a bony tumor"
- May bulge from one or more sides of the bone, Circumferential or expand the bone from within "Enchondroma".
- Fixed to the bone "No Mobility in any direction".
- Hard or Show egg-shell crackling on pressure.

Inspection: Like any other swelling "see the Chapter of examination of swellings".

Site, size, shape surface, special signs, surrounding structure and other swellings.

N.B. Dilated Veins over the swelling indicates a very vascular tumor like Osteosarcoma or rarely a vascular Osteoclastoma.

N.B. Test relation to the muscles "it should be deep to the muscle "It's size has to be smaller on contraction of the muscle" except when the muscle is markedly infiltrated by the tumor where the size of the tumor doesn't change after contraction of the muscle".

Palpation

As in examination of other swellings:

Temperature, tenderness, Site, size, shape, surface, Edge, consistency, Mobility, Special Signs, Surrounding structures "Including skin" and other swellings "of the same nature or enlarged draining lymph nodes".

N.B. Sarcomas and Osteomyelitis have an ill-defined edge "Proceeding from normal bone to the swelling, I cannot sharply demarcate where the pathology starts". On the other hand, in benign lesions there is a well-defined edge "Proceeding with the finger from normal bone to the swelling, I can sharply demarcate where the pathology starts" such as in osteomas and Chondomas.

N.B. Egg-Shell Cracking Sign: This is a sign rarely seen today that can be elicited over an advanced giant-cell tumor, Osteoclastoma, of long bone—a thin cortex only of normal bone remains over the tumor mass and pressure imparts to the fingers sensation.

Examine the Limb Distally and Proximally

For Pulsations, Nerves "sensory and Motor", edema, Veins including DVT and the Limb proximally for secondary LNs.

Examine the Other Lower Limb and Abdomen

Other Bony masses:

- Brodie's Abscess: a subacute osteomyelitis of the bone. It is an uncommon condition, usually mistaken for being a bone tumor and has been frequently observed to involve the metaphysis of bones (especially tibia).
- Sclerosing osteomyelitis: also known as Garre's sclerosing osteomyelitis (GSO) is a rare chronic inflammatory disease that results in the thickening of bony cortices with loss of the medullary canal but lacks any active infection signs.
- Ewing's Sarcoma: Ewing's sarcoma is a rare type of cancer that primarily affects the bones or soft tissues. It most commonly occurs in children and young adults, and is characterized by the rapid growth of malignant cells in the affected area. Symptoms may include pain, swelling, and a lump or mass in the affected area. It is usually accompanied by Local and Systemic manifestations of inflammation.
- Aneurysmal bone cyst (ABC) is a benign bone tumor that typically affects children and young adults. It is characterized by the presence of blood-filled cysts within the bone, which can cause pain, swelling, and potential weakening of the affected bone and pathological fracture. ABCs can occur in any bone in the body, but they are most commonly found in the long bones of the arms and legs, as well as the spine. The exact cause of aneurysmal bone cysts is not fully understood, but they are thought to be related to abnormalities in blood vessels within the bone.

Chapter 31
Peri-Operative Care

Lauren O'Connell

Abstract While some details of perioperative management plans will be specific to the exact procedure being undertaken, there are many elements of pre- and post-operative management which are generalizable and relevant to any surgical intervention. In particular, pre-operative optimization of the patient and preparation by the surgical and anesthetic teams are key to success and will result in enhanced post-operative outcomes.

Keywords Pre-operative · Examination · Sheet · Optimization · Risk · Surgery · Anesthesia · Outcome
While some details of perioperative management plans will be specific to the exact procedure being undertaken, there are many elements of pre- and post-operative management which are generalizable and relevant to any surgical intervention. In particular, pre-operative optimization of the patient and preparation by the surgical and anesthetic teams are key to success and will result in enhanced post-operative outcomes.

Surgical Planning

It is critical to have an awareness of the multiple pre-operative factors which influence and may increase the likelihood of complications. These include general factors applicable to all procedures, such as malnutrition, hypoalbuminaemia, poorly controlled diabetes, immunosuppressed states such as active HIV or patients receiving chemotherapy, as well as factors which increase the risk of specific complications, such as pelvic radiotherapy contributing to increased anastomotic leak rates in the context of rectal anastomoses. The surgeon should also be aware of previous surgeries undertaken, as these will affect pre-operative planning, for example

L. O'Connell (✉)
SVUH, Dublin, Ireland
e-mail: laurenoconnell@rcsi.ie

A. Farag et al. (eds.), *Clinical Surgical Skills Made Easy*,
https://doi.org/10.1007/978-3-031-69158-4_31

previous mesh repairs in the patient undergoing surgery for recurrent incisional hernia, or residual small bowel length in a patient with multiple previous small bowel resections. In the elective setting, up to date cross-sectional imaging should be sought as appropriate to delineate the anatomy and previous operative notes obtained and reviewed if possible. Previous surgical procedures are also an independent predictor of septic complications in patients with Crohn's. Relevant medications should be inquired about, specifically anticoagulants such as warfarin or the family of direct oral anticoagulants; antiplatelet agents; systemic corticosteroids, mTOR inhibitors such as sirolimus, targeted therapies such as bevacizumab, and immunomodulators such as anti-TNF agents; and SGLT2 inhibitors such as dapagliflozin. These may present risks of intraoperative bleeding, wound complications such as seromas and dehiscence, and perioperative ketoacidosis respectively. Close liaison with the anesthetic team, and if appropriate, the primary medical team caring for the patient is best practice to ensure optimal patient outcomes.

Consent and Shared Decision Making

Thorough counselling of the patient with regard to the rationale, risks and benefits of surgery is imperative. Their ideas, concerns and expectations regarding the goals of care and desired long-term outcome to be achieved by surgery should be discussed. This is especially important for procedures being undertaken for a quality of life indication. Ideally, this consultation should be undertaken in the outpatient setting, so that patient queries and clarifications can be explored and addressed outside of the constraints of a busy elective theatre list. The consent process should also ideally be undertaken in the outpatient setting, rather than on the morning of surgery.

In the setting of emergency surgery, decision making regarding the goals of care and anticipated long-term functional outcomes remain paramount. Thorough consideration should be given to the expected effectiveness or futility of surgical interventions, respectively. The next-of-kin and other close family members should be kept apprised of the plan and the patient's condition, as the clinical situation and consequently surgical plan may evolve rapidly. The input of family or next-of-kin should be sought in instances where this may aid in decision-making, for example collateral history regarding the patient's premorbid state and overall condition, presence of frailty and fitness for surgery. However, it is important to recall that while valuable insight may be provided by relatives and family agreement is highly desirable, for those adult patients who lack capacity ultimately decisions regarding appropriate medical care and management rest with the treating team. Exceptions to this include where a family member or other named individual has power of attorney with respect to medical care, and appropriately set out advanced care directives.

Pre-Operative Scoring Systems

Multiple risk calculators exist which can aid in evaluating a patient's pre-operative morbid state and predicting risk of post-operative complications, morbidity and mortality. They may pertain to the elective or emergency setting. These range from general, such as the ACS-NSQIP, P-POSSUM (Physiological and Operative Severity Score for the enumeration of Mortality and Morbidity) and NELA (National Emergency Laparotomy Audit) scores, to those which may be used to predict the likelihood of specific post-operative complications, such as the CeDaR score to predict risk of overall morbidity and hernia recurrence in the setting of incisional hernia repair [1]. These represent useful adjuncts to clinical assessments, and can help inform shared decision-making with patients and their relatives when deciding on the appropriateness or otherwise of surgical interventions.

Prehabilitation

Pre-habilitation, often abbreviated as "prehab", is an increasingly recognized approach in the medical field aimed at optimizing a patient's physical and psychological state before undergoing surgery. This preoperative strategy is designed to enhance the individual's overall health, with the objective of reducing postoperative complications, accelerating recovery, and improving surgical outcomes. The concept of pre-habilitation is grounded in a multidisciplinary approach that encompasses physical optimisation, nutritional optimisation, psychological support, and medical management. The rationale, components, and evidence supporting pre-habilitation are an integral part of preoperative care in modern medicine.

Rationale for Pre-Habilitation

Pre-habilitation is predicated on the understanding that better preoperative health status is associated with improved postoperative outcomes. Surgery represents a significant physiological stressor that can trigger new pathology or exacerbate pre-existing disease states in patients, potentially leading to complications and prolonged recovery times. By addressing these vulnerabilities before surgery, pre-habilitation aims to enhance the patient's resilience to the stress of surgery, thereby facilitating a smoother and quicker postoperative recovery.

Components of Pre-Habilitation

Physical Exercise

A core component of pre-habilitation is a tailored exercise program designed to improve cardiovascular fitness, muscle strength, and endurance. Such programs are often personalized to the patient's baseline fitness level, comorbidities, and the specific demands of the upcoming surgery. Cardiopulmonary exercise testing (typically abbreviated to CPET or CPEX) is frequently utilized in the elective setting for assessment and stratification of fitness for surgery prior to demanding planned operative interventions. In the UK, it is frequently used in patients planned for major gastrointestinal, vascular, urological or cardio-thoracic surgical procedures. Use of CPET assists in providing patients with accurate information regarding their perioperative risk, informs surgical decision-making and helps to plan both perioperative management and post-operative care. It is a dynamic, non-invasive assessment of effectiveness of cardiac and pulmonary function at rest and during exertion. Peak oxygen consumption (VO_{2max}), anaerobic threshold (AT) and ventilatory efficiency are assessed and predict operative fitness. The anaerobic threshold indicates the exertional threshold for an individual at which aerobic metabolism switches to anaerobic metabolism due to insufficient oxygen delivery to the peripheral tissues. An anaerobic threshold of less than 11 ml/kg/min is the limit currently accepted as indicative of significantly increased perioperative risk, although this varies by the particular type of surgery planned.

Nutritional Optimization

Adequate nutrition plays a critical role in preparing the body for surgery and recovery. Nutritional interventions may include oral supplementation to correct caloric and vitamin deficiencies, dietary modifications to support immune function and tissue healing, and strategies to optimize body composition. For specific indications such as bariatric surgery, patients may be placed on a protocolized very low-calorie (400–800 kcal/day) diet in the week preceding surgery, with the goal of achieving rapid weight loss, primarily by reduction of body fat percentage. This has been shown to reduce visceral adipose tissue and liver volume, and is associated with improved surgical outcomes, namely reduced procedure time, reduced estimated blood loss, and shorter length of stay. Conversely, for patients with cachexia arising secondary to malignancy, malnutrition, malabsorption or compromised intestinal function such as may occur in those with obstruction, short gut syndrome or Crohn's disease, additional nutritional support may be required in the pre-operative period. This may range from simple interventions such as high-calorie, high-protein oral nutritional supplements, to enteral feeding via nasogastric tube, to parenteral feeding. Although serum albumin is a poor marker of nutritional status, it is a good marker of overall condition and indicative of likelihood of post-operative morbidity. Pre-operative hypoalbuminaemia is a well described prognostic marker for poorer outcomes and increased complication rate, including wound complications and, particularly in the setting of Crohn's, septic complications.

Sarcopenia

Sarcopenia is the loss of muscle mass along with muscle strength, most frequently observed as part of the ageing and frailty process but also often evident in the context of advanced malignancy. It is frequently underdiagnosed, but is gaining recognition as a predictive marker of post-operative outcomes. The presence of pre-operative Sarcopenia is associated with an increased incidence of late post-operative complications, increased length of stay, increased 30-day mortality and a significantly increased rate of re-admission to hospital after major surgery, including gastrointestinal, orthopedic and cardiac surgeries.

Psychological Support

Psychological readiness for surgery is an often-overlooked aspect of pre-habilitation. Interventions may include stress management techniques, counseling, and education to alleviate anxiety and depression, thereby improving post-operative compliance and outcomes. Direction of patients to patient-centered resources such as support groups for those with a similar history may be of assistance, especially for those with chronic conditions. The need for psychological support is especially the case for complex patients who may have undergone multiple previous surgeries and prolonged intensive care admission, such as those with abdominal catastrophe, longstanding open abdomens and enterocutaneous fistulas. Psychological support, assessment and preparation is also critical for those undergoing bariatric surgery procedures, where long-term success is highly dependent not just upon a satisfactory technical outcome but also sustained patient motivation, compliance and engagement.

Medical Optimization

This involves managing existing chronic conditions such as diabetes, hypertension, and respiratory diseases more aggressively to ensure they are well-controlled and fully optimized at the time of surgery. It may also include smoking cessation programs and alcohol reduction and cessation strategies. If patients are on medications such as systemic corticosteroids, chemotherapy or targeted immunomodulatory agents such as sirolimus or bevacizamab, every effort should be made to discontinue these at least six weeks pre-operatively. Steroid use in the perioperative period is known to increase the risk of wound complications and septic complications such as anastomotic leak, while sirolimus is known to increase the risk of seroma formation and wound dehiscence. Bevacizumab, an anti-VEGF monoclonal antibody used in the setting of neoadjuvant regimens for breast cancer and metastatic colorectal cancer, may similarly increase the risk of wound breakdown and anastomotic leak. For other medications such as anti-TNF biologic agents which may be used in the setting of inflammatory bowel disease and rheumatological disorders, the effect on post-operative morbidity is as yet unknown.

Evidence Supporting Pre-Habilitation

A growing body of research underscores the efficacy of pre-habilitation in various surgical contexts, including orthopedic, gastrointestinal, vascular, urological and cardiothoracic surgery. Studies have demonstrated that patients who undergo prehabilitation programs experience shorter hospital stays, reduced postoperative complications, and quicker return to baseline levels of function compared to those who do not. Furthermore, pre-habilitation has been associated with a significant reduction in healthcare costs due to fewer complications, shorter length of stay and readmissions.

Implementation Challenges and Considerations

Despite its benefits, the implementation of pre-habilitation programs faces several challenges. These include identifying those patients who are likely to derive the most benefit from prehabilitation programmes, developing and standardizing intervention protocols, and ensuring patient compliance. Additionally, there is a need for further research to optimize pre-habilitation strategies, especially for the most co-morbid patients, and to establish individualized guidelines for the various surgical procedures.

Conclusion

Pre-habilitation represents a paradigm shift in preoperative care, emphasizing the proactive optimization of patients' health before surgery. By adopting a holistic approach that includes physical, nutritional, psychological, and medical interventions, pre-habilitation seeks to enhance patients' physical strength and resilience, thereby improving surgical outcomes and facilitating recovery. As the evidence base for pre-habilitation continues to grow, it is likely that such programs will become an integral part of standard preoperative care, tailored to the needs of individual patients and specific surgical procedures.

Reference

1. Fligor J, Lanier ST, Dumanian GA. Current risk stratification systems are not generalizable across surgical technique in midline ventral hernia repair. Plast Reconstr Surg Glob Open. 2017;5(3):e1206. https://doi.org/10.1097/GOX.0000000000001206.

Chapter 32
Management of the Patient in the Post-Operative Setting

Lauren O'Connell

Abstract As in the pre-operative setting, some components of post-operative management will be specific to the procedure undertaken, but many other elements of post-operative care are generalizable and relevant to any surgical procedure. The core considerations include: Management of post-operative pain and provision of appropriate analgesia, via a suitable mode of delivery, venous thromboembolism prophylaxis and others.

Keywords Post-operative · Management · Sheet · Examination · Prophylaxis · Venous · Thrombosis · Pain

As in the pre-operative setting, some components of post-operative management will be specific to the procedure undertaken, but many other elements of post-operative care are generalizable and relevant to any surgical procedure. The core considerations include:

- Management of post-operative pain and provision of appropriate analgesia, via a suitable mode of delivery.
- Venous thromboembolism prophylaxis—mechanical and pharmacological.
- Early mobilization and physiotherapy input as required.
- Management and timing of removal of drains, indwelling lines (such as central, arterial) and urinary catheters.
- Delivery of nutrition in the post-operative period. Consideration of the most appropriate route of feeding (oral, enteral or parenteral) and anticipated interval until return of gut function.

L. O'Connell (✉)
SVUH, Dublin, Ireland
e-mail: laurenoconnell@rcsi.ie

A. Farag et al. (eds.), *Clinical Surgical Skills Made Easy*,
https://doi.org/10.1007/978-3-031-69158-4_32

Role of ERAS Protocols

Enhanced Recovery after Surgery (ERAS) programs have become widely adopted over the past two decades. Initiating with use in elective colorectal surgery, they have now been taken up for a broad spectrum of surgical procedures [1]. Such programs represent a paradigm shift in perioperative care, aiming to optimize patient outcomes through a multidisciplinary, evidence-based approach. These protocols focus on reducing the physiological Sequelae and psychological stress of surgery, with the goal of accelerating recovery, minimizing complications, and shortening hospital stays. This comprehensive discussion delves into the principles of ERAS, with a particular focus on its application in bariatric, colorectal, and esophageal surgeries.

Introduction to ERAS

ERAS protocols encompass preoperative, intraoperative, and postoperative strategies designed to maintain homeostasis, enhance pain control, reduce physiological surgical stress, and facilitate early mobilization and nutrition. The core elements include patient education, optimization of nutrition, minimizing fasting, use of multimodal analgesia to reduce opioid use, early enteral feeding, early mobilization, and early removal of drains and catheters. Prescription of pre-operative carbohydrate containing drinks has been shown to ameliorate the endocrine and metabolic stress response to surgery, as well as reducing the pre-operative discomfort and distress which may be associated with prolonged fasting. Where possible, avoidance of placement of indwelling drains and nasogastric tubes is preferred, in order to facilitate early oral intake and mobilization. Recent data from multiple studies has demonstrated that this approach is safe and does not result in increased patient morbidity. Use of parenteral nutrition and intravenous fluids is minimized, and early post-operative oral intake is encouraged. Early mobilization is similarly encouraged; this improves respiratory morbidity by increasing oxygenation and reducing alveolar collapse, thus minimizing the incidence of atelectasis and consequent lower respiratory tract infections. Early mobilization also has a significant role to play in reducing the risk of venous thromboembolism.

ERAS in Bariatric Surgery

Bariatric surgery presents unique challenges due to the patient population's specific needs, including higher risks of complications due to obesity and metabolic-related comorbidities. ERAS protocols in bariatric surgery focus on:

Patient education on lifestyle changes post-surgery, nutritional assessments, and psychological evaluations are crucial. Prehabilitation, including physical exercises and dietary adjustments, is strongly encouraged in order to enhance postoperative recovery.

Minimally invasive techniques such as laparoscopic or robotic approaches are preferred to reduce pain, wound complications, and length of hospital stay. Intraoperative fluid management is optimized as per a goal-directed paradigm to avoid fluid overload and electrolyte imbalances.

Early mobilization is emphasized to reduce the risk of DVT and PE, which is especially high in the bariatric population, and represents the commonest complication seen in the post-operative period. Twice daily low molecular weight heparin is administered as a weight based regimen. Intraoperatively, thrombo-embolic deterrent stockings (TEDS) and sequential compression devices (SCDs) are used; use of TEDs should continue post-operatively. Multimodal pain management strategies, including the use of non-opioid analgesics, are employed to facilitate early ambulation and reduce pulmonary complications. Early initiation of liquid diets, progressing to solid foods as tolerated over a period of weeks, is recommended to support nutritional needs and weight loss objectives.

ERAS in Colorectal Surgery

ERAS protocols originated for use in the setting of elective colorectal surgery. Colorectal surgery can significantly benefit from ERAS protocols, given the high volume and the potential for complications. Key components include:

Pre-operative counseling and stoma education by a stoma nurse (if applicable) are provided. Combined mechanical bowel preparation with oral antibiotic decontamination is selectively used, typically for left sided rather than right sided resections. This has been shown to result in reduced superficial and deep space wound infections, reduced septic complications, reduced incidence of post-operative C. difficile infection and reduced anastomotic leak rates. As with other ERAS protocols, carbohydrate loading with clear carbohydrate pre-operative drinks is permitted up until 2 h prior to the procedure to maintain an anabolic rather than catabolic state, reduce perioperative insulin resistance and reduce postoperative nausea.

As with bariatric surgery, minimally invasive surgical techniques such as robotic or laparoscopic approaches are preferred where feasible. Active warming is used to prevent hypothermia, and again goal-directed fluid therapy is employed to maintain euvolemia while avoiding volume overload. Early removal of catheters and drains is preferable in order to reduce infection risk and promote mobilization. Indeed, data from the literature suggests that avoidance of routine intra-abdominal drain placement is safe in the setting of colorectal surgery and enhances early recovery due to reduction of pain and facilitation of mobilization. While nasogastric tubes may be utilized Intraoperatively, these may be removed at the conclusion of the surgical procedure. Early oral feeding within 24 h post-surgery is encouraged to stimulate bowel function and minimize the incidence of post-operative ileus, while use of parenteral nutrition and intravenous fluid delivery is preferentially avoided. Multimodal analgesia, avoiding excessive use of opioids, facilitates early ambulation. Patient controlled analgesia is frequently employed, allowing opioid delivery to be tailored to the individual patient's needs. Avoidance of epidural analgesia or the use of 'walking' epidurals again facilitates early mobilization and minimizes the likelihood of prolonged confinement to the bed, thus reducing the incidence of atelectasis and respiratory infections.

ERAS in Esophageal and Gastric Surgery

Esophageal and gastric surgery, given its complexity and the potential for significant morbidity, requires tailored ERAS protocols. As the etiology of esophageal malignancy and many other upper gastrointestinal disorders is strongly linked to alcohol intake and smoking, many of these patients have significant cardiorespiratory morbidity also related to these risk factors. Many patients will have weight loss, sarcopenia and cachexia due to dysphagia or from the presence of advanced malignancy. They may also frequently have undergone neoadjuvant treatment with systemic chemotherapy and/or radiotherapy prior to surgery as part of their treatment paradigm. Components of esophageal surgery ERAS protocols typically include:

Preoperatively, nutritional optimization is crucial due to the high prevalence of preoperative malnutrition and cachexia in esophageal and gastric cancer patients. This may entail supplemental feeding via oral supplements, nasogastric or nasojejunal tube feeding or parenteral nutrition, if feeding via an enteral route is not feasible due to the disease process. Preoperatively, pulmonary function testing and assessment of structural cardiac health via echocardiography and ECG is performed. Patients also routinely undergo cardiopulmonary exercise testing as described above, to assess their capability to withstand operative intervention and predict post-operative morbidity risks. Physiotherapy and respiratory exercises are recommended to improve postoperative pulmonary function.

Intraoperatively, minimally invasive oesophagectomy (MIE) is increasingly favored over open procedures. Open thoracotomy which is required for three-stage esophageal procedures is associated with substantial post-operative pain and thus carries a significant risk of respiratory morbidity due to splinting of the diaphragm and difficulty in engaging with physiotherapy. Minimally invasive approaches result in reduced postoperative pain and thus respiratory complications. Robotic approaches are favored due to the surgical limitations presented by the fixed bony compartment of the thoracic cavity, although laparoscopic approaches are also in use and effective. Careful anesthetic management is essential to maintain hemodynamic stability, identify potential complications such as iatrogenic pneumothorax early and reduce pulmonary morbidity.

Early extubation, when feasible, is pursued to reduce the duration of mechanical ventilation. Early enteral nutrition, typically via a feeding jejunostomy placed at the time of surgery, supports recovery while minimizing the need for indwelling lines for parenteral nutrition and risks associated with anastomotic leaks. Pain management strategies are multimodal, including agents targeting neuropathic pain which may arise after thoracotomy, and focus on minimizing opioid use to facilitate early mobilization and reduce ileus.

ERAS protocols thus represent a holistic approach to perioperative care, emphasizing evidence-based practices to enhance recovery and improve surgical outcomes. The customization of these protocols for bariatric, colorectal, and esophageal and gastric surgeries addresses the unique challenges and needs of these patient populations. By reducing the physiological stress of surgery, optimizing pain management, and encouraging early mobility and nutrition, ERAS programs significantly contribute to improved patient outcomes, reduced hospital stays, and lower complication rates. As these protocols continue to evolve with emerging evidence, they will undoubtedly remain a cornerstone of modern surgical care.

Incorporating ERAS protocols requires a multidisciplinary effort, involving surgeons, anesthesiologists, specialist and ward-based nursing care, dieticians, and physiotherapists, among others. Continuous evaluation and adaptation of these protocols are essential to align with the latest evidence and technological advancements in surgery. As healthcare professionals embrace and refine ERAS protocols, the future of surgical care looks promising, with enhanced patient outcomes and optimized resource utilization.

Post-Operative Complications

Surgical post-operative complications are critical concerns in the medical field, affecting patient recovery, hospital stay duration, and overall outcomes. The incidence and type of complications anticipated after surgery varies by the particular operation type and whether performed in the elective or emergency setting. However, some risk factors are common to many or all complications, and some complications are common to all surgical procedures, although with varying incidences. These include deep venous thrombosis (DVT), pulmonary embolism (PE), respiratory tract infections, wound and deep surgical site infections, anastomotic leak (for gastrointestinal surgeries), and hemorrhage. Knowledge of diagnostic, management, and preventive strategies are crucial to ensure optimal patient care and outcomes. Some of the commonest complications and their diagnosis and management are outlined below.

Unscheduled Care and Emergency Surgery

It is well known that surgery performed during unscheduled care or in the emergency setting is associated with significantly higher morbidity, mortality and poorer patient outcomes than elective surgery. This is in part due to the lack of potential for pre-operative optimization in emergency surgery, and the fact that the condition for which surgery is required may cause substantial deleterious disturbances to the patient's physiological state; for example, electrolyte abnormalities, acute kidney injury, and acidosis with worsening of coagulopathy. Additionally, the trend towards an ageing population worldwide means that there is an increasing proportion of older patients undergoing surgical care, with associated increased pre-operative morbidity and frailty. The UK NCEPOD (National Confidential Enquiry into Peri-Operative Deaths) and NELA (National Emergency Laparotomy Audit) audits, among other data, determined that operative interventions performed at night are further associated with poorer morbidity and mortality outcomes than those emergency procedures performed during the daytime.

Deep Venous Thromboembolism (DVT)

DVT is diagnosed through clinical suspicion initially; typically on findings of new unilateral leg swelling, with erythema, calf tenderness, and pitting edema, potentially in the setting of provoking factors such as immobility, malignancy or recent surgery. They can occur as early as 48 h post-op. The elevated risk of venous thromboembolism persists for up to three months. Clinical assessment tools like the Wells score assist in making the diagnosis. Imaging studies such as duplex ultrasonography are the gold standard with respect to confirming the diagnosis. D-dimer levels can be helpful in low-risk patients. However, this test is highly sensitive but has poor specificity, and is therefore unhelpful in the immediate post-operative setting, as it is inevitably raised in the context of recent surgical intervention.

The management of DVT involves commencement of therapeutic anticoagulation, typically with low molecular weight heparin (LMWH) or direct oral anticoagulants (DOACs). For patients at a particularly high risk of bleeding or where a short half-life is particularly desirable, unfractionated heparin may be used; however, this requires frequent monitoring of therapeutic range with serial APTT measurements. In cases where anticoagulation is contraindicated, inferior vena caval filters may be placed. It is critical to ensure follow up and removal of such filters is arranged, as if left in situ long-term the filter itself may act as a nidus for thrombus formation and embolic complications. Massive DVTs may be treated with interventional methods such as catheter-directed thrombolysis or thrombectomy.

Pulmonary Embolism (PE)

Diagnosis of PE, as for DVT involves primarily clinical assessment initially. Dyspnea, pleuritic chest pain, sinus tachycardia and desaturation are typical symptoms and signs, along with clinical symptoms and signs suggestive of DVT and calculation of a Wells score. Massive PE is associated with the presence of hypotension and shock. As for DVT, D-dimer testing is unhelpful in the post-operative setting. Initial investigations should comprise an arterial blood gas to assess oxygenation and a chest radiograph to exclude infective causes. The gold standard for making the diagnosis is computed tomography pulmonary angiography (CTPA). Ventilation-perfusion (V/Q) scans are alternatives for patients contraindicated for CTPA, for example those with a contrast allergy or significantly impaired renal function.

Management is similar to that for DVT, with commencement of therapeutic anticoagulation. Severe cases may require thrombolytic therapy, surgical embolectomy, or placement of an inferior vena cava (IVC) filter.

Atelectasis and Respiratory Tract Infections

Diagnosis of atelectasis and lower respiratory tract infection is based on clinical signs and symptoms, namely dyspnea, productive cough, chest pain and desaturation, along with typical findings on chest radiograph of atelectasis, consolidation or pleural effusion, and rising inflammatory markers such as white cell count (WCC) and CRP (C-reactive protein). Signs and symptoms of sepsis such as pyrexia and tachycardia may also be present, which should trigger a septic screen including blood and sputum cultures to identify the offending organism. The onset is typically within 72 h of general anesthesia.

For atelectasis alone without signs or symptoms of sepsis, chest physiotherapy and ensuring adequate clearance of respiratory secretions may be sufficient treatment. Management of respiratory tract infection includes initiation of broad-spectrum antibiotic therapy as per local guidelines; these can subsequently be tailored to culture results. Respiratory support with supplemental oxygen is delivered as required based on saturation levels. Occasionally non-invasive positive pressure oxygen therapy such as Airvo or CPAP may be required. Preventative methods are key, and include ensuring adequate analgesia, early ambulation, chest physiotherapy and use of incentive spirometry devices.

Indwelling Line and Catheter Infections

Indwelling lines and catheters such as central lines, peripherally inserted central catheter (PICC) lines and urinary catheters all predispose to colonization and infection. They should be handled using aseptic or sterile technique as appropriate, regularly reviewed to determine the necessity for their ongoing use and removed promptly once no longer required. The development of sepsis may mandate removal of an indwelling line despite an ongoing indication for its use. In this instance, a 24 or 48 h line-free period is required prior to replacement of the line.

Wound and Deep Space Infections

Diagnosis of superficial wound infections involves the identification of signs of infection at the surgical site, such as erythema, fluctuance, presence of purulent discharge, and increased tenderness. Swab cultures help in identifying the causative organism and rationalizing antibiotic therapy. Management includes appropriate antibiotic therapy, wound debridement, and proper wound care techniques. In some cases, negative pressure wound therapy (NPWT) and vacuum-assisted closure (VAC) therapy may be beneficial.

Deep space infections such as intra-abdominal collections or joint infections may present in a more occult fashion, with failure to progress along the normal post-operative course, pain, persistent ileus, reduced range of motion of a joint, increasing inflammatory markers such as WCC, neutrophil count and CRP, and signs of sepsis. While inflammatory markers will inevitably be elevated in the post-operative setting, this follows a predictable trend, where CRP will typically increase up until the third post-operative day, whereafter it should begin to decrease again. Deviation from this pattern, while nonspecific, is typically indicative of some pertubation of the normal post-operative course. Imaging with contrast-enhanced CT or US is typically confirmatory.

Management of deep space infections entails commencement of antibiotic therapy, with the specific choice of antibiotic dependent on the surgical procedure and suspected likely organisms. For clean procedures such as joint replacements, thyroidectomy, carotid endarterectomy and similar, cover should be directed at aerobic Gram-positive organisms, including potential resistant organisms. For clean-contaminated and contaminated procedures such as intra-abdominal and particularly gastrointestinal surgeries, antibiotic therapy with cover for both aerobic and anaerobic organisms should be implemented. For larger collections, typically those greater than 4 cm in diameter, percutaneous drainage may be required. For gastrointestinal surgery, the presence of an abdominal or pelvic collection in the setting of an anastomosis formation should prompt consideration of the development of an anastomotic leak. These typically present between the fifth to seventh post-operative day. Contrast-enhanced CT may suggest the presence of a leak, although in some instances the diagnosis is confirmed with a water-soluble contrast enema. In addition to antibiotics and percutaneous drainage, these may be managed with application of a negative pressure dressing such as the Endosponge, or require surgical re-intervention and revision or takedown of the anastomosis for significant leaks.

Where prostheses such as synthetic permanent meshes or prosthetic joints have developed infections, if antibiotic therapy is ineffective the prosthesis may ultimately require removal.

Hemorrhage

Post-operative hemorrhage is identified by clinical signs of bleeding, such as presence of a hematoma, new or worsening hypotension, tachycardia, and dropping hemoglobin levels. Pain and confusion may be present. Imaging, for example with CT angiography, or endoscopic evaluation may be necessary to locate the bleeding source.

The initial management entails fluid resuscitation with or without blood transfusion. Definitive management may involve surgical re-exploration and direct control of bleeding by suturing or packing, endoscopic intervention with clipping or injection, or radiological localization and embolization to control the bleeding. While historically embolization of gastrointestinal anastomoses carried a risk of rendering the tissue ischaemia in approximately 20–30% of cases, with the advent of superselective embolization techniques this risk has significantly reduced to less than 10%, and thus is significantly more safe. Nevertheless, use of embolization in the setting of anastomotic and staple line bleeding remains highly controversial.

Research suggests that transexamic acid may have a beneficial role in the perioperative setting to reduce the incidence of significant bleeding events and perioperative transfusion requirements. Transfusion of blood products is associated with potential immune-mediated and volume-related complications. It has also been shown to be associated with poorer outcomes in the setting of oncological surgery. The POISE-3 randomized controlled trial investigated use of transexamic acid in a wide variety of non-cardiac surgery settings, including orthopedic, gastrointestinal, vascular, cardiothoracic and urological procedures. It found that administration of transexamic acid at the commencement and conclusion of surgery resulted in significantly fewer major bleeding events and a significantly reduced transfusion requirement, without a concomitant increase in thromboembolic or cardiac events [2]. Discussion is ongoing regarding incorporation of transexamic acid into routine perioperative use for major surgery.

Preventive Measures

Preventive strategies play a crucial role in minimizing post-operative complications. These include risk assessment and prophylaxis for DVT and PE, especially in high-risk patients; utilization of enhanced recovery after surgery (ERAS) protocols to facilitate early mobilization and return of gut function; and strict adherence to surgical asepsis and antibiotic prophylaxis guidelines to prevent wound and respiratory infections.

Conclusion

The diagnosis and management of surgical post-operative complications require a multidisciplinary approach, incorporating evidence-based guidelines, vigilant monitoring, and prompt intervention. By understanding these complications and their management strategies, healthcare professionals can significantly improve patient outcomes and reduce the incidence of adverse events following surgery.

Preparation for Discharge

A critical step in post-operative care is ensuring a safe discharge from hospital and that appropriate follow-up is arranged. The patient should be aware of their follow-up plan and what to expect at the time of their discharge, ideally in a written format. They should also be educated on signs of potential late complications and advised on the appropriate action to take if they experience these. Allied health professionals who have been involved in the patient's care such as physiotherapy and occupational therapy should be similarly satisfied that the patient is safe to be discharged from an acute care facility. There should be an agreed discharge destination which is deemed appropriate by the medical team, allied health care professionals and the patient themselves. While this is often directly to their home, some patients may benefit from a brief period of further recovery in a transitional stepdown setting such a rehabilitation or convalescence facility. The patient and/or their carers should be advised on specific aspects of continued recovery once discharged, in particular wound care, physiotherapy exercise regimens and dietary intake. Dependent on the procedure, the patient may require several weeks of post-operative pharmacological VTE prophylaxis, and they should receive education on this prior to discharge. Again dependent on the procedure, input and training by dedicated stoma care nurse specialists or interventional radiology nurses may be required prior to discharge to ensure patients can independently manage stomas or indwelling percutaneous drains. Finally, the patient should be furnished with an appropriate prescription, ensuring adequate analgesia and including nutritional supplementation as required.

References

1. Ljungqvist O, de Boer HD, Balfour A, Fawcett WJ, Lobo DN, Nelson G, et al. Opportunities and challenges for the next phase of enhanced recovery after surgery: a review. JAMA Surg. 2021;156(8):775–84.
2. Devereaux PJ, Marcucci M, Painter TW, Conen D, Lomivorotov V, Sessler DI, et al. Tranexamic acid in patients undergoing noncardiac surgery. N Engl J Med. 2022;386(21):1986–97.

Chapter 33
Stoma Examination

Enda Hannan, Nicholas Johnson, Tim Harding, and Ehab A. Mansour

Abstract The word ostomy, derived from the Latin word ostium, means mouth or opening. In surgical anatomy, a stoma is any artificial opening in any hollow viscus in the body. The most commonly created stomas are ileostomies and colostomies, which are formed for a wide range of indications and may be temporary or permanent. The first recorded surgical ileostomy was created in 1879 by a German Surgeon, Dr. Baum, to decompress an obstructing caecal adenocarcinoma.

Keywords Ostomy · Ileostomy · Colostomy · Temporary · Permanent · End · Loop · Complications · Siting

Abbreviations

AL	Anastomotic leak
APR	Abdominoperineal resection
CD	Crohn's disease
CRC	Colorectal cancer
FAP	Familial adenomatous polyposis
UC	Ulcerative colitis

E. Hannan (✉) · T. Harding · E. A. Mansour
Department of Surgery, St Vincent's University Hospital, Dublin 4, Ireland

Department of Surgery, The Royal College of Surgeons in Ireland, Dublin 2, Ireland
e-mail: endahannan@rcsi.com

N. Johnson
Department of Surgery, St Vincent's University Hospital, Dublin 4, Ireland

A. Farag et al. (eds.), *Clinical Surgical Skills Made Easy*,
https://doi.org/10.1007/978-3-031-69158-4_33

Introduction

The word 'ostomy', derived from the Latin word *ostium*, means mouth or opening [1]. In surgical anatomy, a stoma is any artificial opening in any hollow viscus in the body [2]. The most commonly created stomas are ileostomies and colostomies, which are formed for a wide range of indications and may be temporary or permanent. The first recorded surgical ileostomy was created in 1879 by a German Surgeon, Dr. Baum, to decompress an obstructing caecal adenocarcinoma [3]. Currently, it is estimated that there are approximately 13.5 million people worldwide living with a stoma [4]. However, despite many advancements in stoma formation and care, complication rates may be as high as 50% [5]. Common complications include high output, parastomal hernia formation, prolapse and stenosis, which serve as a significant source of distress and morbidity to patients [6]. Furthermore, conditions which may require ostomy formation, such as Crohn's disease (CD), diverticular disease and colorectal cancer (CRC), are becoming increasingly prevalent, particularly in younger patients [7]. Thus, the appropriate examination and subsequent management of the patient with a stoma is an essential part of day-to-day surgical practice. The purpose of this chapter is to provide the practicing surgeon with a systemic and structured approach to stoma examination, which will not only allow one to correctly identify the type of stoma and potential indications for its formation, but also to correctly identify its complications, thus empowering the practicing clinician to implement an appropriate management plan based on clinical examination findings.

Background Knowledge

Definition of a Stoma: An iatrogenic opening which connects a hollow viscus to the outside world with a bag to collect its contents.

Indications for Stoma Formation

1. *Resection of a diseased portion of bowel where primary anastomosis is unsafe:*
    - Hartmann's procedure for diverticular disease in the emergency setting (obstruction or perforation).
    - Obstructing sigmoid cancer.
    - Large bowel CD.
    - Subtotal colectomy for medically refractory ulcerative colitis (UC).
    - Acute mesenteric ischaemia.
    - Toxic megacolon.

2. *Resection of a diseased portion of bowel and the anal canal where primary anastomosis is impossible:*
    - Abdominoperineal resection (APR) for low rectal cancer.
    - Panproctocolectomy for UC, familial adenomatous polyposis (FAP) or Crohn's proctocolitis.
3. *Diversion to protect distal bowel or perianal sepsis:*
    - Defunctioning loop ileostomy to protect an anastomosis at high risk of an anastomotic leak (AL), such as following anterior resection for low rectal cancer.
    - Diverting loop ileostomy or colostomy to minimize sepsis and symptoms from a more distal abscess or fistula.
    - Defunctioning loop colostomy to protect a perianal wound, such as following debridement for perianal necrotizing fasciitis or Fournier's gangrene.
4. *Decompression*
    - Loop colostomy or ileostomy (depending on ileocaecal valve incompetence) to decompress large bowel obstruction due to rectal malignancy prior to Neoadjuvant Chemoradiotherapy.
5. *Fecal incontinence:*
    - Loop colostomy for quality of life in patients with conditions with fecal incontinence which is resistant to non-operative measures, such as following obstetric injury or spinal cord injury.
6. Feeding:
    - Feeding jejunostomy to provide adequate nutrition following oesophagectomy where oral feeding is unsafe due to the risk of compromising the anastomosis.
    - Feeding gastrostomy in patients with unsafe swallow to minimize the risk of aspiration.

Classification of Stomas

1. *Anatomical classification*
    - Ileostomy (small bowel stoma).
    - Colostomy (large bowel stoma).
    - Urostomy (following cystectomy and ileal conduit for bladder carcinoma).
    - Jejunostomy (feeding stoma).
    - Gastrostomy (feeding stoma).
2. *Temporary or permanent*

- Any form of loop stoma is technically temporary and may be reversed.
- Any form of end stoma where the anal canal remains in-situ is technically temporary and may be reversed.
- However, it is important to remember that while such stomas may be possible to reverse, it may be unwise or unsafe to do so due to patient factors (such as medical comorbidities which render an increased risk of the frequency or morbidity/mortality as a result of AL).
- Any end stoma where the anal canal is excised (such as following APR or Panproctocolectomy) is a permanent stoma which may not be reversed.

3. End stoma or loop stoma

   - If a single orifice is evident on examination, this is an end stoma.
   - If two orifices are visible at the ostomy site, this is a loop stoma.

Stoma Siting (Table 33.1)

- In the elective setting, it is essential that the patient be seen by the stoma care nurse prior to any operation involving the intestine so that an appropriate location on the abdomen may be identified for optimal stoma placement, should it be required. This should certainly be performed in all operations where a stoma will definitely be created, but should also be done for operations where stoma formation is unlikely but still possible, such as for an elective right Hemicolectomy or sigmoid colectomy where a primary anastomosis without Defunctioning stoma is planned.
- The stoma is typically placed through the rectus muscle slightly below the level of umbilicus and 5 cm away from skin folds, the belt line, bony prominences and the umbilicus.

Table 33.1 Overview of stomas

Type of stoma		Possible procedure
Colostomy – *Usually LIF* – *Hard stool* – *No spout*	**End colostomy** – Single lumen **Loop colostomy** – Two lumens	**Permanent:** APR **Temporary:** Hartmann's procedure, non-restorative anterior resection **Defunctioning loop colostomy:** To protect distal anastomosis **Decompressive loop colostomy:** To relieve distal obstruction
Ileostomy – *Usually RIF* – *Liquid stool* – *Spout*	**End Ileostomy** – Single lumen **Loop ileostomy** – 2 lumens	**Permanent:** Panproctocolectomy **Temporary:** Emergency subtotal colectomy **Defunctioning loop ileostomy:** To protect distal anastomosis **Decompressive loop ileostomy:** To relieve distal obstruction

- Typically, colostomies will be sited in the left iliac fossa (LIF) while colostomies will be sited in the right iliac fossa (RIF). However, this rule is not always followed, but is a good guide to use for approaching stoma examination.

Common Definitions

Hartmann's procedure: Surgical resection of the sigmoid or rectosigmoid with closure of the rectal stump and formation of an end colostomy

- Commonly performed in the emergency setting, such as for perforated or obstructing diverticular disease, or for obstructing or perforated sigmoid cancer.
- While the end colostomy created in a Hartmann's procedure is technically reversible, it is not reversed in as many as 60% of patients due to associated medical comorbidities rending the risk of AL high [8].
- Reversal of Hartmann's procedure is also widely recognized as a highly challenging procedure with significant risk of intraoperative morbidity due to postoperative adhesions.

Panproctocolectomy: Removal of the entire colon, rectum and anus with formation of a permanent end ileostomy

- Commonly performed as a definitive cure for UC.
- Also may be performed for FAP to eliminate the risk of colorectal malignancy.
- This procedure is never performed in the emergency setting due to the significant risks of iatrogenic injury and inadequate resection margins associated with emergency proctectomy.
- In appropriately counselled patients who are stoma-averse, a proctocolectomy where the anal canal is left in-situ and an ileal pouch-anal anastomosis, or J-pouch, is formed may be an alternative (although this will still require a temporary Defunctioning loop ileostomy due to the risk of post-operative AL).

Abdominoperineal Resection: Removal of the lower rectum and anus with formation of a permanent end colostomy

- Most commonly performed for low rectal adenocarcinoma which is either too close to the anal verge to achieve safe resection margins or involving the anal verge.
- May also be performed for benign conditions, such as severe perianal CD.

High output stoma: The normal output from an ileostomy ranges from 300 ml to 800 ml per day. While there is no agreed definition of a high output stoma, it is generally considered to be an output exceeding 1 to 2 L in a 24 h period [9]. Another definition is where the output is at a point where it is causing a physiological compromise for the patient, such as clinical signs and symptoms of dehydration, acute kidney injury or electrolyte imbalance [10].

Preparation

- Wash your hands
- Introduce yourself & confirm patient details (name, date of birth, medical record number)
- Explain the purpose of the examination & gain verbal consent
- Ensure a chaperone is present (Stoma examination is considered an intimate examination)
- Exposure the patient appropriately (from xiphisternum to pubic symphysis)
- Check if the patient is in any discomfort or pain
- Wear non-sterile gloves for the examination
- Ensure lubricating jelly is available
- Ensure good lighting (to appropriate inspect the mucosa of the stoma)
- Check that the patient has a replacement stoma bag with them
- Always use a stoma adhesive removal spray to remove the bag
- Check if the presence of the stoma care nurse is necessary to avoid unnecessary duplicate examinations
- Consider the availability and need for adjuncts to examination, such as stoma dilators in cases where the patient is suffering from stoma stenosis
- Position the patient supine initially for stoma examination, but remember that the patient may need to stand so that you may properly assess for the presence of a parastomal hernia

Clinical Examination

Inspection

- **Mnemonic for stoma inspection:**
- ***S**mall **B**ags **S**hould **L**ay **M**ore **S**nugly **O**n **C**ommitted **P**atients*
- **Site**

  Right iliac fossa: Usually an ileostomy.
  Left iliac fossa: Usually a colostomy.

- **Bag Contents:** Inspect the contents of the bag

  - *Enteric/liquid content:* Ileostomy
  - *Solid/fecal content:* Colostomy
  - Take note if the stoma bag appears to be full or not, as this may represent a high-output stoma

- **Spout:**

  - *Spouted stoma:* Ileostomy

  - *No spout & flushed with the skin:* Colostomy
    - A spout is created in ileostomies to protect the surrounding skin from irritation due to enzymes present in small bowel secretion
- **Lumen(s):**
  - *Single lumen:* End stoma
  - *Double lumen:* Loop stoma
    - In some cases, two lumens side by side may be a 'double' barreled stoma instead of a loop stoma, but this is functionally the same as a loop stoma
    - If there is a visible loop end ileostomy on the right side of the abdomen and a flushed end colostomy on the left side of the abdomen, the left sided stoma likely represents a 'mucus fistula' created from the distal end colon, such as following an emergency subtotal colectomy
    - In the immediate post-operative period following loop stoma formation, a temporary stoma rod is often used to allow the stoma to mature and prevent retraction. This typically should be removed by the stoma care nurse at 72 hours post-operatively
- **Mucosa:**
  - *Pink:* Healthy mucosa
  - *Dusky/blue:* Threatened mucosa, potentially evolving ischaemia
  - *Black:* Necrotic mucosa
  - *Ulcerated/erythematous:* Potential recurrence of the resected pathology, such as CD
    - This step is particularly important in the immediate post-operative period, where potential necrosis may require surgical reintervention with refashioning of the stoma
    - Adequate lighting is essential to assess the mucosa. Consider using a pen torch
    - Necrosis above the Fascial level (determined by digital examination of the stoma) may be managed conservatively with close observation and input from tissue viability services and stoma care nurses
    - Necrosis below the Fascial level will require emergency refashioning due to the risk of dehiscence and intra-abdominal sepsis
- **Scars:**
  - Examine the abdomen for either a midline laparotomy scar or laparoscopic port sites
  - This will help you ascertain whether this was potentially an emergency or elective operation
  - Typically, in imminent life-threatening colorectal emergencies, such as a Hartmann's procedure for obstruction or perforation or subtotal colectomy for

  acute mesenteric ischaemia or toxic megacolon, bowel resection will be performed open or by midline laparotomy
  - Conversely, elective colorectal operations such as for CRC will be performed laparoscopic where possible
  - However, such rules are not rigid and depends on patient status and the challenges posed by the underlying pathology
- **Old sites:**
  - Inspect the abdomen for scars that may represent previous stoma sites
  - In some cases, stomas may need to be re-sited due to complications associated with the original site (such as parastomal herniation) or due to sub-optimal placement of the original stoma
- **Complications:**
  - *Anatomical:* Prolapse, retraction, stenosis, parastomal herniation
  - *Dermatological:* Skin excoriation secondary to small bowel content
  - *Metabolic:* High output stoma resulting in acute kidney injury and electrolyte imbalance
  - *Vascular:* Hemorrhage, ischaemia, necrosis:
  - *Psychiatric:* Depression
  - The above complications may all not be imminently appreciable on inspection and thus may require adjuncts to your examination such as a detailed medical history, inquiring how the patient is coping with their stoma, reviewing previously performed imaging and checking their renal function/fluid balance chart
  - A helpful mnemonic for memorizing common stoma complications is **RIB SPINE** (retraction, infection, bleeding, stenosis/skin excoriation, prolapse/parastomal hernia/psychiatric, ischaemia, necrosis, electrolyte imbalance/high output stoma)
- **Perineum/Anus:**
  - Ask the patient if they still have a back passage or not
  - *Yes & end stoma:* This represents a technically reversible end stoma, such as following a Hartmann's procedure, non-restorative anterior resection or subtotal colectomy
  - *No:* This represents a permanent end colostomy, such as following an APR or Panproctocolectomy
  - In cases where the patient has no anal canal, always inspect the perineal wound for either the presence of wound dehiscence (in the early post-operative period) or perineal hernia formation (in the late post-operative period)
  - In cases where the patient has an anal canal, always perform a digital rectal examination and inquire if they have any perianal discharge or bleeding
  - In non-restorative procedures such as following subtotal colectomy or a Hartmann's procedure, clinicians often forget about the rectal stump, which may serve as a site for potential recurrence of colorectal cancer recurrence or

development of a metachronous tumor. Thus, it is important that the rectal stump is examined endoscopically as part of surveillance for colorectal malignancy in non-restorative anterior resections. Equally, where a subtotal colectomy is performed for ulcerative colitis, the rectal stump requires close endoscopic surveillance for either ongoing proctitis or subsequent development of rectal malignancy

Palpation

- Always inquire if the patient has any pain before commencing palpation
- Always watch the patient's face as you palpate to check for any signs of obvious discomfort or distress as you proceed with the examination
- Feel the contents of the stoma bag to further ascertain if the contents are solid (faeces) or liquid (small bowel content)
- While wearing non-sterile gloves and using lubrication, gently insert your finger into the lumen(s) of the stoma to assess patency
- Typically, if a stoma will admit one digit easily on examination, this likely represents a patent stoma
- It may be necessary to use a stoma dilator gently for this step with patient consent
- Assess for the presence of a parastomal hernia by placing both hands around the stoma and asking the patient to cough while you feel for an obvious protrusion or impulse
- If a parastomal hernia appears to be evident, deep palpation of the abdomen at this point may allow you to appreciate the Fascial edges to ascertain the size of the potential defect
- If a parastomal hernia is not evident on this step with the patient in supine position, you now must ask the patient to stand up (and thus increase intra-abdominal pressure) and repeat this step

Auscultation

- Using the diaphragm of your stethoscope, auscultate for the presence of absence of bowel sounds just below the umbilicus
- This step is particularly important in the immediate post-operative period in the context of either low/absent stoma output, which may represent either a post-operative ileus or a bowel obstruction
  - *Absent bowel sounds in the post-operative period:* Ileus
  - *Hyperactive or 'tinkling' bowel sounds:* Concerning for bowel obstruction

Adjuncts to Clinical Examination

- Consider performing a full gastrointestinal/abdominal examination
- Review the patient's bedside vitals, fluid balance chart and recent blood tests (including renal function/electrolytes) for evidence of a high-output stoma
- Consider involving the stoma care nurse if required
- Perform a detailed review of the medical chart including the operation note
- Consider the need for scheduling an endoscopic examination, particularly in the context of post-operative CRC or CD/UC surveillance
- Consider the need for arranging further imaging investigations, such as computed tomography of the abdomen and pelvis, such as for assessing potential parastomal herniation of for post-operative CRC surveillance
- If the patient has a parastomal hernia, a detailed history is required. Parastomal hernia repair is highly challenging and associated with a high risk of recurrence and post-operative morbidity. It should only be considered as a last resort in the elective setting. Consider the use a stoma support belt, which may alleviate may symptoms associated with parastomal hernia
- Consider the need for measures to address a high output stoma, such as the use of loperamide, codeine phosphate, intravenous fluids, electrolyte replacement or oral rehydration solutions
- In some cases, where patients are struggling to manage to live with a stoma, it may be necessary to involve psychiatry services, clinical psychology and linking the patient in with stoma support groups
- If the patient has a temporary Defunctioning ileostomy, such as following an anterior resection for CRC, consider if it is an appropriate time to consider stoma reversal (typically 3 months following the postoperative period and/or completion of potentially necessary adjuvant chemotherapy). Prior to reversal, it is essential that the patient undergo a gastrograffin study to ensure patency of the anastomosis.

Summary

- The presence and necessity for stoma formation is increasingly common in surgical practice, particularly with the increasing incidence and prevalence of diseases of the intestinal tract, such as CD, UC, diverticular disease and CRC.
- Despite improvements in surgical techniques and post-operative care, the presence of stoma-related complications remains unfortunately high.
- Thus, it is essential that the practicing surgeon be appropriately equipped with the knowledge and skills required to approach the patient living with a stoma.
- In this chapter, we have provided a systematic and structured approach to stoma examination, which not only aims to allow the clinician to correctly identify the

type of stoma present and to ascertain its likely indication, but to also recognize the presence of potential complications which may require prompt intervention.

- Preparation prior to examination is essential, such as ensuring that the patient has replacement stoma bags available and that you have all necessary relevant equipment available prior to commencing.
- A structured approach using inspection, palpation and auscultation may be applied to stoma examination, similar to clinical examination of other systems.
- As part of inspection, the mnemonic 'small bags should lay more snugly on committed patients' (site, bag contents, lumen(s), mucosa, scars, old sites, complications, perineum).
- With regards to palpation, this key step will allow the clinician to ascertain for the presence of other potential complications, such as stoma stenosis, high output or parastomal herniation.
- Auscultation will allow the clinician to assess for the presence of potential ileus or bowel obstruction in the post-operative period.
- While performing the clinical examination, it is important to maintain awareness of potential stoma complications (including anatomical, dermatological, metabolic, vascular and psychological complications) and potential interventions that may be required following completion of the clinical examination.
- Remember to utilize appropriate adjuncts to clinical examination where indicated, such as a complete gastrointestinal examination, involving the stoma care nurse, reviewing the patient's blood results, fluid balance chart, operative notes, endoscopic investigations and radiology.

References

1. Martin ST, Vogel JD. Intestinal stomas: indications, management, and complications. Adv Surg. 2012;46:19–49. https://doi.org/10.1016/j.yasu.2012.04.005. PMID: 22873030.
2. Cataldo PA. Intestinal stomas: 200 years of digging. Dis Colon Rectum. 1999;42(2):137–42. https://doi.org/10.1007/BF02237118. PMID: 10211488.
3. Kennedy HJ, Al-Dujaili EA, Edwards CR, Truelove SC. Water and electrolyte balance in subjects with a permanent ileostomy. Gut. 1983;24(8):702–5. https://doi.org/10.1136/gut.24.8.702. PMID: 6347830; PMCID: PMC1420234.
4. Morss-Walton PC, Yi JZ, Gunning ME, McGee JS. Ostomy 101 for dermatologists: Managing peristomal skin diseases. Dermatol Ther. 2021;34(5):e15069. https://doi.org/10.1111/dth.15069. Epub 2021 Aug 4. PMID: 34309140.
5. Krishnamurty DM, Blatnik J, Mutch M. Stoma Complications. Clin Colon Rectal Surg. 2017;30(3):193–200. https://doi.org/10.1055/s-0037-1598160. Epub 2017 May 22. PMID: 28684937; PMCID: PMC5498161.
6. Malik T, Lee MJ, Harikrishnan AB. The incidence of stoma related morbidity - a systematic review of randomised controlled trials. Ann R Coll Surg Engl. 2018;100(7):501–8. https://doi.org/10.1308/rcsann.2018.0126. Epub 2018 Aug 16. PMID: 30112948; PMCID: PMC6214073.
7. Loomans-Kropp HA, Umar A. Increasing Incidence of Colorectal Cancer in Young Adults. J Cancer Epidemiol. 2019;2019:9841295. https://doi.org/10.1155/2019/9841295. PMID: 31827515; PMCID: PMC6885269.

8. Roig JV, Cantos M, Balciscueta Z, Uribe N, Espinosa J, Roselló V, García-Calvo R, Hernandis J, Landete F; Sociedad Valenciana de Cirugía Cooperative Group. Hartmann's operation: how often is it reversed and at what cost? A multicentre study. Colorectal Dis. 2011;13(12):e396–402. https://doi.org/10.1111/j.1463-1318.2011.02738.x. PMID: 21801298.
9. Nightingale JMD. How to manage a high-output stoma. Frontline Gastroenterol. 2021;13(2):140–51. https://doi.org/10.1136/flgastro-2018-101108. PMID: 35300464; PMCID: PMC8862462.
10. Baker ML, Williams RN, Nightingale JM. Causes and management of a high-output stoma. Colorectal Dis. 2011;13(2):191–7. https://doi.org/10.1111/j.1463-1318.2009.02107.x. PMID: 19888956.

Chapter 34
Conclusion

Ahmed Farag

Abstract Starting my medical career as a house officer in 1981 and as a resident of Urology for 6 months and a resident of General surgery since 1982 and practicing surgery till now made my generation and myself the lucky generation of surgery and medicine in general. We witnessed the evolution of Surgery and Medicine from the almost 90% Clinical skill based practice to the Modern era of investigations and Practice.

Keywords Clinical · Skills · Lives · Resources · Health · Care · Errors · Examination

Starting my medical career as a house officer in 1981 and as a resident of Urology for 6 months and a resident of General surgery since 1982 and practicing surgery till now made my generation and myself the lucky generation of surgery and medicine in general. We witnessed the evolution of Surgery and Medicine from the almost 90% Clinical skill based practice to the Modern era of investigations and Practice. I operated on the first urine flow-meter introduced in our hospital as a resident of urology in 1981 it was a gas flow-meter and witnessed the introduction of Ultrasonography, CT scan, MRI, Isotopic scans, and finally the PET-CT and the evolution of intervention radiology, interventional Urology. Laparoscopic.

Surgery and Recently the Robotic Surgery

We are the bridge between the Clinical based diagnosis where the generation of our professors used to have the plain X-rays and the IVU and Ba studies as their all what they have to reach a clinical diagnosis and take a decision in their patients. We studied from books where the sound and through history taking had been thoroughly addressed hand in hand with the modern technology in investigating and treating patients [1].

A. Farag (✉)
Kasr Alainy Hospital, Cairo University, Cairo, Egypt

A. Farag et al. (eds.), *Clinical Surgical Skills Made Easy*,
https://doi.org/10.1007/978-3-031-69158-4_34

The declining interest in clinical examination and relying on modern investigations is spreading like a fire in a stack of hey among the new generation of doctors practicing medicine and surgery. There is a consensus that physical examination skills have been greatly deteriorating during the past twenty years [2].

Clinical Surgery Save Resources

In an article written in 2018 by Faustinella and Jacobs [2] they presented 3 cases of misdiagnosis of the case due to the lack of history taking and physical examination5. One of those cases they mentioned is a case of a woman diagnosed of fever of Unknown origin admitted from the A&E department by the residents. She had an evident cellulitis in her leg. Apparently she was not examined or even had a history taking at all.

In my practice I face frequently similar situation where the patient had not been diagnosed because the examining doctor didn't ask the relevant question or do the proper test correctly or even at all.

One of those examples are a case of acute abdominal Pain who presented into my clinic referred from a senior physician with one week history of acute abdomen and absolute Constipation. She can walking to my clinic apparently not severely ill "An important Finding", walking, talking and breathing normally during History taking "Another important finding" with history of Left Loin and Left lower quadrant pain in the abdomen, She had no urinary symptoms "Another important finding" and absolute constipation since one year. She had Chemotherapy 2 years ago for blood malignancy and recently she is on corticosteroids for autoimmune vasculitis. She had a battery of blood investigations with normal CBC and Normal white cell Count. Normal abdominal ultrasonography apart from fatty liver and normal CT abdomen with contrast.

Her husband told me that few days before presenting to me she had skin rash and her physician on her follow-up visit didn't examine this rash and told her most probably it is an allergic reaction to one of the medicine she had. I asked for her permission to examine her and the diagnosis was Simply Varicella Zoster infection in an immune-compromised patient causing reflex ileus (Fig. 34.1). I referred her back to her physician, pain clinics and prescribed a prokinetic medication "Prucalopride" 2 mg once per day for her. 12 h later she had her first bowel motion since 1 week.

Another case during my clinical rounds diagnosed as a neck.

Mass at the right supraclavicular area in a 30 years old male. He Was admitted since a week waiting investigations including Ct scans. During examination I told them it is a straightforward hemangio-lipoma. CT proved the diagnosis. They failed to examine the mass for "Compressibility", as another example of a diagnosis which could have be done in any outpatient clinic. It is an example of wasting the resources in our modern health care systems. Simply due to the lack of clinical skills [2].

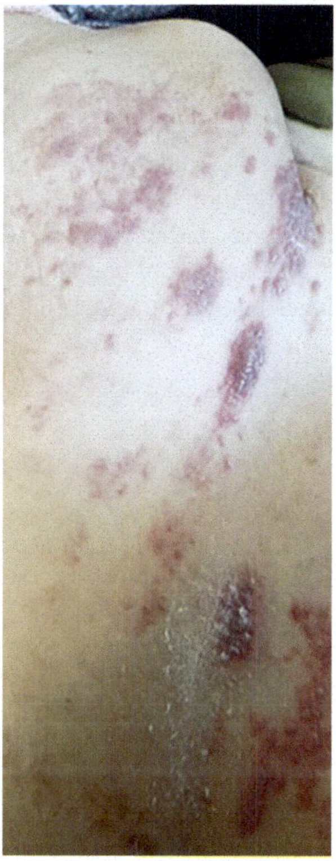

Fig. 34.1 Varicella Zoster rash in the patient mentioned above

Clinical Skills Save Lives

The First case as an example is a 5 years old boy presented to me when I was a resident in the A&E department in our University hospital accompanied with the resident of pediatrics who diagnosed him as acute appendicitis. When I examined him he has all the textbook picture of acute appendicitis including tenderness, rebound tenderness over McBurney's point and Roving's sign. I did smell acetone in the room it was the Child's breath. I asked for blood Sugar analysis and acetone in Urine. It was a case of Diabetic ketoacidosis. Without this smell the child may have died under anesthesia, not only have an un-necessary operation.

The second example In one of the rounds at the out-patient clinic in our University hospital, I was explaining to the students the value of through though swift general examination in a 35 years old lady who came to repair her post-Cesarean section incisional hernia, and during her general examination, while feeling her pulse, she had an unexplained tachycardia 105 per minute, which proved later-on to be a case of unreported "Asymptomatic" thyrotoxicosis. I she did have the operation directly she may had a thyrotoxic crisis and even died during surgery [2].

Being Senior Surgeons we are asked to diagnose cases not otherwise diagnosed since, weeks, months or even years with a lot of un-necessary investigations and un-necessary medications with loss of precious money, working days and Joyful life for our patients.

I always say "The Key for Proper treatment is the proper diagnosis" which has to start or can be only verified by our Clinical skills.

If I am responsible for the health care in any part on earth I will not allow any investigation to be requested without through Clinical examination where the investigations can be ignored if we diagnose the case with 100% accuracy in our Clinic "Like the case of hemangio-lipoma mentioned above or we can ask for the relevant investigations in case of DD. Or in preparation for surgery.

References

1. Farag A. Health errors in the era of declining clinical skills and rising whatsapp medicine. Acta Sci Gastron Disord. 2019;2(7):1–2.
2. Faustinella F, Jacobs RJ. The decline of clinical skills: a challenge for medical schools. Int J Med Educ. 2018;9:195–7. https://doi.org/10.5116/ijme.5b3f.9fb3.

The manufacturer's authorised representative in the EU is Springer Nature Customer Service Centre GmbH, Europaplatz 3, 69115 Heidelberg, Germany. If you have any concerns regarding our products, please contact ProductSafety@springernature.com

Printed and bound by CPI Group (UK) Ltd, Croydon, CR0 4YY

01/10/2026

02225935-0008